Patricia M. Davies, Steps to Follow, 2. Edition

Springer

Berlin
Heidelberg
New York
Barcelona
Hong Kong
London
Milan
Paris
Singapore
Tokyo

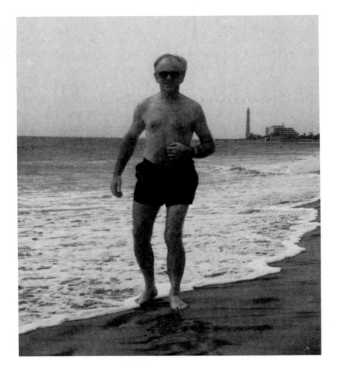

*Free to choose where, when and with whom
he would like to be, or even to be on his own*

(Chapter 10)

Patricia M. Davies

Steps to Follow

The Comprehensive Treatment
of Patients with Hemiplegia

Second, Completely Revised Edition

With a Foreword by Prof. Jürg Kesselring, M.D.

With 401 Figures in 740 Separate Illustrations

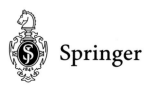 Springer

Patricia M. Davies, MCSP, Dip. Phys. Ed.
Switzerland

Photographs:
David J. Brühwiller Foto Fetzer, CH-7310 Bad Ragaz
Rainer Gierig, D-82362 Weilheim, Germany

ISBN 3-540-60720-X Springer-Verlag Berlin Heidelberg New York

Library of Congress Cataloging-in-Publication Data
Davies, Patricia M.: Steps to follow : the comprehensive treatment of patients with
hemiplegia / Patricia M. Davies. – p. ; cm. – Rev. ed. of: Steps to follow / Patricia M.
Davies. 1985. – Includes bibliographical references and index. – ISBN 3-540-60720-X
(alk. paper) – 1. Hemiplegics–Rehabilitation. I. Title: Steps to follow. II. Davies, Patricia M. Steps to follow. III. Title. – [DNLM: 1. Hemiplegia–rehabilitation. 2. Rehabilitation–methods. WL 346 D257s 2000] RC406.H45 D38 2000 – 616.8'42–dc21

Springer-Verlag is a company in the BertelsmannSpringer publishing group.
© Springer-Verlag Berlin Heidelberg 1985, 2000
Printed in Germany

Cover Design: design & production GmbH, Heidelberg, Germany
Typesetting, printing and binding: Appl, Wemding, Germany

SPIN 10494845   22/3133Sy - 5 4 3 2 1 0 – Printed on acid-free paper

Foreword

A true paradigm shift is taking place in the field of neurology. Earlier it was regarded as the science of exact diagnosis of incurable illnesses, resigned to the dogma that damage to the central nervous system could not be repaired: "Once development is complete, the sources of growth and regeneration of axons and dendrites are irretrievably lost. In the adult brain the nerve paths are fixed and immutable – everything can die, but nothing can be regenerated" (Cajal 1928). Even then this could have been countered with what holds today: rehabilitation does not take place in the test tube, being supported only a short time later by an authoritative source, the professor of neurology and neurosurgery in Breslau, Otfried Foerster. He wrote a 100-page article about therapeutic exercises which appeared in the *Handbuch der Neurologie* (also published by Springer-Verlag). The following sentences from his introduction illustrate his opinion of the importance of therapeutic exercises and are close to our views today (Foerster 1936):

> *"There is no doubt that most motor disturbances caused by lesions of the nervous system are more or less completely compensated as a result of a tendency inherent to the organism to carry out as expediently as possible the tasks of which it is capable under normal circumstances, using all the forces still available to it with the remaining undamaged parts of the nervous system, even following injury to its substance. This happens spontaneously, when neither a reversal of the damage nor a regeneration of the destroyed tissue is possible, simply by means of a reorganisation of the remaining parts of the nervous system, which is not a machine composed of individual parts that stands still when one part fails; rather, it possesses an admirable plasticity and exhibits an astonishingly extensive adaptability, not only to changed external conditions but also to disruptions of its own substance. Therapeutic exercises influence the course of spontaneous restoration; they support it, strengthen it. Not infrequently, in fact, they actually set it in motion when the forces essential to restoration lie fallow and are not deployed by the organism . . . ."*

Due to new findings about the above-mentioned plasticity of the nervous system (Stein et al. 2000), and thanks to new pharmacological possibilities, but above all through the systematic application of neurorehabilitation, neurology has in fact become a therapy-driven speciality

(Kesselring 1997). Research into cells and their connections as well as into neurotransmitter systems, the description of functional changes by means of imaging procedures (Frackowiak et al. 1997), and the (albeit difficult) measurement of the effects of rehabilitation show that the central nervous system of the adult has an astounding potential for regeneration and adaptability, which can be specifically enhanced. Translated to the level of the physiology of the organism as a whole, and of psychology, this can be understood as the basis of learning. Whereas a previous main objective of neurology was to describe the deficits and their pathogenesis as precisely as possible according to the lesions, interest today has shifted more to identifying the potential still available and promoting it through a learning process.

When this pioneering work by Pat Davies, which was to become one of Springer-Verlag's most successful titles, first appeared in 1985, the field of neurorehabilitation was regarded as a marginal discipline. Neurologists who wished to follow her methods, were disregarded by their academic colleagues with a contemptuous smile, or at most were thought to be moving in a direction which could only lead to a dead end. With very few exceptions, rehabilitation at that time was not a subject for the university; it was neither taught nor studied there. However, under the self-confident direction of just such practised and didactically experienced therapists as Pat Davies it has become possible to study particular aspects of behaviour following disturbances of brain function, allowing a broader understanding of the field of clinical neurology. This therapeutic approach promotes more extensive training to improve function, with more comprehensive guidance and care of patients with chronic sequelae of diseases and injuries of the nervous system, thus enabling them to cope with the problems of everyday life. This is what is truly relevant.

Neurorehabilitation can become an outstanding example of the urgently needed attempt to unite under one roof the two cultures within which medicine is developing. The one is the scientific side and the other the practical, or what has on occasion been called the "humanistic aspect" (Wulff 1999). The famous English haematologist Sir David Weatherall used the dilemma as the title of his book, which is well worth reading: *Science and the Quiet Art. Medical Research and Patient Care* (Weatherall 1997). He searches for the complement to his own occupation as a scientist, which he experiences as being one-sided despite his success. He finds it in a quotation from Virgil's *Aeneid*, which speaks of the "quiet art" which should be practised "regardless of fame". It is the esteem and the respect, however, shown by such a famous scientist and director of an institute of molecular medicine to those who practise the quiet art in their daily work, which lend a special significance to this book and its basic approach.

Man's basic intellectual interests point in two main directions. On the one hand are the technical interests, which have developed into modern scientific medicine, and with which objective facts are collected, described and tested. These can be likened to the way in which man earlier had to learn to hunt, gather edible food and distinguish it from that which was poisonous, seek shelter, and warm himself. On the other hand, we are also social beings and in order to survive we must be capable of communicating with one another which is the interpretative or hermeneutic interest. It has a horizontal orientation, in that we must understand and interpret what others say here and now and how they behave in relation to the current situation, as well as a vertical orientation learned from earlier experiences and from those of previous generations.

Karl Popper (Popper and Eccles 1982) takes a more radical view, referring to two different worlds in which we move and to which he assigns numbers. "World 1" is the objective world, the playing field of the natural sciences and all too often the only area of interest to one-sided physicians. "World 2" is the subjective world of our feelings, memories and thoughts. Each one of us is part of "world 1" but there is always a small, subjective "world 2" within each of us, to which no one else has direct access. In this world our moods, our state of health, suffering and sickness, and fears of the future interplay – they with us and we with them. Medical science belongs to "world 1", but the aim of every medical and therapeutic effort lies in "world 2". In her book, Pat Davies concerns herself with this aspect.

Popper distinguishes still another world – "world 3": the cultural achievements of many generations. Examples are languages, works of art, scientific theories, Zeitgeist (the feeling of that generation) and, of particular significance in this connection, ethical values, norms and rules of behaviour.

Clinical considerations usually begin in "world 1" if we work from theoretical knowledge and regard the patient firstly as a biological organism, a natural phenomenon with its healthy or restricted functions. In every case considerations from "world 3" play a role here as well, from the cultural context in which these aspects of medicine are learned and practised. In particular, we must learn to take also the "world-2" aspects of an illness into consideration – the way in which the patient experiences and interprets his illness or disability within the framework of his life experience, and how he himself contributes to changing the situation.

One of the most remarkable occurrences of today is the way in which earlier trust in progress is turning into a fear of progress. Grateful appreciation of medical success is being replaced by a suspicious and radical criticism of medicine. The dramatic growth of our ability to conquer diseases is condemned as increasing dehumanisation of medicine and as exploitation of the patients. What was once welcomed and celebrated as a chance for healing is now looked upon as an instrument of inhumanity. This grave re-evaluation of progress as an agent of destruction is sustained by the tendency to forget. It is easy to forget man's earlier captivity in disease, pain and suffering, which have been relieved and reduced through medical progress. Progress has led to advantages in life, the absence of which would not only be unpleasant but even inhumane. Why is it that the more successes medicine achieves, the more criticism it attracts? Progress is often said to be Janus-faced, because it not only eliminates evil, but also engenders it. Why is it that we are interested only in the latter of the two faces? The increasing rational control of our environment, our reality, necessitates a greater division of labor and, in turn, a greater need for mutual trust. But it is exactly this aspect which is questioned today and changed into mistrust. Where progress really succeeds and does eliminate evil, the newly attained state of affairs is quickly taken for granted but the negative aspects which remain become increasingly exaggerated. Just as goods which are scarce become more and more expensive, so the vestiges of evil become ever more tormenting and finally unbearable, to the point where people suffer from precisely that which spares them from the other kinds of suffering. The current criticism of medicine speaks not for its failure but rather for its success, even if there is, unquestionably, still much room for improvement in order to allow further progress. Medicine's inadequacy can just as well be explained by excessive expectations and demands as by any lack of accomplishment. Because absolute demands are always disappointed, we should learn to dispense with them.

Perhaps the claim that medicine is a science is unrealistic to begin with. Even today it can fulfil only some of the criteria which define a mature scientific discipline such as mathematics or biology (Kuhn 1965). Medicine is still partly at the stage of lists of descriptions, partly at that of competing theories; little of daily practice is indeed evidence-based. One reason for the crisis in which modern Western medicine finds itself may be that the various paradigms on which it was founded, and which were held to be unshakable, have begun to falter simultaneously and are drifting apart, without any force in sight which might hold them together. One of these paradigms is the reductionist path of molecular medicine and genetics. Undeniably great results have been obtained along this road, particularly in the field of clarifying disease mechanisms and their pathogenesis, and more are being achieved at breakneck speed. Many valuable qualities pertinent to the practice of medicine are lost, however, in the attempt to understand the mechanisms of diseases instead of the troubles and needs of sick people. One problem with reducing medicine to a molecular level lies in the fact that personality, experienced by us directly as "I" and "you", disappears or goes astray. As in the study of space, we have no organ which allows perceptions in the molecular field without instruments. Spectacles, a cane or even a wheelchair are accepted immediately as personal aids because they are of obvious advantage. The extension of basic technology to the astronomical dimensions of space and time is even more easily tolerated because these are domains far beyond our own temporal and spatial horizons. The aids which permit indirect perception at the molecular level, however, are complicated and rather difficult to visualise, so that they are mastered by only a few expensively trained specialists. Nevertheless, in the field of medicine, there is the feeling and the assumption that the object of investigation is ourself or someone close to us. Lack of knowledge of the area of perception always causes anxiety, which is probably one reason why many people are sceptical about scientific knowledge gained from areas which are not accessible via direct experience and straightforward examination. In philosophy, and thus in the minds of those affected, reducing interpretation to the molecular and genetic level leads, despite the use of the most modern technology, to a return to the days when anxiety ruled because all life was interpreted as being predestined – at that time by either fate or God.

A second paradigm shift in medicine is manifested by the impetus of so-called alternative medicine, which profits precisely from its standpoint opposing scientific medicine. A "holistic" view of the human being is advocated here, the factual basis of which is often accessible only to the initiated. This type of medicine is no longer content with trusting in the ability of the body to heal itself and in recommending a healthy way of life and physical exercise; rather, it has now caught up with classical medicine with regard to costs. An essential contrast to scientific medicine lies in the fact that, in the alternative scene, an improvement in the subjective assessment of a given case is judged to be proof of the success of the therapy. Scientific medicine, although concerning itself, as a safeguard, with elements from "world 3", requires statistical support based upon parameters of measurement which have been established with sufficiently large numbers of patients examined over an adequate period of time, before a treatment may be considered useful. In the area of "hands-on" therapy which is of the greatest importance in neurorehabilitation, other criteria for judging effectiveness than those used in scientific studies of the efficacy of medication have to be applied. If these therapies are to induce a learning effect, they must be compared with pedagogic or training effects. It would not occur to anyone to test the efficacy of education or of a sports training camp in a double-blind study. Of course, prejudices, a lack of readiness for change, and authoritarianism have delayed progress in every age. Medicine is still an art, but one which has become more difficult to practise because the knowledge of our ignorance and our unawareness is increasing.

A further paradigm change in our society is having an effect on medicine as well. Suddenly, the till which for so long had been able to finance all desires for development and reform is empty, but the demands that everything which can be done must be done have not ceased and these demands have not become quieter or more modest. From this point of view, neurorehabilitation should be compared less with other therapeutic methods in medicine and more with other cultural services and educational functions, and financed accordingly. A fourth problem of modern medicine, one which is only very reluctantly addressed, lies in the realisation that work to preserve and prolong life, which is beneficial per se in the individual case, has catastrophic consequences in the overriding, more general and politically relevant aspect of demographic evolution. Neurorehabilitation, however, is concerned not with prolonging life, but rather with improving the quality of life, and this is justified from all points of view.

Pat Davies' fundamental clinical (practical-humanistic) approach, so comprehensively reflected in this book, is a fitting example of how the "uneasiness with modern medicine" (Kesselring 1998) can be countered. In addition to her original, practice-relevant views on the physiology of the nervous system as it manifests itself in behavior patterns seen daily in clinical practice, her instructions for direct, practical treatment of patients preclude the danger of concentrating only on diseases in the abstract instead of on the people who suffer from them.

There is no fundamental contradiction between a scientific understanding of disease mechanisms and their influence, on one hand, and providing good care and attention to sick or disabled persons on the other. Certainly, the prerequisites for clinical work and research are not identical; they are, in part, even opposite. Clinicians should radiate self-confidence and assurance, should convey trust and hope – qualities which enhance the healing process and make it easier to deal with sickness and disability. They will do some things without being aware of any exact scientific basis for them; they often have to assess and treat on a basis of limited information, and this skill tends to be called intuition. Discussions related to the extent of our ignorance and unawareness cannot be carried out at the bedside. To endure the uncertainty and insecurity and nevertheless convey assuredness and take action is one of the clinician's most difficult tasks, one which can never be completely resolved. Characteristic of the researcher, on the other hand, is a fundamental skepticism which involves repeated questioning and answer-seeking, because only such an approach can give rise to further studies and to a critical appraisal of the results. Of course, much in science serves more the self-glorification of the researcher than a practicable path or aim.

Pat Davies is one of the very few persons who win wide recognition through their clinical work, who come up again and again with creative possibilities for solving problems relevant to daily life, and who are also, at the same time, didactically skilled and charismatic teachers. Clinical researchers and academic teachers need to be able to enter into communication and be able to understand problems and suggested solutions, even when these are proposed by persons who do not come directly from their field of work. Only then can they integrate theoretical findings into daily practice. Leadership of a team in which people from various fields of training work together, indispensable for the complex task of neurorehabilitation, can only succeed if proof can be presented of successful work in both scientific medicine and clinical practice, and especially of a willingness to cooperate. In contrast to the days of George Bernard Shaw, the "Doctor's Dilemma" today consists of resolving the contradiction between scientific medicine and clinical practice and in forming a synthesis of the two. This requires new educational curricula and the practical instruction which stem from critically reviewed experience such as presented in this book and also a continued willingness to be active in both medical cultures and to promote communication between colleagues on both sides.

March 2000

Prof. Jürg Kesselring, M. D.
Professor of Clinical Neurology and Neurorehabilitation, Universities of Bern and Zurich.
Chairman of the Scientific Panel Neurorehabilitation of the European Federation of Neurological Societies.
Head of the Department of Neurology, Rehabilitation Clinic, 7317 Valens, Switzerland

References

Cajal R (1928) Degeneration and regeneration of the nervous system. Oxford University Press, London
Condrau G (ed) (1976) Vom Januskopf des Fortschritts. Benteli, Bern
Foerster O (1936) Übungstherapie. In: Bumke O, Foerster O (eds) Handbuch der Neurologie, vol VIII, Allgemeine Neurologie, pp 316–414
Frackowiak RSJ, Friston KJ, Frith CD, Dolan RJ, Mazziotta JC (1997) Human brain function. Academic, San Diego
Kesselring J (1997) Neurologie – ein therapeutisches Fach. Schweiz Med Wochenschr 127: 2140–2142
Kesselring J (1998) Warum dieses Unbehagen an der modernen Medizin? Schweiz Arztezeitung 79: 1552–1554
Kesselring J (1999) Kontroversen der neurologischen und neuropsychologischen Begutachtung – vom objektiven Befund zum Versuch, Befindlichkeit zu objektivieren. Schweiz Arztezeitung 80: 1439–1442
Kuhn TS (1965) The structure of scientific revolutions. University of Chicago Press, Chicago
Marquard O (1993) Medizinerfolg und Medizinkritik: die modernen Menschen als Prinzessinnen auf der Erbse. Manuscript of speech, May 1993
Popper KR, Eccles JR (1982) Das Ich und sein Gehirn, 2nd edn. Piper, Munich
Stein DG, Brailowsky S, Will B (2000) Brain-Repair. Das Selbstheilungspotential des Gehirns oder wie das Gehirn sich selbst hilft. Thieme, Stuttgart
Weatherall D (1997) Science and the quiet art. Medical research and patient care. Oxford University Press, London
Wulff H (1999) The two cultures of medicine: objective facts versus subjectivity and values. J R Soc Med 92: 549–552

Preface to the Second Edition

In the hurly-burly of clinical practice, it is easy for us to lose sight of the fact that each and every patient is unique, a person with individual wishes, memories, habits, likes and dislikes, ways of moving, dressing and conversing. There is not a typical picture of hemiplegia, characterised by paralysis of certain muscles, spastic limb postures and loss of sensation, as some textbooks persist in describing, and therefore no treatment recipe which is suitable for all patients. In fact, no two patients manifest exactly the same symptoms, nor do they demonstrate the same degree of dysfunction because of similar symptoms. The way in which they respond to treatment procedures may also vary, so that comparing the success of one patient with that of another should be avoided, as it can be most demoralising. Instead, for successful rehabilitation in the true sense of the word, the specific problems experienced by the individual patient need to be carefully analysed and the treatment must be aimed at solving them.

In the 15 years since I wrote the first edition of *Steps to Follow* there have been exciting advances in treatment that offer us additional possibilities for helping patients to overcome both motor and perceptual difficulties. It would be professionally irresponsible if we did not take advantage of these developments, because none of us can be completely satisfied with the rehabilitation outcomes achieved with present practices. It is for this reason that I have undertaken the task of rewriting *Steps to Follow*, to include valuable new activities while retaining many of those from the first edition which have proved to be most effective. I hope very much that therapists will include the activities which I recommend in their treatment and see for themselves how well their patients respond. Unfortunately, some doctors and therapists have introduced theories and therapeutic procedures which tend to block progress, while still others are afraid to incorporate new ideas and are inclined to pass on their fears. Most of the theories are unsubstantiated and the fears unwarranted, but Cowley (1997) points out that "most of us harbour beliefs for which hard evidence is lacking", and that "beliefs that survive are not necessarily true". We must therefore be aware when we read a new publication, listen to someone speaking with apparent authority or are taught a new treatment modality that, although it may sound like "God talking for eternity" in fact "it is never anything other than just one person talking from one place in time and space and circumstance" (Pirsig 1989). Only by trying out for ourselves what we have learned or discovered and evaluating the results honestly and objectively can we really be sure of its functional value.

Many such misbeliefs or "viruses of the mind", as Cowley terms them, are prevalent today, and while some are harmless, others are actually harmful, in that they prolong the period of rehabilitation, may prevent a more successful outcome and can even be the reason for treatment being discontinued.

Harmless "viruses" are those that do not interfere with the actual treatment of the patient. Many involve neurophysiological explanations regarding which area of the brain or which cortical tract is being stimulated and is responsible for movements in the extremities. But neurophysiology is based on ever-changing hypotheses, usually emanating from animal studies or human laboratory experiments which have little if anything to do with a person's ability to function in real-life situations. Some of the other questionable beliefs will also not detract from the therapy, for instance, the misconception that sight is important for posture and balance even though blind people participate in sport, climb mountains, sing on the stage and use public transport.

Far more worrying are the detrimental or harmful "viruses" that not only limit the treatment which the patient receives but cause those caring for him to have a less positive and hopeful attitude towards his rehabilitation. These widespread but erroneous beliefs are potentially so harmful that I should like to draw attention to the most frequently encountered and contradict their validity.

→ *All recovery of activity or improvement following a stroke takes place within the first 3–6 months.*

Reflections on validity: Recovery of activity and improved functional ability have been reported in patients more than 5 years after their stroke. With informed therapy and diligent performance of a home exercise programme, the chances of later recovery are far greater.

→ *Patients who suffer from epileptic attacks following a stroke have poorer rehabilitation outcomes.*

Reflections on validity: An outstanding international cricket player has epilepsy but nevertheless participates in test matches with skilled movements and quick reactions. Therefore, other reasons for the poor outcomes should be considered, such as the quality of the rehabilitation itself, members of the therapeutic team having a less positive attitude towards patients who develop seizures, or diminished expectations on the part of the carers.

→ *Elderly patients with hemiplegia are poor candidates for rehabilitation because they are unlikely to benefit or achieve independence in the activities of daily living.*

Reflections on validity: Even older patients can make a remarkable recovery with appropriate treatment, but they often are not given the chance of intensive rehabilitation simply because they are considered to be too old. Age has not proved to be a significant factor in determining the success of rehabilitation.

→ *Moving treadmill training is a quicker and better way to teach patients with hemiplegia to walk independently than skilled hands-on physiotherapy.*

Reflections on validity: There is far more to walking than merely moving the legs on an obstacle-free surface. Human beings walk because they have intentions, goals that they wish to achieve, and because they need to maintain balance and move out of the way to avoid other people and objects in their path. No mechanical aid could ever help to re-establish such a complex performance. A physiotherapist is able to adapt her support, help the patient to regain the lost components of gait and practise walking with him in the great variety of situations required for truly functional independence (Davies 1999).

→ *Clasping the hands together with the fingers interlaced in order to protect the paralysed hand and prevent loss of mobility will injure its joints and soft tissues.*

Reflections on validity: On the contrary, if the patient is taught how to clasp his hands together correctly, the hemiplegic hand is less liable to sustain injury, and by this simple procedure, deformities that are unsightly and painful and make personal hygiene difficult can be prevented even after cessation of therapy (see pp 116–118).

→ *Standing with a rolled bandage placed beneath the toes can cause subluxation of the metatarsophalangeal joints.*

Reflections on validity: Anatomical structures in the sole of the foot are so arranged that subluxation of these joints does not occur when the foot is dorsiflexed and the toes extended as they are during phases of normal walking. Instead, the therapeutic procedure prevents shortening of the calf muscles, ankle clonus and painful clawing of the toes, and the patient will later be able to maintain the mobility of his hemiplegic foot by performing the exercise on his own at home (see pp 152–155).

→ *Standing with the patient's knee supported by a splint is passive.*

Reflections on validity: Activity in the extensor muscles of the hemiplegic leg is actually stimulated by weightbearing. With the aid of the splint, the patient can stand with all his weight on the affected limbs, which he begins to feel as a result, and active, selective control is facilitated. In addition, the therapist has her hands free to help the patient to move his trunk actively as well.

→ *Subluxation of the glenohumeral joint causes pain in the hemiplegic shoulder.*

Reflections on validity: Subluxation of the hemiplegic shoulder is in itself not painful, but without the relevant muscular activity to protect them, the joint and the surrounding structures are extremely vulnerable and can easily be traumatised (see Chap. 12). The patient's arm should not be immobilised in a sling or other form of support because these will not correct the subluxation or alleviate the pain but can cause additional problems. Surgical intervention or fixation should be avoided at all costs.

All such false notions must be guarded against because if they are believed and allowed to spread, they will limit development in treatment and block the progress of countless patients. "The fate of a thought contagion depends on several factors, including how much fervor it inspires, how long each host stays infected and how much resistance it encounters in the population" (Lynch 1996). It is therefore incumbent on all of us in the rehabilitation team to halt the spread of erroneous ideas by offering sufficient resistance in the form of improved treatment measures and more convincing results.

We must remain open to new ideas and continue to search for additional treatment possibilities. Berta Bobath herself provides a wonderful example of a therapist who never stopped searching. Although her concept had already proved to be most successful and was widely accepted internationally, right up to the time of her death at the age of 83 she was constantly seeking new ways to overcome the patients' problems and find explanations for the efficacy of her treatment. It was her sincere wish that her concept be built upon and enlarged but nevertheless remain intact. In the introduction to her last book, which she sent to me personally, she wrote: "We all learn and change our ways of treatment according to our growing knowledge and experience of the reactions of our patients during treatment, for better or for worse. Such changes are good and necessary and will continue" (B. Bobath 1990).

My work with patients and the activities which I recommend when teaching and writing adhere to the principles inherent in the Bobath concept, and indeed, it was through working with the Bobaths many years ago that I first learned how to treat patients with upper motor neuron lesions more successfully. Like Sir Isaac Newton, to quote his famous statement from 1676, I acknowledge fully that, "if I have seen further, it is by standing on the shoulders of giants." Now, with "growing knowledge and experience" gained through continued searching, good fortune and the opportunity to learn from many experts in the field of rehabilitation, I hope that I have been able to build upon and enlarge the Bobaths' original concept in the way they wished by incorporating new ideas. With knowledge and understanding being a cumulative affair, sometimes, according to Burton (1621), "Pygmies placed on the shoulders of giants see more than the giants themselves."

But we should not become complacent or be content with the present status quo, because there is still an urgent need to improve the treatment of neurologically impaired patients even further. We certainly have not found all the answers yet, and my sincere hope is that the activities and the philosophy contained in this book will stimulate others to search for additional ways to facilitate future progression.

In his brilliant seminar, Roger Nierenberg (1999) explains how focusing on the client, the customer or, in our case, the patient can make our work more meaningful and successful. He demonstrates how internal focus isolates us from the patient (customer or client) because we then focus solely on the correctness and alignment of everything that we are doing, while external focus encourages us to create, gives meaning to our work, why we are doing it and towards whom it is directed, namely, the person for whom it was designed. Nierenberg also stresses the importance of teamwork with communication both ways, because as he says, the lines of communication are "the heartbeat and pulse" of an organisation's effectiveness and the ability to reach a consensus of opinion. No one professional within the team can have complete success if he works on his own. One hour of correct treatment will be of little or no avail if for the rest of the day or night the same principles are not followed. All members of the team will need to be convinced and encouraged to carry out their treatment procedures along similar lines, and of course the patient's relatives are an integral part of the team. They should never be excluded from participating, from learning and being shown how they too can contribute by assisting in more therapeutic ways.

We should avoid being discouraged by negative prognostications and predictions based on statistics relating to rehabilitation outcomes because, in the words of Gegax and Hager (1994), "Statistics are confusing, misleading, often abused. So why use them?" Instead, we must strive to achieve the best possible return of function for each and every patient while at the same time preventing secondary complications that could cause additional suffering or limit the chances of recovery. Recent advances in treatment will certainly help us to achieve these goals, but the basic tenets of positioning the patient correctly in bed and chair and careful handling when he is being helped to move are still as important as ever.

I sincerely believe that the recommendations and therapeutic activities which I have included in this new edition will lead to more successful rehabilitation outcomes and enhanced quality of life for patients. Certainly, for them and for those of us involved in their treatment, a successful rehabilitation outcome is a very worthwhile reward for all the time spent and the hard work entailed.

March 2000   Pat Davies
                                                             Switzerland

Preface to the First Edition

People need hope,
People need loving,
People need trust from a fellow man,
People need love to make a good living,
People need faith in a helping hand.

Abba

For the last 7 years my professional time has been divided roughly in half, between treating patients and giving courses on the treatment of neurological disorders, mainly adult hemiplegia, for members of the medical and paramedical professions. Both the patients and course members alike frequently ask me if there is not a book which contains all that they have learnt, so that they can read more to deepen and stabilise their knowledge. I have found it difficult to advise them what to select from the enormous amount of rather theoretical literature, which often fails to give practical guide-lines on just how to cope with the manifold problems which confront them.

I hope that this book will fill the gap, and in writing it I have tried to be practical and at the same time as scientific as possible. But essentially it is a book about people, the patients and those who care for them, and people are not made up of facts and figures as the literature tends to imply. Furthermore, I hope that all the many therapists, nurses and relatives of patients who do not have the opportunity to attend special courses will also find the book useful. As Sagan (1977) writes, it has been possible to learn from a book since the invention of writing and not be entirely dependent on the "lucky accident" that there is someone nearby to teach us in person.

Apart from caring for or treating the patient in the hospital or rehabilitation centre, it is important to see how he manages in the world outside, with all its variety and challenge. It is part of rehabilitation to observe the patient in as many and as various situations as possible. Many judgements as to the success of the rehabilitation programme are made solely on the patient's performance in a very sheltered environment. Because of the pleasant custom in Switzerland, where by the patient at the end of a period of treatment invites his therapists and his doctor to a meal, I personally have learnt a great deal and have been forced to alter many preconceived ideas. There is an enormous difference between "can walk 45 m unaided" and walking to a table in a crowded restaurant. Eating together also provides a valuable time for listening to what the patient says, time which is often missing in a busy department.

For the therapists and others who read this book I should like to offer a few thoughts which could be of help, especially for those who may have had little experience in treating patients with hemiplegia before, or in using the concept described.

1. Because it is a concept rather than a technique, there is no absolute prescription which would suit every patient. Anything which results in a new ability for the patient, or enables him to move in a more normal way, can be used without hesitation.
2. The treatment of hemiplegia is not a series of isolated exercises performed in a set order, but is a sequence of activities in preparation for an actual function.
3. Rehabilitation starts on the day when the patient suffers a stroke, and not only when he is fit enough to attend a rehabilitation centre.
4. All who work with the patient must be very convinced of the importance of each position or activity used, because if we are not convinced he certainly will not be.
5. Not all hemiplegic patients are old and decrepit, and they will have expectations from their rehabilitation which extend way beyond just independence in self-care in the home, or managing to walk 45 m slowly even if unaided. It is important to try to achieve far higher goals for each patient. And even if the patient is old, his age should not exclude him from a full and active treatment programme. Age has been shown to be no deterrent to rehabilitation or recovery (Andrews et al. 1982, Adler et al. 1980).
6. The patient should be spoken to in a normal adult way and care must be taken to avoid a singsong voice and the use of the "we" form when he alone is being asked to do something. Much can be asked of him as long as we talk and discuss matters with him seriously. Hemiplegia is, after all, a very serious event in his life, and he has a right to be involved in decisions concerning his future. Particular care must be taken when addressing the patient who has aphasia. Being able to watch the speaker's face and the use of short, concise sentences will help him to understand what is being said.
7. When ever possible, negative feedback should be avoided, as the patient's day can otherwise be filled with "nos" and "don'ts". Merely by changing a few words the same correction can be given in a positive form.

Patients of all ages and at different stages of their rehabilitation have been used for the illustrations in the following chapters, to try to give an idea of the great diversity of people suffering from the effects of a stroke. The ages of the patients shown in the book range from 30 to 80 years.

For purposes of clarity, the masculine pronoun has been used in the entire text to refer to the patient, and the feminine form for the therapist or assistant. In the legends the correct form of the pronoun is used according to the sex of the person in the photograph.

Bad Ragaz, November 1984   Pat Davies

Acknowledgements

Writing a book is no easy task, as anyone who has written for publication will agree. The practical help given me by many people and their moral support and encouragement have made an enormous difference and lightened the load considerably. Advice from colleagues and stimulating discussions with them have been most valuable with regard to the different chapters and what should be included in them. The response of the therapists who attend the courses that I teach and the questions they repeatedly ask have also been a useful guide. I should like to express my thanks to everyone who has contributed in any way to this new and up-to-date edition of *Steps to Follow*. In particular, though, I am indebted to those who have been involved personally and practically in its production and publication. It is difficult to decide just who should head the list!

Perhaps I should start with my publishers, because it was Bernhard Lewerich, still today my gifted mentor, who convinced me to undertake the revision in the first place. I thank him for inspiring me to write and share my knowledge and experience with others, for his creative ideas and for his sound advice on publishing matters. I am most grateful to Springer-Verlag for allowing me to include the many additional figures in this revised edition, which illustrate clearly the new developments and therapeutic activities. I should like to thank Marga Botsch at Springer for her constant encouragement, help and advice throughout the publication of the book. Mary Schaefer has been a skilled and patient copy-editor, and I greatly appreciate the way in which she has corrected and arranged the text. My thanks go to Jaroslaw Sydor as production manager, for the modern layout and for the laborious work entailed in placing the many new figures and rearranging the original ones to coincide with the revised text in a meaningful way.

I have been most fortunate to have Rainer Gierig as photographer, and I thank him not only for taking such clear and exact photographs of patients in action, but also for his kindness to them and the interest he took in their progress. I am grateful to him for his patience during the shooting of the treatment sequences and for the speed and accuracy with which he worked, thus eliminating the need for retakes. My thanks go to his parents, Clara and Manfred Gierig, as well, for developing and organising the many new photographs so promptly and professionally.

Because the illustrations of patients play such an important role in explaining the treatment, I am extremely grateful for the hospitality and help which I received at the two centres where the majority of the new photographs were taken. My sincere thanks go to Professor Hans-Peter Meier-Baumgartner, MD, Medical Director of the Albertinen-Haus, Medical Geriatric Clinic in Hamburg, for enabling me to photograph patients at different stages of rehabilitation in his up-to-date and yet very humanistic centre. He not only placed a large room at my disposal for this purpose but also allowed Marianne Brune, who is the Bobath instructor in his clinic, to be free to help me for the whole time I was there. I thank Marianne for her invaluable assistance in selecting suitable patients, ensuring their punctual and willing attendance, organising all the necessary equipment and checking the finer details of the activities during shooting.

Likewise, I thank Dr Martin Rutz, Medical Director of the Rheinburg Clinic in Walzenhausen, Switzerland, wholeheartedly for granting me permission to select and photograph his neurological patients. I cannot thank his wife, Louise Rutz-LaPitz, enough for the way in which she supported, advised and encouraged me during my stay, despite her enormous work load as superintendent therapist, senior Bobath instructor and director of postgraduate studies at their excellent rehabilitation centre.

Sheena Irwin-Carruthers, who, by sorting out and numbering the many new photos, spurred me on to complete the final chapters, deserves a special word of thanks. With her excellent command of the English language, she also proved to be of inestimable help with finer points of grammar and style, giving up precious holiday time to assist me with the text. Sue Adler was a help in this respect, too, and the scientific discussions with both these leading physiotherapists were most stimulating and productive.

Hans Sonderegger has helped me to understand the inextricable relationship between movement, function and perception. I thank him for teaching me how patients can be helped to overcome problems arising from perceptual disorders and thus to re-establish a more normal interaction with their environment.

It was David Butler who first opened my eyes to the way in which abnormal tension in the nervous system affects movement, and I am grateful to him for showing me how increased tension, with its many adverse effects, can be reduced through mobilisation and neural mobility thus restored.

I am most grateful to my partner, Gisela Rolf, who has stood at my side throughout the planning and writing of this book. She has once again, as with the previous books, been prepared to suffer the numerous inconveniences which having an author in the house entails, ranging from papers littering the place to taking on extra household duties. Above all, though, I must thank her most sincerely for her invaluable advice, for the stimulating discussions about patients and for teaching me so much about neurodynamics. Based on her considerable experience, which includes certification as an international Bobath instructor and her in-depth knowledge of the pioneering work of David Butler and

Geoffrey Maitland, Gisela has developed a concept for overcoming the problems of pathoneurodynamics for neurologically impaired patients. Her concept has enabled me and many other therapists to assess such problems more accurately and to achieve more successful treatment results.

I cannot thank Jürg Kesselring enough for his unstinting support and encouragement throughout the years since we first met, for his appreciation of my work and for the way in which we have been able to exchange knowledge and experience with one another. He has indeed been a veritable "fountain of knowledge", answering my questions, searching out literature for me and sending me fascinating new books on related subjects. I greatly appreciate the fact that despite his many international commitments he found the time to read the manuscript and write the thought-provoking and philosophical foreword for this book.

Last but certainly not least, I should like to thank the many patients whom I have been privileged to meet and treat, because it is they who have convinced me that my treatment really works and they who have encouraged me to keep searching for new and better ways to overcome their difficulties. In particular, I am most grateful to all those patients who were willing to be photographed while working with me so that additional useful activities could be clearly illustrated in the book.

March 2000

Pat Davies
Switzerland

Contents

1 Problems That Cannot Be Seen Directly

In the rehabilitation of patients who have suffered a stroke or some other unilateral brain lesion there is a widespread tendency to focus attention only on those problems which can actually be seen. Observing the patient, the therapist immediately notices the position of his spastic arm, his inability to move his fingers or use his hand. She can see at a glance if he walks with his knee hyperextended and is unable to dorsiflex his foot to clear the ground. Most contemporary treatment concepts therefore concentrate on reducing spasticity, stimulating activity in the paralysed muscles and teaching the patient how to perform daily tasks independently with his sound hand. The word "hemiplegia" itself emphasises the motor problems in its original meaning – a paralysis of half (of the body).

Unfortunately, for many patients with hemiplegia the problems are far more complex. The dynamic interaction of the brain as a whole and the diffuse effect which a lesion in one area will therefore have on other areas is underlined by Ruskin (1982), who explains that

> The largest amount of the central nervous system white matter is utilised not by direct pathways, as was previously thought, but by internuncial neurons participating in feedback and feed-forward types of communication, interrelating all of the cells in a highly integrated whole and uniting the two sides of the central nervous system at every level of the neuraxis.
>
> When damage occurs in any portion of the brain, not only are those functions which might be the primary concern of that region disturbed, but the entire brain suffers from the loss of communication with the injured portion. The remaining normal portions of the brain are deprived of input from the damaged area, and they are also subject to abnormal messages and misinformation generated as a result of a lesion.
>
> From this basic understanding of the neuron, it is seen that there is no such thing as a simple stroke with only hemiplegia. The victim of the stroke will have significant difficulties with both sides of the body, and these difficulties will extend in some degree to all functions of the brain. Motor function will be impaired on both sides. Balance and coordination will not be the same. Sensory perception and spatial orientation will be impaired with far-reaching and often disastrous effects. Memory, cognition, and behaviour will all be altered, often presenting the most formidable challenges of rehabilitation.

Unlike the obvious motor loss in the limbs, perceptual disorders cannot be observed per se. Their presence can only be presumed by observing and interpreting the difficulties which the patient reveals during the performance of actual tasks, in the way he behaves in different situations or adapts to his changing environment. Failure to recognise and understand such problems will lead to disappointment and frustration for both therapist and patient in the rehabilitation programme. In a survey of the long-term outcome for patients and their families, Coughlan and Humphrey (1982) found persisting problems of self-care in two thirds of 170 surviving stroke patients who had been treated during an 8-year period.

Jimenez and Morgan (1979) gave a figure of only 59 % of patients with a stroke who were able to care for themselves independently when they were discharged from hospital. In a study involving over 2000 patients, Satterfield (1982) described only 46 % as having been taught independence in dressing at the time of discharge.

The reasons which are generally given for stopping the active treatment of patients who have not yet achieved complete independence vary. Adams and Hurwitz (1963) wrote:

> *Some patients are said to have been confused or uncooperative; others to have had no drive or initiative; and yet others to have had inadequate mentation or lack of motivation. These terms, however expressive or elegant, imply only that the patient was getting nowhere. They do not say why, and sometimes they attach a misleading label of impending dementia to a patient whose true disability is a focal cerebral lesion causing impaired comprehension, loss of recent memory, postural imbalance, apraxia, or loss of body-awareness with neglect, anosognosia, or denial of ownership of the affected limbs.*

Such difficulties can be said to result from disturbances of perception and constitute some of the problems which cannot be seen directly. They can be observed only indirectly by studying many different performances, making inferences about their prerequisite perceptual processes and then comparing them (Affolter and Stricker 1980). Successful rehabilitation outcome is dependent upon not only recognising the problems but also including specific therapy to overcome the difficulties arising from them.

Problems Related to Disturbed Perception

Disturbances in the way in which patients perceive their own body, the world around them and the interaction between the two can cause a great variety of problems and to very different degrees. Some patients may be unable to move their limbs, while others may move well but be unable to use the movements for functional tasks. Still others may have difficulties in making choices and decisions in real-life situations despite having done so successfully during laboratory testing (Damasio 1994). Many problems are, in fact, so subtle that they elude detection by any presently available form of test. As Sagan (1977) writes: "For example, lesions in the right hemisphere of the cerebral cortex may lead to impairments in thought and action, but in the nonverbal realm, which is by definition difficult for the patient or the physician to describe."

Reporting on his own experiences following an acute left-sided hemiparesis, Brodal (1973) notes:

... the patient has found that destruction of even a minor part of the brain causes changes in a number of functions, which are difficult to study objectively. They are, however, very obvious to him. They are what one might call general defects in the functions of the brain: loss of powers of concentration, reduced short-term memory, increased fatigue, reduced initiative, incontinence of movements of emotional expression and other phenomena.

It has also been astonishing to note how long it takes for these symptoms to improve visibly. Even after ten months, if the patient seems to be as he was before, apart from his slight remaining pareses, he is painfully aware himself that this is not so.

Brodal gives an interesting example of his difficulties by showing the changes in his handwriting after his stroke, despite his being right-handed and, on conventional assessment, having only left-sided symptoms.

It is important to realise that disturbed perception affects the whole body and is not unilateral as the motor deficits may appear to be. One example of the bilateral effects is the finding that, "Discriminative sensory disturbances, which often occur bilaterally in some modalities, are common in patients with unilateral stroke, even in those with intact sensory function on routine examination" (Kim and Choi Kwon 1996).

More often, though, therapists will be treating patients whose perceptual disorders have led to far more obvious difficulties. It may help to understand the nature and effects of such disorders by using a concrete example of one which is frequently encountered. Patients with hemiplegia often have considerable difficulty in learning to dress themselves. If a patient is observed as he struggles unsuccessfully to get dressed, an insight can be gained as to the complexity of the problems. The movements do not flow; he cannot put on his clothes in the correct order; he may not find the armhole and sometimes ends up with the garment on back to front. The activity is slow and laborious, and very often the patient will be unable to complete the task at all and will resign after a few unsuccessful attempts. By comparison, a normal subject simulating a total paralysis on one side of the body can dress himself with one hand easily and efficiently in less than 5 min. The activity proceeds effortlessly, and the model adjusts quickly to the new experience. After a few practice runs the person will have no difficulty in carrying out the task. The same applies to a patient whose disability is primarily a motor one. Even without specific training, he too will learn to dress himself with one hand in a very short time, as indeed many do.

Failure to learn to dress independently can therefore be assumed to be the result of perceptual problems and not due to the motor deficit. Although failure to dress independently has been used as an example, it must be taken into account that such problems are never isolated or specific to one particular function.

The relationship is not always as obvious as it is when a patient is struggling unsuccessfully to put on his clothes. It is therefore often not realised that disturbed perception is in all probability the underlying cause of many other difficulties which patients demonstrate during their rehabilitation. Such difficulties can be frustrating and even irritating for therapists, nursing staff and relatives alike if the reason for their occurrence is not properly understood.

Some Common Problems Associated with Disturbed Perception

Hypertonicity

If the patient is not receiving adequate information about his body, from the fine changes in sensation from within, he tries to enhance what he feels. One way is by increasing the tension in muscles, much as we would do when walking on a slippery or unstable surface, which in his case presents as hypertonicity. Examples:
- While he is lying flat in bed, the patient's leg demonstrates marked extensor hypertonicity and resists the therapist's attempt to flex it passively.
- His arm flexes when he is in upright positions.
- His wrist and finger flexors show markedly increased tone whenever he is off balance.

Adopting End-of-range Joint Positions

In his attempt to feel more accurately the position of his limbs, the patient may hold certain joints at the limit of their mechanical range, so that he feels an absolute resistance which provides him with more distinct information as to their present position. Examples:
- When he is lying supine on an anti-decubitus mattress, his scapula retracts, and his elbow, wrist and fingers flex strongly.
- The patient's knee hyperextends during weightbearing although he has sufficient active control of the relevant muscles in his leg.
- His foot pushes into plantar inversion, the strain on the lateral structures of his ankle joint allowing him to feel its position more clearly.

Pressing Too Hard Against Supporting Surfaces

If the patient has difficulty in feeling where he is, he pushes with his hands and feet against hard supporting surfaces. Examples:
- In sitting, his sound hand presses so hard against the plinth that his fingers become quite white, even if he is not being asked to move or maintain his balance.
- When he is seated, his feet press down so strongly against the floor that the heels are seldom in contact with the supporting surface.

Hyperactivity, and Inordinately Quick Responses to Commands

If the patient is better able to perceive kinaesthetic information than tactile, he will tend to move parts of his body even when there is no demand for the movements. Examples:
- The patient turns over constantly in bed, and does not stay in the position in which the nurses have carefully placed him.
- When sitting, he moves from side to side or his sound hand may keep moving about aimlessly. If he is able to move his hemiplegic hand, then it too moves constantly, sometimes in bizarre patterns.

The patient may react so quickly to the therapist's instructions that she has to ask him to wait until she is ready and has finished what she is saying. Examples:

- The nurse is helping the patient to transfer from his bed to the wheelchair, and he tries to move across before his feet are placed on the floor or before his seat has been lifted off the bed.
- The therapist starts to prepare the patient for coming to a standing position, and he leaps to his feet before she has her hands in place to support him.

Use of Far Too Much Effort When Performing Simple Activities

When asked to do a relatively easy activity the patient uses an inappropriate amount of effort, tenses his muscles and holds his breath, despite the therapist's quiet instructions to the contrary. Examples:

- The therapist asks the patient to sit up straight, and he immediately elevates his shoulder girdle, extends his neck vigorously, pushes his chest forwards and breathes in loudly.
- Even if asked just to breathe quietly, forced inspiration and expiration follow with exaggerated movements of his thorax.

Inability to Perform Tasks Despite Adequate Muscle Activity

The patient may have recovered considerable selective movement in his affected limbs but still be unable to use them functionally. He is often reproached for not doing more for himself. Examples:

- In sitting, the patient can extend his knee and dorsiflex his ankle fully. The physician complains that he is not trying hard enough because he is not yet able to walk.
- Despite the return of voluntary activity in his affected limbs the patient requires help with the activities of daily life.
- At home the patient does nothing to help his partner with the cooking or other household chores, although he is able to move his hemiplegic arm and hand selectively on command.

Inability to Remember Appointments, Instructions or Corrections Which Have Been Given Previously

The patient misses various therapy appointments because he fails to attend or arrives too late. Other patients may arrive far too early and fret because they have to wait. The patient makes the same mistakes constantly despite repeated admonitions from the therapist and nursing staff, and despite repeated practice of the correct movement. Examples:

- At the start of the physician's ward round the patient is nowhere to be found, although the nurse has asked him to wait beside his bed.
- He forgets to put on the brakes of his wheelchair before standing up or transferring to his bed.

- When putting on his pullover, he places the sound arm in the sleeve first, pulls the garment over his head and is then unable to manipulate the affected arm into its sleeve.
- Each time he stands up from sitting, he does so by taking all the wait on his sound leg with his hemiplegic foot much too far forward and his leg pushing back in extension.

Failure to Perceive Stimuli on the Affected Side

Failure to perceive stimuli is condition sometimes termed hemi-inattention (Kinsella and Ford 1985). It is as if the world on his affected side does not exist for the patient any more. He fails to see objects on that side, does not hear when someone speaks to him and may injure his hemiplegic limbs because he does not realise that they are in danger of being trapped in the wheelchair or crushed against the doorframe. Examples:
- The patient fails to acknowledge the greeting of someone approaching him from his affected side and is thought to be deaf or unfriendly.
- When attempting to leave his room, he pushes his wheelchair against the side of the door and cannot fathom why it will not move. He may bump into other patients who are on that side when he is moving about in his chair.
- He may continue to push his chair forwards, although his affected hand is caught in the spokes of the wheel.
- Because he fails to see the words on one side of the page, the text makes no sense and the patient no longer enjoys reading.

Urinary Incontinence

The patient with marked perceptual difficulties is likely to be incontinent, particularly during the night. His inability to control his bladder is not due to sphincter weakness alone or to loss of sensation in the area, but rather to the fact that he cannot cope with the complex planning and timing involved in being continent. Examples:
- The patient has wet trousers when he comes to physiotherapy after a session with the speech therapist, because he has not thought of visiting the toilet with so much else in mind.
- During the night he wets his bed because there are no events to act as cues to visit the toilet.

Nonvalid Explanations for Failed Task Performances

As most people tend to do, the patient will try to find an explanation as to why he cannot perform some activity successfully. In his case, the reasons he gives may not seem logical or relevant. Examples:
- If he is unable to take weight on his affected leg, he may tell the therapist that he suffered a gunshot wound in World War II, even though he walked normally during the intervening years before his stroke, or he may say that he is very tired, having not slept well.

- When he cannot tie his shoe laces, he explains that his wife has always done that for him, ever since their marriage.

Failure to Carry Over into Daily Life Activities Performed Successfully in the Treatment Sessions

It is often frustrating for the therapist, after a successful treatment session, to observe the patient moving in an abnormal way once he has left the gymnasium. Examples:
- The patient was able to move his arm and hand during therapy and dressed himself using both hands. Later at the swimming pool, however, he is observed using only his sound hand to put on his clothes.
- Under the therapist's watchful eye the patient walks without hyperextending his knee or hitching up the side of his pelvis to take a step. Outside, he is seen to walk with a marked limp, with his leg held rigidly in total extension.

Apparent Loss of Initiative

Many patients can perform activities or make decisions only when instructed to do so by another person. Without instructions or suggestions, the patient sits immobile and expresses no desire to go out and about. Examples:
- The therapist holds an object for the patient to grasp, but she has to tell him to extend his elbow before he does so.
- If the nurse (or his wife, if he is at home) does not ask him to get out of bed in the morning he just lies there and waits.

Inability to Recall Words or Form Sentences of Normal Length, i.e. Aphasia

The whole subject of aphasia is very complex and involves many factors. It is, however, dependent upon perceptual processing of a high order and will not be a problem related solely to language and the ability to speak (Sonderegger 1997).

Social Behaviour Differs from That Expected in a Given Situation

In comparison to his previous life style, the patient behaves differently to the way he did before his stroke. He may talk excessively and inappropriately, interrupt others who are talking or use crude language. Examples:
- The patient tells a dirty joke in the middle of a team meeting, when his future is being discussed.
- He interrupts the therapist while she is busy treating another patient, to tell her about his grandchild's birthday party.

Inability to Adapt Behaviour to Different Situations or Tasks

Some patients have difficulty in performing a task which they have learned to complete successfully if they are in another place or if the situation differs in some way. Examples:

- The patient can dress himself independently when seated in his room next to his bed. After being examined in the doctor's office, however, he is unable to put on his clothes again.
- Having practised a certain activity many times with one therapist while seated on a particular plinth in the department, the patient is unable to do the same activity when he is in the hands of another therapist, working on a different plinth. He may say that he has never attempted that activity before, and appears to be confused about what is expected of him.

Inability to Inhibit an Immediate Response to a Stimulus, Particularly a Visual One

The patient reacts immediately when he perceives a stimulus and is unable to prevent the reaction from occurring. He continues to react until the stimulus is no longer there. Examples:

- While walking with the help of the therapist, the patient sees a chair and immediately starts to sit down, even though the chair is still too far away from him and he has not yet turned around appropriately.
- Seated at the dining-room table, the patient eats a whole kilo of grapes, which happens to be in a fruit bowl in the middle of the table.

Apparent Lack of Motivation

Because he is unable to perform relatively simple tasks independently, makes excuses, forgets instructions and cannot initiate movements, the patient is often unfairly labelled as being unmotivated and uncooperative. Every patient desperately wants to make progress and improve his condition; thus, any apparent lack of motivation is far more likely to be due to inadequate perception than to failed compliance. It must be taken into account that there is no single "centre" in the brain responsible for motivation, nor, in the words of Wall (1987), referring to pain and its mechanisms, should it be "considered as a separate special system bolted on to the outside of the real brain". Motivation is dependent upon the environment and the amount of help the patient is given to achieve realistic goals.

Reciprocity of Perception and Learning

It may be easier to understand the difficulties the patient has if certain relevant features of normal perception and memory or learning are considered first. Our ability to learn and to adapt continually to our ever-changing environment is dependent upon intact perceptual processes. The concept of perception is very complex, and as Affolter and Stricker (1980) state: "Perception includes all mechanisms used in processing the stimuli of an actual situation, including the different sensory modalities, supramodal organisation levels, respective storage systems, and recognition performances." Similarly, Carterette and Friedman (1973) have defined perception as "understanding the way in which the organism transforms, organises and structures information arising from the world in sense data or memory."

In normal life, from the time we wake up till the time we go to sleep we are constantly solving problems and making decisions for the necessary adaptation to movement, to happenings and to other people around us. The tactile-kinaesthetic sensory system is the perceptual process essential for adaptation and also for the development of more complex performances. Visual and auditory information is secondary and qualitative, as is repeatedly demonstrated by the ability of blind people to live independently, raise a family and work in a variety of professions to earn a living. The same applies to those who are deaf, even if they have been so since earliest childhood. It has sometimes been suggested that posture and balance are dependent upon vision, a hypothesis which seems illogical in view of the fact that many who are blind participate in sports and use public transport. Boccelli, the famous Italian tenor who has been blind since childhood, stands unsupported on the stage to give recitals. Dennet (1991) explains the tendency to overemphasise the importance of vision in his inimitable way: "Vision is the sense modality that we human thinkers almost always single out as our major source of perceptual knowledge, though we readily resort to touch and hearing to confirm what our eyes have told us." In addition," Sight so dominates our intellectual practices that we have great difficulty in conceiving of an alternative." He feels that the habit of "seeing everything in the mind through the metaphor of vision" is a major source of distortion and confusion.

Describing visual perception as being "a feeling of the body as we see", Damasio (1994) explains that, "When you see, you do not just see; you feel that you are seeing something with your eyes." When an object is seen, its shape, form, weight and meaning are recognised not merely because signals are transmitted to the retina but because it has been experienced in other ways before. For instance, a bottle, from a purely visual point of view, appears as straight lines, but we know that it is round because we have handled many bottles and thus recognise the shape we see and can also anticipate how heavy it would be to lift. "When we estimate how much effort has to be spent on a task, we reach back to previous experience for the answer because our perceptions of the present are rooted in the past" (Brooks 1986). The same applies to the way in which we move because, according to Brooks, "The CNS generates motor actions on the basis of correlations of peripheral sensory motor information with central models based on past experience".

During active movements, there is a natural association between the efferent motor patterns and the (re)afferent patterns that measure their sensory consequences (Morasso and Sanguinetti 1995). This "sensory-motor dialogue", as it has been termed by Paillard (1986), is the way in which we learn sensory-motor transformations by active exploration of the environment during our whole life, particularly during our early development.

The efference-reafference cycle "can be seen as a self-organizing or self-supervised strategy for learning the association between sensory stimuli, taken as targets, and the movements that are able to acquire the targets" (Morasso and Sanguinetti 1995).

The authors reject the idea that motor behaviour is the inevitable response to a set of explicit sensory-motor transformations, a unique motor pattern for any given stimulus which does not allow any kind of task-dependent adaptation. They suggest instead a concept of body schema which represents implicitly a number of input-output transformations and can be used differently in the context of different tasks. "In our view, a body schema is therefore an internal model, necessary for the initiation and planning of goal-orientated movements", one that "is not a mere association of kinesthetic and somesthetic cues but rather a framework where the cues are integrated".

The term for such motor programs can be replaced by "learned motor routine or motor sequence memory", and "voluntary motor acts are the result of either ideas or goals formulated by other brain areas or reactions to events in the surroundings". (Roland 1993). In addition, this author explains how motor structures are coactivated with nonmotor structures to produce patterns of activations (and deactivations) under the demands of the task.

"Perception is essential to action just as action is essential to perception", and "motor control emerges from the interaction between the individual, the task and the environment" (Shumway-Cook and Woollacott 1995). In other words, "Perceiving is as much about acting on the environment as it is about receiving signals from it", as Damasio (1994) explains. Brooks (1986) also emphasises the correlation between the two: "Learning from previous experience thus depends on sensing and moving, not just on sensing. The two processes are facilitated by unceasing communication between the sensory and motor systems."

The structural changes which occur in the formation of long-term memory, learning, and also in development are similar, and for all of these "a target is necessary – a feature that makes for plasticity, or the all-important ability to change in response to the environment" (Ackerman 1992).

Bach-y-Rita (1981) writes that "it is now clear that neuronal dendritic growth results from functional demands. Furthermore, extensive growth of dendritic arborizations occurs in man even in old age. This growth is evidently accompanied by new synapse formation."

In summary, learning is task orientated and requires moving and feeling.

Together with the internal representation of the goal and the motor program that initiates the neural commands to the muscles, position sense will be shown to be part of a complex, proactive rather than retroactive mechanism, which acts not only in the short term for steering movements, but also in the longer term in processes like motor learning and motor memory (Jeannerod 1990).

As Moore (1980) says:

The nervous system learns by doing. Active involvement has repeatedly been shown to be superior to passive participation in order for the nervous system to learn, mature and remain viable. Granted one can learn by observation but this has never been as effective as learning actively. The organism needs to 'get into the act' so to speak, and go through the process of an activity before permanent memory engrams are laid down.

In fact, it has been proposed that "the process of observation cannot develop the appropriate sensory corrections for movement control, which are very important in bringing about change in movement" (Newell 1996). Vision can actually detract from the performance of a large number of learned skills because practised movements which are usually corrected by muscular-articular sensation are disrupted by the interference of a distracting visual control (Bernstein 1996).

Disturbed Perception and Learning

Adaptation is dependent upon intact perceptual processing, so that the hemiplegic patient, who has a disturbance of the perceptual processes due to the lesion, will fail to behave and adapt adequately in his daily life as a result. It has been postulated that patients who fail in complex human behaviour receive inadequate or distorted tactile/kinaesthetic information (Affolter and Stricker 1980). Damasio (1994) also stresses the importance of feeling with regard to the patient's learning or relearning: "Somehow what does not come naturally and automatically through the primacy of feeling cannot be maintained in the mind", and he explains that new facts presented verbally or through direct visual confrontation are soon forgotten.

Many terms, such as "apraxia", "agnosia" and "psycho-organic syndrome", have been attached to the perceptual problems experienced by hemiplegic patients, but such words describe only a group of symptoms. They do not explain the underlying cause of the difficulty, which the therapist needs to know in order to treat the patient appropriately. Whichever of these problems the patient demonstrates, they will be related to his inability to feel. The findings of a recent study revealed, for example, that visual field defects do not exacerbate neglect, but that, "poor functional recovery in many patients with visual field defects is due to the association of sensory loss with the underlying causal factor of neglect" (Halligan et al. 1990).

Proprioception is essential for movement and learning. According to Bernstein (1996), "Muscular-articular sense is definitely the primary and most essential sense in most cases of motor control. All the various organs of this type of sensitivity are termed in physiology the proprioceptive system. (Proprioceptive sense means 'sensing itself', that is, having a sense of one's own body)." The effects of losing this modality are graphically illustrated by Sachs (1985) in a description of a patient who lost all proprioception permanently as a result of an exceptional type of polyneuritis and felt that she was "disembodied." Sachs quotes how this patient described her state in her own words, using analogies derived from other senses: "I feel my body is blind and deaf to itself ... it has no sense of itself." Bannister (1974) describes such a state as being "perhaps the most disturbing and disorganizing experience that man can undergo", because, as he says, to live in an inexplicable world is frightening enough, but to be inexplicable to oneself must be even more frightening.

Patients who have loss of proprioception and thus of the "sense of their own body" and its interaction with the world around them will therefore experience a profound disruption of mental processes (Damasio 1994). The tactile/kinaesthetic system is unique among the sensory systems, in the sense that it is the only one that relates directly to reality.

To reiterate, it must be remembered that as a result of such disturbances, the patient who has difficulty in performing one task will also fail to perform successfully other tasks of a similar complexity. For example, as has been mentioned, the patient's unsuccessful attempt to dress himself will not be an isolated failure but only a visible symptom of the whole problem. No area of the brain is so specialised as to control only one function. As Mountcastle (1978) writes, ". . . one can localise a lesion but not a function", and Ruskin (1982) describes how even "the simplest of activities such as taking an apple from a bowl requires the participation of a near totality of the central nervous system as well as the entire musculoskeletal system".

Similarly, the ability to remember and store information, in other words, to learn, is not dependent upon any one part of the brain, as was previously believed. For example, present-day research with positron emission tomography (PET) imaging has demonstrated that in fact many different brain regions and not specific clusters of nerve cells are at work for even the simplest acts of recollection. According to Prof. Steven Rose (cited by Geary 1997), it is impossible to say where in the brain a particular memory is located: "Memory is a dynamic property of the brain as a whole rather than of any one specific region."

Bach-y-Rita (1981) stresses the importance of utilising the brain's potential for recovery in therapy:

Traditionally neurology has emphasised the correlation between the localisation of the lesion and the deficit of function. While certainly essential to an understanding of neurological symptoms and syndromes, this approach has frequently been accompanied by therapeutic nihilism. Greater emphasis on this plasticity of the brain (specifically on its capacity to mediate recovery of function) should lead to increased efforts to obtain the maximum recovery and reorganisation of function that the damaged nervous system is capable of sustaining.

Implications for Therapy

The aim of therapy is that the patient learn maximally, and learning takes place through repeated interaction with the environment. Affolter and Stricker (1980) describe how "interaction between the environment and the individual requires contact. Contact means to be 'in touch with'. To be in touch or in contact with can be realised only through the tactile kinesthetic sensory system."

Damasio (1994) describes the importance of the skin with regard to interaction with the environment: "The first idea that comes to mind when we think of the skin is that of an extended sensory sheet, turned to the outside, ready to help us construct the shape, texture and temperature of external objects, through the sense of touch". He goes on to explain that, "A representation of the skin might be the natural means to signify the body boundary because it is an interface turned both to the organism's interior and to the environment with which the organism interacts".

It is easier for patients to learn in real-life situations, where they can draw on past experience to assist them. "And of course, it should be realized that the mechanism of forming a new memory must be inherently more complex than recalling an old one

. . ." (Russell and Dewar 1975). "Learning occurs only from successful performance. Attempts resulting in non-performance or inaccurate performance do not train the sensorimotor system to perform the desired task. Repeated erroneous responses only train the performance of that erroneous task" (Kottke 1978).

The patient who is unable to move and feel adequately will be deprived of the opportunity to learn or relearn through experiencing the successful performance of tasks and the sensory-motor enhancement which moving to solve problems provides. It is the desire to solve a motor problem which leads to meaningful corrections for the whole movement, according to Bernstein (1996).

During treatment, therefore, the patient cannot learn through separate sensory stimuli being applied in isolation to the different senses, such as loud noises, pain, being stroked with soft materials or smelling aromatic spirits, as has been suggested in some coma-stimulation concepts (Le Winn and Dimancescu 1978), as well as by advocates of sensory integration therapy. It must be remembered that normally "we perceive events, not a successively analysed trickle of perceptual elements" (Dennet 1991).

Guided Movement Therapy (Guiding)

Because learning has been shown to be task orientated and dependent upon handling and feeling in order to solve a problem, the treatment of choice must certainly be that of guiding the patient's hands and body during the performance of real-life, problem-solving tasks. Such a concept helps the patient to interact with the environment and the objects required for an actual task and to search for the necessary information about his body in relation to the environment (Affolter and Bischofberger 1996).

"Perception of objects incorporates active motor components to provide the necessary searching movements" (Luria 1978). If the patient is unable to move adequately on his own, he will need to be assisted in his search. The therapist cannot take the patient's eyes and move them in such a way as to be sure that he is seeing, nor can she turn his ears towards a sound and know that he is hearing its meaning. As Affolter (1981) so rightly says:

> There is only one sensory modality which one can activate directly and that is the tactile-kinaesthetic system. By taking the hands or the body of the patient, and by guiding them to explore stimuli of the situation, some input can be assured. In addition to allowing input, the tactile-kinaesthetic system is unique among the sensory systems because it is the only sensory system that relates directly to reality.

Guiding enables the patient to obtain more information than he would be able to on his own, due to his inability to move and feel adequately. Guiding thus provides him with what has been termed "augmented information", i.e. information which is not otherwise available to the learner when learning and performing a task (Newell 1996). The author explains how, "augmented information provides the support for facilitating the search of the perceptual-motor work space, the construction of attractor dynamics, and the realization of the task."

Therapists and other caretakers can guide the patient, either as an intensive therapeutic measure or when he is being helped to carry out an activity in his daily life which he is unable to perform on his own. As Werner (1996) points out, when helping a patient (in this case a little girl) to learn a new skill, the ensuing movements are better if her hands are guided than if she is told how to do something. The author's advice is, "Do not to try to 'make her learn' but give her many learning opportunities."

Therapeutic or Intensive Guiding

When the therapist is guiding the patient intensively as a treatment procedure, she aims at ensuring the following:
- An enhanced interaction with the environment
- Activity which is goal orientated, with the goal recognised by the patient
- That the goal is provided by a real task of a problem-solving nature
- Active exploration of the objects relevant to the task by handling and touching and moving them
- Assisted searching and organisation of the search for information to obtain augmented information about the supporting surfaces and the task itself
- Changing the sources of the information from those within the patient, i.e. kinaesthetic, to those provided by contact with the environment, i.e. tactile

The therapist can guide the patient in a variety of positions, and whether he is lying, sitting or standing, these aims can still be fulfilled. However, it is usually easier for her to ensure that the patient explores the stability of the different supporting surfaces and is in contact with them with his body if he is seated at a table. Guiding in sitting will nevertheless improve his ability to stand and walk, because of the enhanced tactile/kinaesthetic information which he experiences during the guided task performance. Regardless of the starting position and the task to be performed, to guide the patient successfully, the therapist should know exactly how she will guide the various movements and in which different ways the problem could possibly be solved. It is well worth her while to practise the guided task beforehand, with a colleague or a relative of the patient acting as a model and imitating his symptoms, thus avoiding unexpected difficulties that might arise in the actual treatment situation. Certain objects can prove very difficult to manipulate without such careful preparation, for example, picking up a knife with the patient's hand or peeling a banana if he has hypertonicity in the finger flexors.

Using Verbal Instructions

If the problem which requires solving is clear because all the objects required are in front of the patient, the therapist does not need to explain verbally what he has to do. Instead, she commences to guide him in his exploratory movements, beginning with those objects which present the problem. For more advanced patients, the therapist may choose a problem which is not directly within their visual field and which therefore requires a short verbal explanation.

While guiding, the therapist does not give the patient verbal instructions or feedback. Her voice would only distract him from the activity, as he would need to stop and listen to her, or the words would provide a clue to the next step, a clue which would not be there when he is trying to carry out a similar task on his own. However she talks to him spontaneously during intervals in the actual performance, when a part of the activity has been completed and both are catching their breath before continuing. The therapist will definitely need to speak to the patient if, for any reason, something goes wrong or the patient reacts in a negative way and the task has to be interrupted or changed.

How the Patient is Guided Therapeutically

Having chosen an appropriate task, the therapist presents the problem to the patient in such a way that he understands the eventual goal. She starts at once to guide him as he explores the objects, recognises the problem and strives to find possible solutions.

Whatever the task, the patient is guided in a similar way, according to the principles explained in the following example: Slicing a cucumber and putting the slices in a salad bowl (**Fig. 1.1**).

The therapist arranges appropriate articles on a table, in a way designed to encourage the patient to look and reach out in a certain direction, or in order to overcome other particular difficulties which he may have. The patient is then helped to sit down on a stool at the table.

■ **Fig. 1.1 a.** The therapist guides his hands to draw the table closer to him. Standing well to one side of the patient, with her thigh against the outside of his, she places one of her hands over his and presses it down gently but firmly to test the stability of the table surface. First with her finger tips directly over his, and then with the whole of her hand on the dorsal aspect of his, the therapist helps him to make contact with the surface by moving her hand slightly from side to side, as if feeling the table through his hand. She then does the same with her forearm over his. Once the patient's arm and hand are resting in contact with the table, the therapist moves his other hand slowly sideways towards the far edge of the table, holding his arm lightly from above the wrist. She does not move his hand all the way, but takes only a small step in that direction. Then she moves round to that side of the patient until her other thigh is against his, and places her hand over his in the same sequence as she did previously, searching for information through his fingers, hand and forearm before moving his contralateral hand. Step by small step, she guides the patient's hands one after the other, until she can grasp the edge of the table with his hand and help him to pull it nearer to his body.

■ **Fig. 1.1 b.** Moving from one side of the patient to the other and feeling the table through his hand and arm with each step, the therapist moves the patient's hands gradually towards the opposite side of the table, and draws that towards him as well. Once it is close to him, she uses her body to move his trunk forwards until his chest is in contact with the table in front of him, a contact that she can feel through his body. She does not just press him against the table but tests its stability by using slight searching movements of his trunk.

From this moment onwards, the therapist never moves both the patient's hands in the air at the same time. Instead, she always guides one of his arms first to make contact

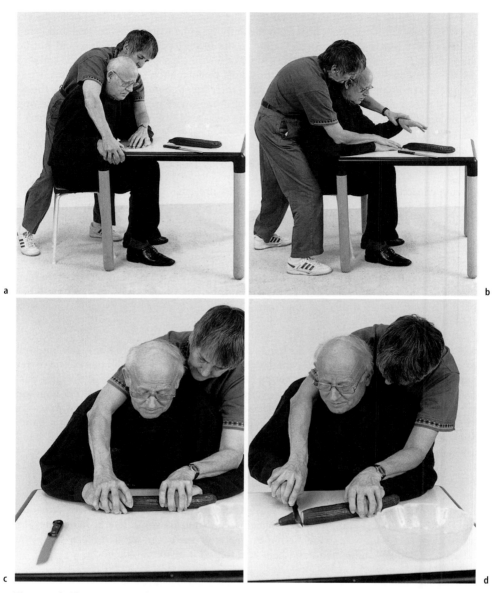

Fig. 1.1 a–i. Therapeutic guiding (right hemiplegia). **a** Drawing the table towards the patient. **b** With his trunk and arm in contact with the table the patient's other hand is free to reach for the cucumber. **c** Exploring the cucumber to discover the problem. **d** Cutting the cucumber and feeling the resistance through the knife

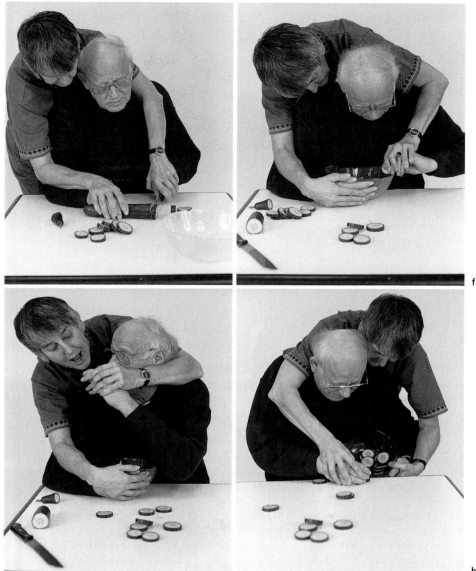

Fig. 1.1 e–h. e Feeling the table with the other side of his body while slicing. **f** Putting the slices in the bowl. **g** Introducing an unexpected variation. **h** Holding the bowl between trunk and table while putting in the slices

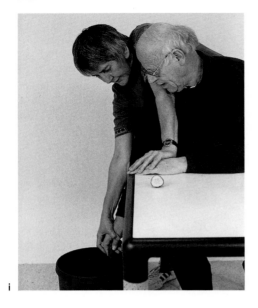

i

Fig. 1.1 i. Reaching down to throw the remains in the bin

with the supporting surface and test its stability, before his other arm moves or is moved to make the next step in the task performance. The patient's arm should feel light and easy to move if the overall support is adequate. The guided movements should be performed slowly to allow the patient time to adapt to each new position, to feel secure and be able to follow the movements of his other side. If the moving arm becomes hypertonic or demonstrates increased tremor, the therapist immediately guides an intensified search for a stable support as she did before, only then moving the patient's other hand towards the goal by taking a small step. For additional information about the supporting surfaces, the therapist can also help the patient to feel the seat on which he is sitting by pressing down over his thigh and moving her hand slightly from side to side. While guiding, she tries to bring as much of his body as possible into close contact with stable, palpable surfaces in the immediate vicinity. It is of no help to the patient to press down over a part of his body which has an empty space beneath it, for instance pushing down on his knee to bring his heel onto the floor, because the supporting seat does not extend that far.

■ **Fig. 1.1 c.** The cucumber is brought towards the patient and the problem explored; an instrument is required in order to slice it.

■ **Fig. 1.1 d.** The patient is guided as he reaches out for the knife, grasps it and begins to cut the cucumber. The therapist guides the activity in such a way that the blade remains in contact with the cucumber as the knife is moved up into position for cutting the next slice.

■ **Fig. 1.1 e.** Within a very short time, the hand which is in contact with the table will cease to perceive the underlying surface and the therapist changes her position and guides the patient's other arm down onto the surface. Guiding first one of his hands and then the other, the therapist adjusts the position of the objects appropriately and the patient continues to cut the cucumber, but with the knife held in his other hand.

■ **Fig. 1.1 f.** Once the cucumber has been sliced, it would be appropriate to pause briefly before continuing, because a part of the task has been completed and both the therapist and the patient can relax for a moment or two. The therapist then guides the patient to reach for the salad bowl, bring it towards him and hold it firmly in place against his chest. With his other hand he begins to put the slices into the bowl. He does not move his hand though the air but is guided so that the slice maintains contact with the hard surface of the bowl.

■ **Fig. 1.1 g.** It is important that the activity does not become too repetitive, with no change in the motions. The therapist therefore guides the patient to introduce some new and unexpected variation to the task. For example, instead of the next slice being placed in the bowl, it can be brought up to her mouth for her to eat.

■ **Fig. 1.1 h.** Another change can be introduced, for example, by placing the bowl between the patient's chest and the edge of the table and using his other hand to slide the slices into it. The therapist guides the patient's trunk forwards to maintain a firm contact, sufficient to keep the bowl in place.

■ **Fig. 1.1 i.** Once the task has been completed, the patient can also be guided while he clears the table. To place the ends of the cucumber in a bin on the floor, the therapist guides his hand towards it, maintaining contact with the leg of the table on the way, thus avoiding his having to move down through an open space, which could be alarming for him. The surface of the table can be wiped clean, and if the patient is able to walk with help, the salad bowl can be taken and put in the refrigerator or on the kitchen counter.

The completion of a task provides a very good opportunity for the therapist and the patient to discuss the work which has just been done. Important features can be emphasised and incidents recalled, which will be of great help both for patients with aphasia and for those with short-term memory problems.

Choosing a Task

Kottke (1978) is convinced that optimal learning takes place when the patient is practising just below the peak of his best performance. "It is only when practising near the peak of performance that the level of performance increases."

The therapist may have difficulty in deciding what the patient's best level of performance is. Patients who have suffered a brain lesion may often be functioning on a far lower level of planning, as described by Affolter (1981), than they did prior to their stroke. Because some patients have such a high level of speech performance, their actual planning and performance level is often overestimated. A patient may be able to speak in detail about Beethoven or Picasso, whereby he is merely drawing on previously stored information. Retrieving such verbal information from memory requires no new planning or decision-making. It can be likened to a stored computer programme. The same patient, however, may be unable to find his way to his own room or open the door if he has a cane in his hand.

The therapist can estimate the patient's actual performance level more accurately by observing his attentiveness and general behaviour when she is guiding him during a problem-solving task. That the task is on the correct level can be assumed if:
- The patient is quiet while working and does not speak or move restlessly.
- The tone throughout his body is felt to normalise and remains adequate, regardless of whether hypertonicity or flaccidity is the problem.
- There is an intent expression on his face.
- The eye contact for the task is appropriate; i.e. he does not look around vaguely, but will either be looking at what he is doing or tensing the muscles around his eyes intently, to the point of closing them, as we do when we are sensing something finely.

Patients react in characteristic ways when the task confronting them is too complex or too easy, just as we all do. The patient with a brain lesion only reacts more strongly!

That too much is being demanded of him is interpreted if:
- The patient shows panic or fear. He cries out or clutches desperately at someone or something.
- His tone increases markedly.
- He talks exaggeratedly about irrelevant matters, e.g. old family history, or tells repetitive jokes.
- He makes constant requests to visit the toilet.
- He complains of other symptoms which could account for his lack of success, e.g. backache, old war wounds or lack of sleep.
- He shows signs of aggression directed towards the therapist or nurse.

When too little is demanded of him:
- The patient appears bored and disappointed.
- He chatters inconsequentially, or makes repetitive jokes.
- He is inattentive and keeps looking at other stimuli, e.g. at fellow patients or out of the window.
- The patient fiddles with his clothing or scratches his face or other parts of his body.

When working at his individual peak performance level the patient recognises his successful performance and is motivated to continue working at the task. "It does not help the patient to tell him a given step has been performed (well or not well) as long as he cannot experience the success of that step of the event himself" (Affolter 1981). "When we are working intensively we feel keenly the progress of our work; we are elated when our progress is rapid, we are depressed when it is slow" (Polya 1973). "And the typical consequence of prolonged or frequent failure is a general feeling of apathy. In the world of children, the concept is expressed as an I-don't-want-to-play-any-more attitude. The game is too hard. The rewards, while attractive, are too far removed to be a strong motivating force" (Jeffrey 1981).

Motivation is dependent upon the suitability of the task and the way in which the therapist guides the patient. By guiding the patient the therapist can enable him to work at his correct level of planning, irrespective of his motor ability. She can ensure that he completes the task successfully and does not experience repeated failure as he might otherwise do.

Some clinicians feel that it is belittling for adult patients to be guided during task performance, but experience has shown that this is not the case at all. Patients who are professors, doctors, teachers and farmers, to name but a few from clinical practice, have enjoyed the experience and verbalised the beneficial effects on their condition. In fact, patients at all stages of their rehabilitation are only too willing to be guided if they understand that voluntary movements in their hand, their speech or their ability to walk independently can be improved through such guided activities.

Additional Considerations When Choosing a Task

Other factors will influence the therapist's choice of a suitable task and also her decision as to how she can best guide the patient.

Size of the Patient

Ideally, the patient sits on a stool at the table, as shown in **Fig. 1.1 a**, to allow the therapist to guide his trunk and limbs from behind him and to either side. Even if he is still in a wheelchair, she can transfer him onto the stool and, through her close proximity, ensure that he does not lose his balance. If the relative sizes of the patient and therapist allow, she may prefer to sit immediately behind him with her legs on the outside of his while guiding his trunk and arms. Usually, though, she will need to stand when she guides, to allow her more freedom of movement during the activity. The therapist will certainly have to stand if the patient is still too weak to sit safely on a stool and has to be guided while seated in the wheelchair, because she will need to adapt to the restrictions of its arms and the backrest.

Mechanical Factors

The therapist must also take into account what objects and instruments are required for the task and whether she will be able to manage their manipulation from a purely practical point of view. For example, if the patient's hand has flexor spasticity, a zucchini or a cucumber is far easier to deal with than a banana, and picking up a knife will be difficult if he cannot help actively. Cutting an orange and pressing it is an ideal problem to solve manually, but guiding the patient's hands when they are slippery from the juice is no easy task. The same applies if a juicy fruit has to be peeled and sliced.

For a patient who has painful limitation of range of motion, the therapist will need to choose objects which are not too big for him to hold, and the objects must be placed near enough for him to reach them without pain being elicited.

The Patient's Stage of Progress

When working with a severely disabled patient in the early stages, the therapist tries to select tasks which can be performed with his hands and body and do not involve manipulating one object with another (Davies 1994). Using an intermediary tool such as a knife, a fork, a screwdriver or a corkscrew constitutes a more advanced stage than direct contact with the objects themselves, as does placing a cup on a saucer, because the user has to "feel" through the instrument. Gibson (1966) explains how, "when a man touches something with a stick he feels it at the end of the stick, not in the hand". This ability, which allows the performance of countless skilled tasks, ranging from eating with a knife and fork to performing intricate brain surgery, has been termed the "stick" phenomenon (Affolter and Stricker 1980) or "wand" phenomenon (Dennet 1991).

The number of objects on the table also plays a significant role in increasing the degree of difficulty of the task from a perceptual point of view, the simplest being just the two essential things required to present and solve the problem For example, a bottle of mineral water and a glass standing on the table directly in front of the patient indicate that the bottle will be opened, water poured into the glass and a drink taken.

For very severely affected patients the goal may even then be too far removed and not clearly understood. The therapist will sometimes have to place the key object in the patient's arm against his body from the start, or on the wheelchair table immediately within his grasp. When working with a patient who has made further progress, objects other than those actually required can be added, and he can be guided to explore and discover which are really necessary for the task in hand.

Still more complex are tasks where all the objects and instruments necessary for solving the problem are not within the patient's visual field and he has to move and look for them. For example, the patient is making a pizza in the occupational therapy kitchen and needs the rolling pin to smooth out the pastry. He has to open various cupboards and drawers to find it, with the therapist guiding him during the search.

Location

The place where the patient is to be guided will influence the therapist with regard to the task she chooses. For instance, preparing a ham sandwich in the gymnasium would not be appropriate, whereas opening a bottle of mineral water and having a drink after exercising would be.

While the patient is still in the intensive care unit, finding a suitable task becomes difficult. He is lying in bed, space is limited, and in all probability he is not yet able to eat or drink. It is most important, however, for the patient to be guided during the acute phase, even if he appears to be unconscious, because otherwise he is deprived of any meaningful stimulation. Surrounding him are monitors and machines, and all he hears are the repetitive noises which they make and the voices of those who are performing routine procedures while caring for him. He sees only the ceiling and surrounding walls, and the soft anti-decubitus mattress offers him no reliable information as to his whereabouts. Despite the limitations, the imaginative therapist will always find possible tasks and be able to guide the patient. For example, with the patient lying on is side, the therapist guides him as he applies his aftershave lotion (**Fig. 1.2**).

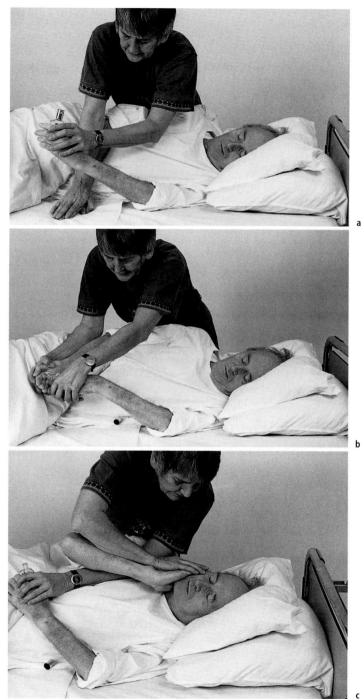

Fig. 1.2 a–c. Guiding the patient in bed (left hemiplegia). **a** Lifting the bottle of after-shave lotion; **b** placing some lotion in the palm of his hand; **c** rubbing the lotion on his face

■ **Fig. 1.2 a.** The therapist first guides one of the patient' hands to search for a stable contact with the surface beneath him, before moving his other hand to lift the bottle of aftershave lotion.

■ **Fig. 1.2 b.** With the bottle pressed firmly against the patient's body, it is opened and the lotion is put on one of the patient's hands.

■ **Fig. 1.2 c.** The therapist guides the patient's hand towards his face and he rubs the lotion onto his cheek.

Some other tasks which the therapist could guide the patient to perform in the intensive care stage include brushing his hair, taking a Kleenex from a box and cleaning his nose, holding a pot of hand cream and applying the cream to his hands. A portable radio held close to his body can be switched on and a programme chosen which interests him.

The Time Available for the Guided Activity

With present-day restrictions on the amount of time allotted to individual patients, the therapist may feel under pressure and try to complete the whole task with the patient in a relatively short period. She therefore needs to consider the time she will be able to spend guiding the patient when she is choosing a task for him and adapt accordingly. It is important that the patient be guided slowly and carefully in order for him to adapt to each new position, understand the problem confronting him and have time enough to anticipate and follow the subsequent movements. On no account should the therapist try to hurry him along in order to complete the whole task. The guiding is seldom too slow, although sometimes the therapist imagines that she is moving at a snail's pace. On the contrary, all too often, when reviewing videos of her guiding she discovers that she has in fact moved far too quickly for the patient. Once again, it is the patient's responses which tell her whether or not the speed is correct for him. It is not essential that a task be completed on any one day. If the therapist feels that time is running out, instead of rushing to finish, she should rather complete just a part of the task and tell the patient that they will continue during their next session together.

Guiding When Giving Assistance

All those who are involved in caring for the patient can follow the principles of guiding whenever they are helping him to do something he cannot manage on his own. Even if the patient is guided for only a few moments each time it will be most beneficial, because there will be many such occasions arising quite spontaneously during the day when someone can assist him in this therapeutic way. All members of staff should therefore know how to guide and be prepared to step in whenever they observe that the patient is in difficulty. It does not matter to which professional group they belong; even the enlightened medical superintendent of a large hospital in Munich guides patients as a matter of course during consultations in his office!

The following example illustrates how the principles of guiding can be applied in everyday situations in the hospital or rehabilitation centre. It frequently happens that a patient pushes his chair against a fixed object and cannot continue further. If the therapist reverses the chair for him and steers it away from the hindrance so that he can push the chair further she will have taken over and made the necessary plan for him. He will then have learned only that when the chair becomes wedged he must have someone to help him. And so he calls for help the next time it happens, or waits expectantly for someone to come to his aid. In a similar way, if the therapist tells the patient what he must do each time, she is actually doing the planning for him. Her verbal instruction is the next step required before he can complete the task.

Instead, the therapist or a nurse, finding the patient in the situation, should take his hand and guide it to the wheel of the wheelchair and then reverse the chair by guiding his hand on the wheel. In this way he learns the necessary sequence, through feeling and storing. Later he will be able to produce the steps on his own in any situation where his wheelchair becomes wedged against an object.

Whatever the task confronting the patient may be, e.g. turning over in bed, dressing himself in the morning or trying to take the elevator to the dining room, guiding is the most beneficial way to assist him. The following examples demonstrate how guiding can be used spontaneously and therapeutically as a way of assisting the patient during everyday activities:

Example 1: Washing Face and Hands

■ **Fig. 1.3 a.** The wash basin provides a stable surface, and the therapist guides one of the patient's hands to make firm contact with it. His other hand moves to put on the tap and then to test the temperature of the water.

■ **Fig. 1.3 b.** Because the arm will no longer perceive the underlying surface if it stays too long in one position, the therapist guides his other hand to search for a stable support while he moves to switch off the tap when the basin is sufficiently full.

■ **Fig. 1.3 c.** With one arm firmly in contact with the basin, the patient reaches for the towel when he has finished washing and brings it towards him.

■ **Fig. 1.3 d.** He dries his hands, one after the other.

■ **Fig. 1.3 e.** When he has washed his face the therapist helps him to dry it by pressing firmly against the skin, rather than by rubbing the towel back and forth.

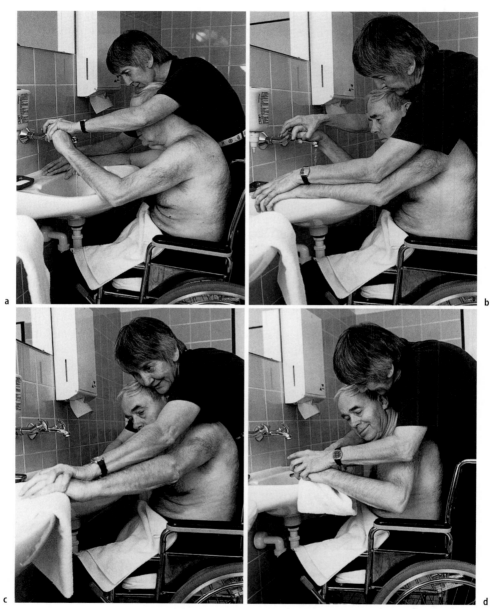

Fig. 1.3 a–e. Helping the patient to wash his hands and face (right hemiplegia). **a** Putting water in the basin; **b** one arm stays in contact with the basin while he switches off the tap; **c** reaching for the towel; **d** drying his hands

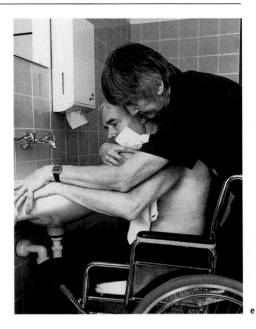

Fig. 1.3 e. Drying his face

e

Example 2: Eating Yogurt for Breakfast

■ **Fig. 1.4 a.** The patient is seated on a stool at the table with the yogurt jar, the basin and a spoon in front of him. The therapist guides his right arm and hand to test the stability of the surface of the table before helping him to reach for the yogurt with his other hand and draw it towards him.

■ **Fig. 1.4 b.** With the yogurt jar clasped firmly against his body and in contact with the table, the patient is helped to lift off the lid.

■ **Fig. 1.4 c.** With one arm remaining firmly in contact with the table, the patient pours the yogurt into the bowl which he has just brought towards him.

■ **Fig. 1.4 d.** The patient's left arm and hand are guided to feel the table surface and to hold the jar in place while, with his right hand, he replaces the lid and pushes it down firmly, moving it slightly from side to side to check that it is properly closed.

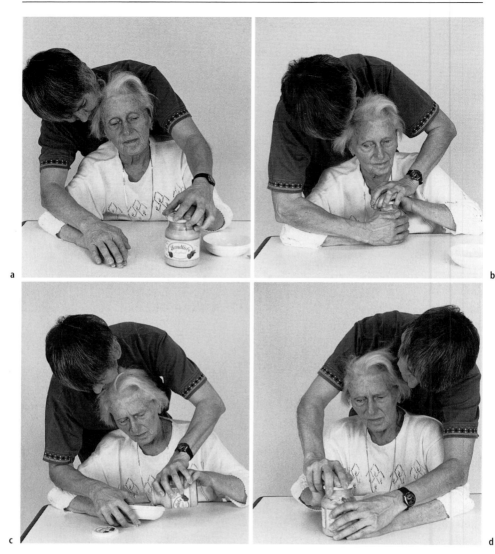

Fig. 1.4 a–d. Having a yogurt for breakfast (right hemiplegia). **a** Reaching for the yogurt; **b** yogurt jar firmly stabilised and then opened; **c** placing some yogurt in a bowl; **d** putting the lid on again

■ **Fig. 1.5 a.** With his left arm the patient feels the underlying surface and keeps the bowl steady as he takes the spoon in his right hand and starts to eat.

■ **Fig. 1.5 b.** Once again the supporting or searching arm is changed so that he can hold the spoon in his left hand

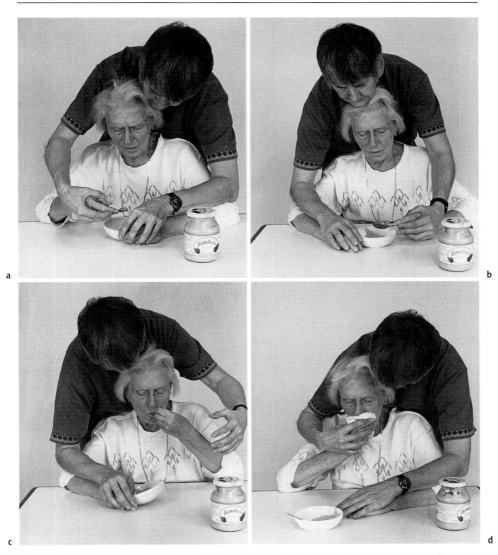

Fig. 1.5 a–d. Eating yogurt (right hemiplegia). **a** Holding the bowl steady; **b** testing the surface with one hand; **c** the patient eats alone; **d** being helped to wipe her mouth with a napkin

■ **Fig. 1.5 c.** Eating with his unaffected hand, the patient starts to manage without help and the therapist allows him to continue on his own for a while.

■ **Fig. 1.5 d.** When he has finished eating, the therapist guides his left arm and hand to check the stability of the table and he wipes his mouth with the napkin held in his right hand.

Example 3: Putting on the Wheelchair Brakes and Lifting the Footplates Prior to Standing Up or Doing a Transfer

■ **Fig 1.6 a.** The therapist guides the patient's right hand and forearm firmly onto the arm rest of his wheelchair, to ensure that it is stable and can support him. Then his left hand moves to put on the brakes.

■ **Fig. 1.6 b.** With his hands clasped together he encircles his knee with them and lifts his affected foot off the footplate to place it flat on the floor.

■ **Fig. 1.6 c.** The therapist guides his right arm to press against the side of the chair, his hand in contact with the upright bar which supports the footplate. The patient then bends forwards and, with the therapist's other hand guiding his, tips the footplate up and out of the way.

Guiding the Patient in a Standing Position

The therapist can also guide the patient when he is standing up from a chair and when he is performing a problem-solving task which requires that he stand upright. However, in standing she will need to guide other parts of his body as well, to enable him to be in contact with the supporting surfaces in his immediate vicinity, be they in front, behind or to the side. Generally speaking, that part of the patient's body which is being brought into contact with the surrounding, stable surfaces is guided by the equivalent part of the therapist's body; i. e. his knee is moved by hers, his head with her head against it, and her trunk feeling the amount of pressure against the firm surface through his trunk.

The principles for guiding in standing are explained in the following example, where the patient is guided as he prepares a tray for serving coffee to his visitors.

The patient stands up in the kitchen in order to reach for the crockery in a cupboard. The therapist has placed the thermos of coffee on the counter beneath the relevant cupboard. The patient stands up from his chair right in the corner so that there is a fixture to one side of him as well as right in front.

■ **Fig. 1.7 a.** The therapist guides one of the patient's hands onto the counter top, presses his knees forwards with hers to make contact with the cupboard doors, and shifts his pelvis to the right so that his hip and thigh are firmly against the cupboard there. She guides the patient as he reaches for the cups and saucers, etc., and also when he is arranging all the necessary items on a tea trolley.

■ **Fig. 1.7 b.** Having changed his shirt and brushed his hair before welcoming his guests, the patient wheels the trolley towards the table where they are seated.

It is interesting to note that previous attempts to walk this patient, even with the assistance of the therapist, had proved unsuccessful. He had been very frightened, with a marked increase in flexor spasticity in both his arm and his leg. However, immediately after standing in the kitchen and being guided, and then pushing the trolley as part of the task, the patient was able to walk confidently and with no increase in tone.

When a patient is walking or standing away from walls, cupboards or other fixed objects, guiding in the true sense is not possible The therapist's body is a soft and moving

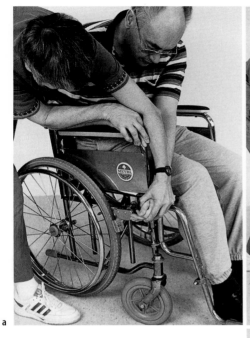

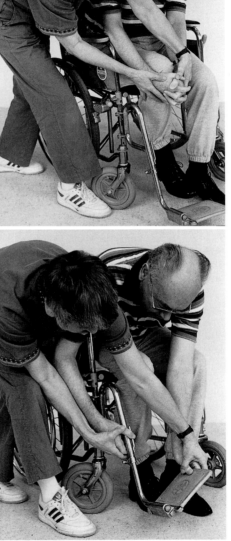

Fig. 1.6 a–c. Preparing to stand up from the wheelchair (right hemiplegia). **a** Putting on the brakes; **b** placing the patient's foot on the floor; **c** lifting the footplate out of the way

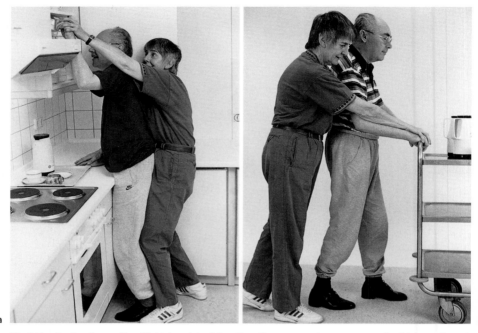

a   b

Fig. 1.7 a, b. Serving coffee (right hemiplegia). **a** Standing to get the cups out of a high cupboard; **b** pushing the loaded tea trolley to the table

support which does not provide an absolute resistance. Although she cannot guide the patient in such situations, the therapist can facilitate the correct gait pattern while he is walking by using her hands in whichever way necessary as he, for example, carries a tray to the kitchen or goes to the washbasin to brush his teeth. Once he arrives at a table on which to place the tray or reaches the basin where his toothbrush is, she can then commence guiding him again.

Considerations

The successful rehabilitation of patients with perceptual problems may be long and arduous, but their improved independence and quality of life justify the time and effort.

It is often noted in the literature on neurology and rehabilitation that virtually all the recovery from stroke that will take place occurs during the first 6 months. Many laboratory and some clinical studies do not support this view, and the possibility exists that the cessation of recovery after 6 months may well be the result of a self-fulfilling prophecy: the clinician's attitude in this regard may influence the outcome (Bach-y-Rita 1981).

Laboratory studies have demonstrated that recovery of function continues to occur more than 5 years after a stationary lesion. Bach-y-Rita and other authors have reported several cases where continuing recovery of function occurred up to as long as 7 years after the onset of stroke.

Many patients with comparatively slight hemiplegia also suffer from perceptual disorders which are often not recognised on routine clinical examination. Even if it is not possible to overcome all the patient's difficulties, care must be taken to preserve his self-respect. The problems arise from the lesion, and the patient should in no way be blamed for his failure to achieve the desired rehabilitation goals. Because of the constant problem-solving and decision-making which are necessary for adaptation in normal daily life, behaviour-modification approaches do not equip the hemiplegic patient for his life outside the rehabilitation centre. Such approaches train only habits which the patient is not able to modify or use in other situations. The patient may be easier for the staff to manage and be "good" and more amenable, but the profound advice of Jacobs (1988) should be carefully and honestly considered before any system involving punishment and reward is introduced.

Programmes and procedures must always be for the benefit of the client and not the convenience of the programme. It is always necessary to consider whether it is the client's behaviour or the programme's procedures that need modification. In many cases ambiguities or problems in the overall rehabilitation programme may be responsible for the noted aberrations on the part of the client. In such situations intervention must focus on programme modification rather than modification of the client's behaviour to conform to a substandard programme.

The principles of learning described in this chapter should be borne in mind during all activities aimed at improving the patient's sensory/motor abilities because perception and movement are dependent upon one another. As Luria (1978) emphasises, "Human voluntary movements and actions are complex functional systems, carried out by an equally complex dynamic 'constellation' of concertedly working brain zones, each of which makes its contribution to the structures of the complex movements. For this reason, a lesion of one of these zones, by blocking one component of the functional system, disturbs the normal organization of the functional system as a whole and leads to the appearance of motor deficits".

It would be impossible to treat a patient's motor and perceptual problems separately. They are inextricably interrelated, there being no motion without perception and, without movement and interaction, no possibility to perceive. Our hand is, after all, much more than merely a grasping organ! (Zittlau 1996). As Latash and Anson (1996) point out, "Brain plus redundancy makes the design of our bodies, including the system for production of voluntary movements, flexible and able to adapt not only to changes in external conditions but also, at least to some extent, to changes within the body itself".

Further ways in which the patient can be helped to meet the demands of his daily life again and enjoy his leisure hours as well are described in the following chapters.

2 Normal Movement Sequences and Balance Reactions

The treatment of patients with hemiplegia is a process of teaching and learning. The therapist teaches, the patient learns. When teaching, it is always important that the teacher should know her subject very well, and in this case, where it is movement and reactions that are being taught, the therapist must know exactly what should take place, i.e. how people move and react normally. It should be remembered, however, that "actions characteristically consist of two components; a mental component and a physical component" and the two are closely related, because "The bodily movements in our actions are caused by our intentions" (Searle 1984) Once a person decides to put a plan into action, he has an intention to act, and "the organization of voluntary action, from the intention to the execution, is dependent on the type of voluntary behaviour the subject wants to express" (Roland 1993). Referring to different levels of intentions, Woodworth (1899) explained that, "When I voluntarily start to walk, my intention is not of moving my legs in a certain manner; my will is directed towards reaching a certain place," and that "I am unable to describe what movements my arms and legs are going to make; but I am able to state what result I design to accomplish". There will therefore always be some variation in how movements are performed, depending on the surrounding conditions and the person who is moving. "In all cases in which motor initiative or adjustment is required, there is a certain tuning of the movements to an emergent task" (Bernstein 1996). In addition, not only do the nature of the task and the environment alter the body movements; anatomical differences also play a role. Referring to the influence which an individual's constitution has upon how he or she moves, Klein-Vogelbach (1990) explains that, "deviations of the lengths, widths, depths and weights of certain body segments from hypothetical norms alter a person's motor behaviour in a predictable manner, particularly when the long axis of the body is inclined out of the horizontal."

Despite the many individual variations and possibilities, however, we all move in basically similar patterns, common to us all. These patterns start developing from earliest childhood and become automatic in adult life, so that they occur throughout the day without our being aware of them. How we get out of bed in the morning, how we stand up, walk, sit down, drink a cup of coffee and even how we speak, all are carried out in a certain pattern of movement. Each of these activities has been learned, and we notice at once when someone else performs them in an unfamiliar or strange way. The background of automatic movement is such that we do not have to think consciously about how we have to move – the movements occur spontaneously. For example, when writing we do not think how to form each letter but concentrate on the content. The same applies when we speak to someone. When we walk we do not consider the act of moving each leg but can admire the surroundings or concentrate on our destination, or even hold a conversation on the way (**Fig. 2.1**).

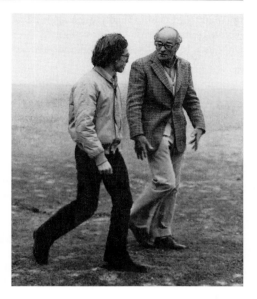

Fig. 2.1. Walking and talking

If we consider the action of walking, we see that every person walks in a similar way, one foot moving forwards and then the other, arms swinging and the body upright. Yet small individual differences enable us to recognise someone in the far distance, or even when we can only hear his footsteps approaching. Such individual variations can be observed whenever we move and are usually related to the following:

- Our constitution – whether we are short or tall, fat or thin, long-legged or not
- What we have learned by imitation from a very early age, from the customs or habits of those around us
- Our personality, with its variety of inhibitions or lack of them, and the situation in which we find ourselves at the time
- Concentrated training for a particular sport, dance form or profession
- The presence of any stiffness or pain which causes us to move differently. Even a corn on the little toe changes someone's walking pattern considerably, as does a stiff neck or shoulder. Certainly, as explained in Chap. 15, increased tension in the nervous system impedes normal neurodynamics, with altered sensory/motor activity as a result (Shacklock 1995).

Although there are indeed such variations, so similar are the normal patterns of movement that they can be used diagnostically, if someone is seen to do something very differently from everyone else. For adults the repertoire of movement possibilities is enormous, but a few everyday examples have been selected which are very important in the treatment of hemiplegic patients. People generally perform these activities in the same basic economic way. If a patient cannot perform one of the activities in this way, the therapist must discover why he cannot do so. The answer to the "why" will later become the basis of the treatment. She will try to enable the patient to carry out the movement normally and economically once again. To do so she will have to analyse very carefully which component of the movement is preventing him from carrying out the activity. Only as a result of such careful analysis can the treatment be appropriate and exact.

Analysis of Certain Everyday Movements

The analysis is not highly detailed. For each example, it is important to decide which observations led to the conclusion that a person was moving normally. The therapist needs to observe how these activities are usually performed so that she can facilitate or guide a patient correctly, enabling him to relearn the movement by feeling it.

Rolling Over from Supine to Prone (Fig. 2.2)

When starting to roll over we lift our head from the supporting surface and turn our face to the side towards which we are rolling. The head never bangs against the floor, changing from being held in some flexion to being held in some extension appropriately, in order to protect the face or back of the head alternately. When the movement is completed, the head returns to rest gently on the supporting surface.

The arms move out of the way so as not to impede the movement. They may do so in a variety of ways, either by being held above the head or by moving in front of the body, but never appearing to be in the way or remaining trapped beneath the body. Our arms sometimes swing to add momentum to the movement. During normal rolling we do not use our hands to pull ourselves over, nor do we push on the floor behind or in front of us to assist the movement, or to prevent ourselves from falling forwards or backwards.

Trunk rotation takes place so that the movement is smooth and harmonious, and the body does not jerk forwards in one piece, en bloc, while rolling forward or thud backwards when moving from the side to the supine position. Although the rotation is sometimes almost imperceptible, the fluidity of the movement is dependent upon it.

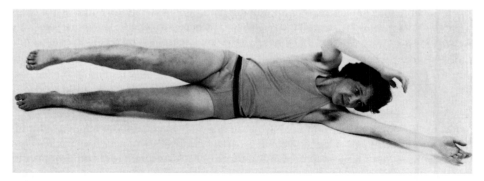

Fig. 2.2. Rolling over from supine to prone

Our legs move as if a step were being taken, the size of the step altering from person to person. The upper leg moves forwards while the lower leg rolls into outward rotation, until it lies flat on the supporting surface. Rarely do we push off with one foot behind us, nor do we attempt to pull ourselves forwards with the underneath leg. When we roll right over to lie prone, our legs are extended before we reach the prone position, as flexion at the hips would impede the movement, and the moving leg comes to rest on the floor only after the turn has been completed.

The activity of rolling is effortless, rhythmic and smooth, and we roll along a fairly straight line, even with our eyes closed.

Sitting, Leaning Forwards to Touch the Feet (Fig. 2.3)

When we sit, our feet rest on the floor without pushing down actively against it and with only the passive weight of the inactive legs taken through them. If we lean forwards to touch our toes or to pick up something from the floor, our feet still do not participate by pushing against the floor or the heels lifting. The same applies when we return to the upright position again. Our head comes naturally forwards as we lean forwards or return to an upright sitting position again, without being held fixedly in extension. We can, however, hold it in different positions or let it relax forward without interfering with the overall movement.

Standing from Sitting on a Chair

When we stand up from a chair both feet are flat on the floor when weight starts to be taken through the legs. Usually, the feet are parallel to one another or one foot is slightly in front of the other, but many variations occur spontaneously under certain circumstances. For example, if the hostess rises quickly from the dinner table without pushing

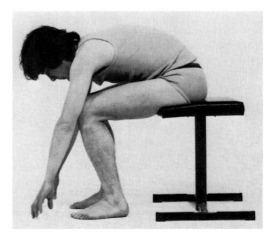

Fig. 2.3. Sitting, leaning forward. The feet remain flat on the floor and show no activity

her chair back to fetch a missing item from the kitchen, she will probably place one leg sideways in abduction and turn towards that side as she stands up.

We draw our feet sufficiently far back towards the chair to allow our knees to move forwards over our toes when weight starts to be taken through our legs. Our hips flex to bring the trunk forwards until our head is approximately over our toes or even further. With back and neck held fairly straight we rise to our feet, with our arms swinging forwards reactively (**Fig. 2.4**). (If the seat is very low, or when we stand up very slowly, the arms come actively forwards in extension, or we may use our hands to assist us by pushing down on the seat.)

As a result of increasing dorsal flexion at the ankle, our knees are able to move forwards over our feet. Both thighs maintain the same angle relative to the midline because our hips stay in the same position, neither abducting nor adducting as we come to standing (**Fig. 2.5**). Our trunk and limbs move symmetrically unless we are avoiding furniture or reaching out sideways to grasp something while standing up.

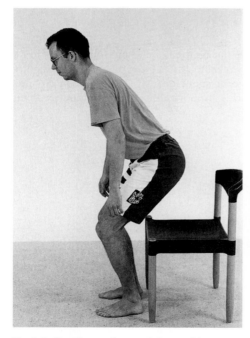

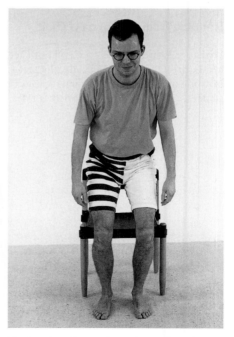

Fig. 2.4. Standing up from a sitting position (lateral view) The head leads the way, as the trunk extends to bring the weight forwards over the feet

Fig. 2.5. Standing up from sitting (frontal view) Weight is taken equally through both legs and the whole body is symmetrical

Standing up from the Floor (Fig. 2.6)

We can get up from the floor in many ways, one of which is through the half-kneeling position. From kneeling we place one foot in front and the knee moves forwards over the toes. Our weight comes forwards so far that our head is over the foot in front with the back straight. We then stand up, the arms moving slightly forwards as we do so.

Going Up and Down Stairs (Fig. 2.7, 2.8 and 2.9)

When climbing stairs we place one foot flat on the stair above, and the knee moves forwards over the toes as weight is taken through that leg. We transfer our weight forwards with a straight back until our head and trunk are over the foot in front, and then we bring the other foot up onto the step ahead. Active plantar flexion of the ankle is not required but is an option dictated by our mood and the speed of the movement. The supporting leg never extends fully at the knee, but remains slightly flexed as the other foot is placed on the step above (**Fig. 2.8**). When the steps are smooth and regular we do not look at them, but look ahead to where we are going or to the steps further ahead of us. Because we do not need to see the steps, we can carry objects up and down stairs, for instance the tea-tray to a room on the next floor.

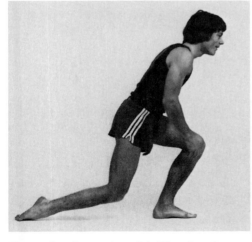

Fig. 2.6. Standing up through half-kneeling. Considerable dorsiflexion of the foot in front allows the knee to move forwards

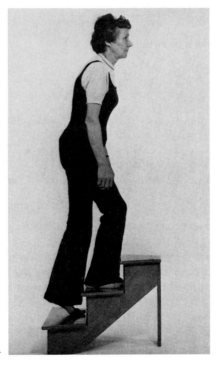

Fig. 2.7. Going upstairs ▷

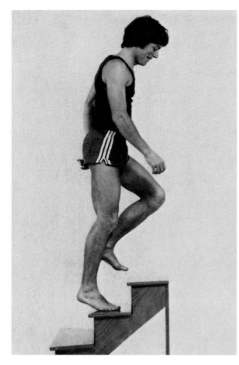

Fig. 2.8. Going upstairs, the legs are in constant motion as in bicycle-riding and the knees are never fully extended

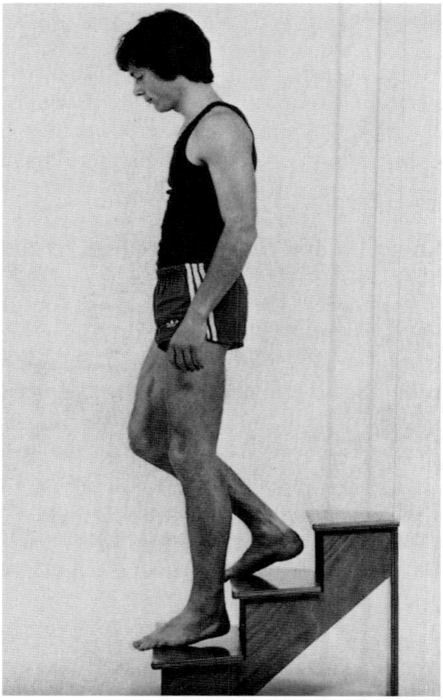

Fig. 2.9. Going downstairs. The weight keeps moving forwards over the leg in front

When we are going down stairs one foot moves forwards and downwards, and even before it reaches the step below we transfer our weight forwards by lifting the heel of the supporting leg behind (**Fig. 2.9**). The heel must come off the step above, as we would otherwise not have sufficient range of dorsal flexion at the ankle to allow the movement of the weight forwards, which takes place before the other foot reaches the next step. Once the leg below has taken our weight with the foot flat on the step, the other leg swings forwards with momentum and the sequence is repeated.

Walking

Walking has been often and most fully analysed by many authors. To gain an overall impression it is sufficient to consider the following points:
- The action of walking is rhythmic and apparently effortless. We can walk easily for an hour without being out of breath or exhausted.
- Walking is not dependent on a specific position of the head, so that we are able to look around freely while we walk and even wave to someone (**Fig. 2.10**).

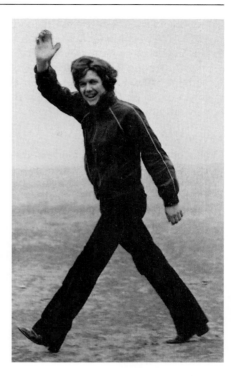

Fig. 2.10. Head and arms are free to move independently even when the subject is walking fast

- The trunk remains upright over the pelvis with the thorax dynamically stabilised to provide an anchorage for the abdominal muscles and, through them, for the muscles which move the legs (Davies 1990).
- Both our hips move forwards continuously while we walk, never going backwards or remaining stationary. When we take a step, the hip flexes to only about 30° and remains in that position until the heel reaches the floor in front.
- Our knees are never fully extended when we are taking weight on one leg during the stance phase but remain mobile and ready to relax for the initiation of the subsequent swing phase. At the end of the swing phase the knee is more extended than at any other time during walking, in order to carry the swinging foot far enough forwards for an adequate step length.
- Our arms swing alternately forwards or backwards, due to the rotation between pelvis and shoulder girdle which takes place below the level of about the 8th thoracic vertebra. As one foot comes forwards, the arm on the opposite side swings forwards. We do not consciously move our arms; their movement is reactive as a result of momentum caused by the weight transference. The arm swing is dependent on the speed of the walking and will vary accordingly. In fact, if the speed is reduced to less than 70 steps per minute the arms no longer swing at all.
- The strides are of the same length and speed. The mean step length is 78 cm, and most people take between 108 and 120 steps per minute (Basmajian 1979; Klein-Vo-

gelbach 1995). The feet make the same noise when they make contact with the floor. We each have an individual rhythm when we walk.

- It is important to notice that the heel strikes the floor first in front and the big toe behind leaves the floor last (**Fig. 2.11**), and that for a short period both are in contact with the ground. We do not lift our leg actively from the hip to take a step; it swings forwards as we push off with the supporting foot by active plantar flexion, which generates the most important impulse of energy (Winter 1988). Our weight is transferred forwards before the heel makes contact with the ground in front. It is as if we are losing our balance and are saved only by the foot reaching the ground in time. The position which the foot assumes on the ground varies slightly from person to person, but it is important to notice that normally the angle from or towards the midline is the same for both feet (**Fig. 2.12**).

- The distance between the feet, or stride width, is less than the distance between our hip joints. In the study by Murray et al. (1964), the mean stride width was found to be 0.8 cm, while Klein-Vogelbach (1995) describes there being just enough distance between the feet to allow the swinging leg to pass the other without being impeded. If the feet are too far apart there would need to be excessive and uneconomical lateral shifting of weight over each supporting leg (Saunders et al. 1953).

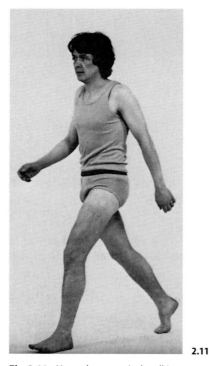
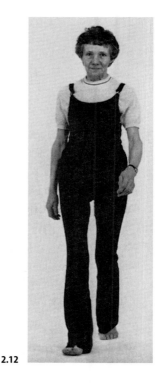

2.11   2.12

Fig. 2.11. Normal economical walking

Fig. 2.12. Both feet assume the same position relative to the midline when they meet the ground in front. Their angle is determined by the rotation at the hip as the leg swings forwards

The movements involved in walking are automatic, and recent research has indicated that central pattern generators (CPGs) play a certain role in their production, but only that of the basic, rhythmic movements. Although CPGs can produce stereotyped locomotion patterns, control from higher centres and sensory feedback from the limbs is essential for walking to be refined and varied, or adapted to task performance or to the ever-changing environmental conditions. "The most complex controls, emanating from the cerebral cortex, the cerebellum and the brain stem, initiate and maintain patterns of optimal activity by making predictive adjustments based on the circumstances of the moment" (Brooks 1986). Without such controls, stimulation of spinal pattern generating circuits can produce only what has been described as being "at best, a bad caricature of walking" (Shumway-Cook and Woollacott 1995). Certainly, such complex control from higher centres is necessary for us to maintain our balance while walking, which is perhaps why it has been difficult if not impossible to construct a computer-controlled robot capable of walking on two legs (Raibert and Sutherland 1983) Walking is a far more complex process than merely moving the legs in a certain way, "so complicated, in fact, that muscle experts are still arguing today over the finer points of how it operates, and how we manage to stride along so successfully" (Morris 1987).

Balance, Righting and Equilibrium Reactions

Every activity we carry out requires that we react to gravity, and our body has to adjust accordingly in order to maintain balance. The adjustments are anticipatory, in that the postural muscles are activated in advance of a skilled movement or task which we are about to perform or before an expected perturbation or disturbance of balance. Postural control involves not only controlling the body's position in space for stability, which means controlling the centre of gravity within the base of support, but also maintaining an appropriate relationship between the body segments and between the body and the environment (Shumway-Cook and Woollacott 1995). Originally, K. Bobath (1980) described this ability as the "normal postural reflex mechanism". Today however, because it has been established that the mechanism is not in fact a reflex one, the term "the normal postural control mechanism" is used instead. As described earlier by Bobath, it is dependent upon:

- Normal tone in the musculature, which needs to be sufficiently high for us to support ourselves and move against gravity but not so high that it impedes movement
- Reciprocal innervation or reciprocal inhibition, which enables us to stabilise certain parts of our body while we move other parts selectively
- Patterns of movement common to us all

The normal postural control mechanism presupposes an intact adult brain and provides the background for skilled movement. "Posture is safeguarded by multiple inputs and outputs. It reflects the care that evolution has bestowed on the capability to adjust the body to the direction of gravity, and parts of the body in relation to each other" (Brooks 1986). In the upright posture, particularly when standing, we need very highly developed balance reactions which must be adaptive as well as anticipatory. Equilibrium reactions make possible the maintenance of balance while sitting, standing and walking.

As a result, the upper limbs are released from their early function of support so that they may become the tools for skilled manipulative activities (Fiorentino 1981). The reactions are automatic, although we can control or modify them voluntarily for functional use. They range from tiny invisible tonus changes to gross movements of the trunk and limbs. When we consider that posture is arrested movement, that if we stop at any stage of any movement and hold the position we have adopted a posture, it becomes clear that the combinations and possibilities are infinite.

In our daily life we have to react to gravity in countless different situations where balance is required.

- We move to perform an activity while the supporting surface remains stable and level. For example, while sitting in a chair we reach out for a required object, or while standing we put on a shoe or step out of the way to avoid something. No matter how small the movement, there will be an adjustment in the tone, activity and position of many other parts of the body. We see the need for this adjustment most clearly when working with patients with complete spinal cord lesions above the level of C-5. With the help of the therapist, it is possible to find a position in which unsupported sitting is achieved, but even turning to look at something causes the patient to fall over because the necessary adjustment cannot take place.
- The supporting surface moves and we react to maintain our balance, as when sitting in a moving motor car or standing in a crowded train.
- We move on a stable but uneven supporting surface and the body reacts appropriately, as when we walk in a meadow of long grass, climb stairs or walk along a winding path.

The following examples of balance and equilibrium reactions require careful study, because their re-education is an integral part of the treatment of hemiplegia.

Lying on a Surface That Tilts Sideways

Although balance in lying is seldom required, it is interesting to note that the pattern of the reactions which develops in babyhood in this position will also occur, although in a modified way, in sitting and standing. The reactions can be observed when a normal person lies supine on a tilt board that is being tilted up on one side (Fig. 2.13).

- The neck flexes laterally to the upper side of the surface, i.e. the side working against the pull of gravity.
- Almost simultaneously there is lateral flexion of the trunk, concave on the side which is uppermost.
- The arm and leg of the uppermost side abduct and extend.

If the board is tilted further trunk rotation takes place, the lower arm coming forwards across the body. The lower leg also comes forwards, and finally the person turns completely over into prone lying.

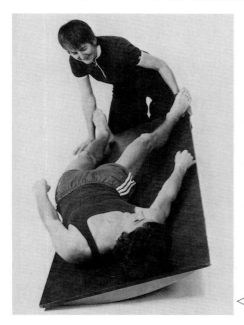

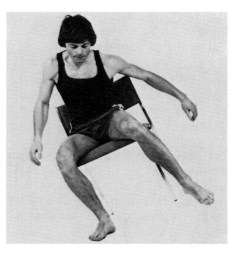

Fig. 2.14. Balance reactions in a sitting position when the supporting surface tilts

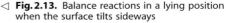

◁ **Fig. 2.13.** Balance reactions in a lying position when the surface tilts sideways

Sitting on a Surface That Tilts Sideways

The same sequence of movement which takes place in lying will also occur in sitting if the chair is tilted to one side (**Fig. 2.14**). When the chair tips towards the right, the head flexes to the left, so that the eyes are horizontal and facing forward. The right side of the trunk elongates as the weight comes over the right buttock. The arms abduct in extension. The lower leg rolls outwards from the hip. The uppermost leg abducts in some extension and leaves the floor.

If the chair tips further, the right shoulder and arm move forwards across the body with trunk rotation, or otherwise the right leg makes a quick protective step sideways in abduction.

Sitting, Being Drawn Sideways by Another Person

If the surface remains stationary but the body is moved sideways, the pull of gravity changes. The sequence of the reactions is therefore much the same as when the surface moved (**Fig. 2.15**). However, the shoulders remain on one level because the braking action of the abdominal muscles on the weight-bearing side serves to prevent that side of the trunk from lengthening. The contraction of the abdominals is necessary to provide sufficient hold for the muscles on the contralateral side, which have to support the

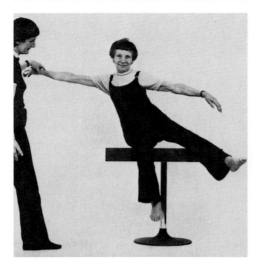 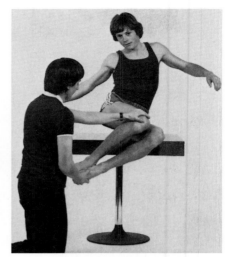

Fig. 2.15. Balance reactions in a sitting position when the supporting surface is stationary

Fig. 2.16. Increased head and trunk reactions when the legs are not participating

weight of the body as well as that of the lifting leg against gravity. The lower leg rolls outwards at the hip to allow the weight to be transferred right over to the side, adjusting to the changed alignment of the trunk. The upper leg, freed from weight, lifts off the supporting surface to provide a counterweight by moving further and further into abduction with the knee in relative extension. The arm on the uppermost side abducts and elongates through the elbow extending. Throughout the lateral movement, the shoulder girdle and pelvis remain parallel to one another, rotating neither backwards nor forwards on one side. In fact, there is no rotation of the trunk until just before the person finally loses his balance, when the lower side rotates forwards. At the same moment, the foot on the uppermost side dorsiflexes with pronation.

Sitting with Both Legs Flexed and Turned to One Side

The head, trunk and arms react in the same pattern, but the movements are exaggerated, requiring more activity because the leg can no longer extend and abduct to act as a counterweight. The trunk rotation therefore occurs earlier (**Fig. 2.16**).

Sitting, Reaching Out to Grasp an Object

In order to perform a task such as reaching to lift a book, the same reactions would take place but must be modified (**Fig. 2.17**). The head-righting reaction is inhibited to allow the subject to turn and look at the book. The trunk side flexion and elongation are re-

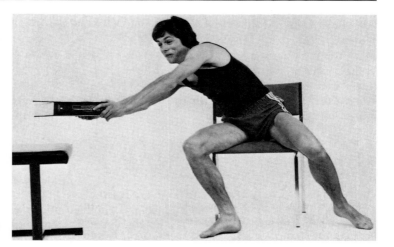

Fig. 2.17. Balance reactions modified to allow function

versed, as is the trunk rotation. The arms cannot react in abduction and extension, because the hands must grasp the book.

Standing, Tipped Backwards

Small intrinsic muscles in the foot coordinate to adjust to the first slight change of posture. As the weight moves further back, the feet and toes spring into dorsal flexion, and the trunk is brought forwards by the hips flexing slightly. The extended arms move forwards from the shoulder as the spine flexes and the head comes forwards, all acting as a counterweight **(Fig. 2.18)**.

Standing, Tipped Forwards

The toes flex and the foot pushes firmly against the floor until, as the weight continues to be brought forwards, the heels rise. Rapid extension of the hips and spine follows, and the arms move backwards in extension **(Fig. 2.19)**. The head also extends strongly. In normal circumstances only the first events occur, because it would then be more economical for us to take a quick step or steps to regain our balance. The whole sequence would occur only if we were not able for some reason to take a quick step forwards or back, e.g. when standing fully clothed on the edge of a swimming pool in winter, when stopping abruptly at the pavement edge to avoid an oncoming car, or if a tiny child or kitten were on the floor immediately behind us.

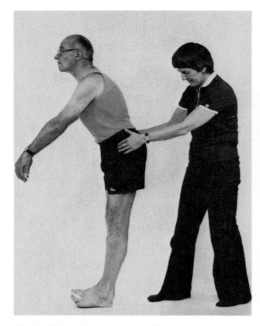 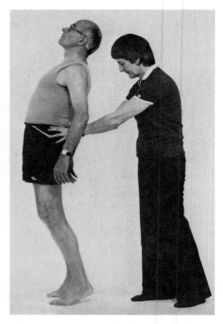

Fig. 2.18. Standing, tipped backwards   **Fig. 2.19.** Standing, pushed forwards

Standing, Tipped Sideways

The reactions which take place closely resemble those which occur in supine lying when the supporting surface is tilted. The whole side elongates over the weight-bearing leg, with the trochanter the most lateral point. As the weight is brought sideways the supporting foot rolls outward until eventually only its lateral border is in contact with the ground (**Fig. 2.20**). The toes flex strongly. The head rights to the vertical, maintaining its normal relationship to the shoulder girdle. The opposite side shortens, with the leg moving into abduction. Both extended arms move into abduction.

Standing on a Tilting Surface, Such as a Tilt-Board

The reactions which occur when the subject is lying supine on a tilt-board are repeated in much the same way when he is standing and tilting the board sideways (**Fig. 2.21**). The trochanter moves laterally to the side of the board which is lower, and the trunk elongates on that side. The head rights to the vertical. The feet remain in contact with the board, with the knee on the uppermost side flexing somewhat. The arms abduct at the shoulder and the elbows extend.

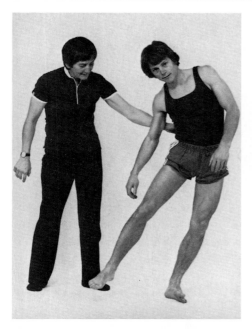

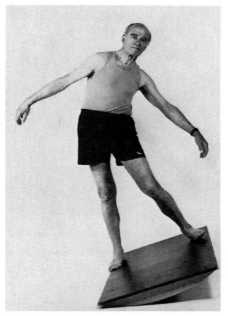

Fig. 2.20. Standing, tipped sideways until only the lateral border of the foot is on the ground. The head has righted beyond the vertical

Fig. 2.21. Balancing while tilting the board sideways

Automatic Steps to Maintain or Regain Balance

Normally, when reacting quickly and economically to maintain or regain our balance, we take a quick step in whichever direction is necessary: forwards, sideways or backwards. If we are still off balance, these steps are repeated as often as is necessary to prevent our falling, one foot following the other in quick succession. When we step forwards the arms extend in front, as if in preparation to save our face should we fall **(Fig. 2.22 a, b)**.

Stepping sideways, one foot crosses in front or behind the other **(Fig. 2.23)**. When we take quick steps backwards to regain balance, the trunk and head move forwards from the hips **(Fig. 2.24)**.

Steps to Follow

When someone blocks our path and we have to avoid colliding with them we take quick steps in any direction which is necessary. The ability to do so enables us to walk in a crowded street or supermarket without losing our balance as we step around and out

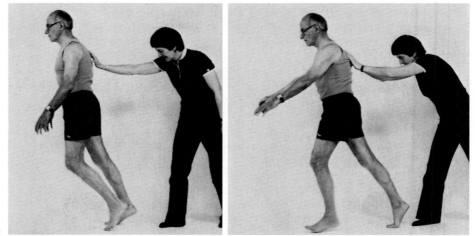

a   b

Fig. 2.22 a, b. Steps to regain balance. **a** About to fall forwards; **b** protective steps forwards

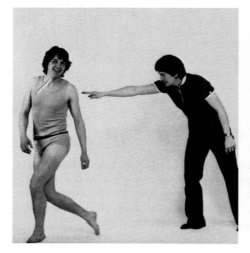

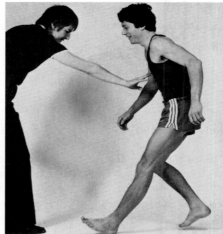

Fig. 2.23. Protective steps sideways   **Fig. 2.24.** Protective steps backwards

of the way of objects or other people. If someone takes us by the hand or guides us from our shoulders, we follow at once and without resistance, turning and stepping rhythmically in whatever way that person is leading us. The automatic steps to follow in the direction which the other person is indicating occur without our having to think consciously about them at all and are an integral part of the normal postural control mechanism.

Balancing on One Leg

When we stand on one leg, the supporting foot moves pliantly and coordinatedly, adjusting to the changing shifts in weight (**Fig. 2.25 a**). As the weight is shifted further in one direction, we move by pivoting on the foot, with the heel moving medially and laterally in quick succession, a rapid movement alternating between weight being taken through the heel and then through the ball of the foot (**Fig. 2.25 b**). If the weight is transferred even further, and too rapidly to allow the pivot, we hop on that leg in the direction required to regain our balance (**Fig. 2.25 c**).

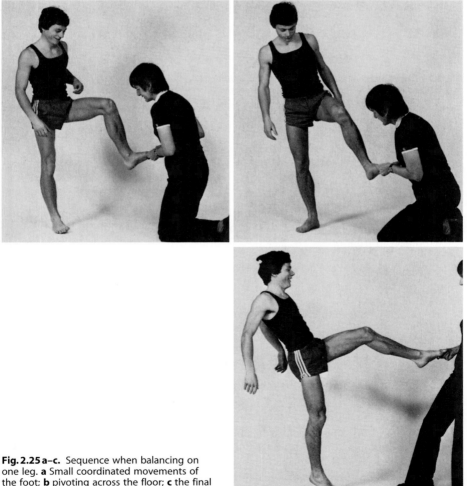

a

b

c

Fig. 2.25 a–c. Sequence when balancing on one leg. **a** Small coordinated movements of the foot; **b** pivoting across the floor; **c** the final hop

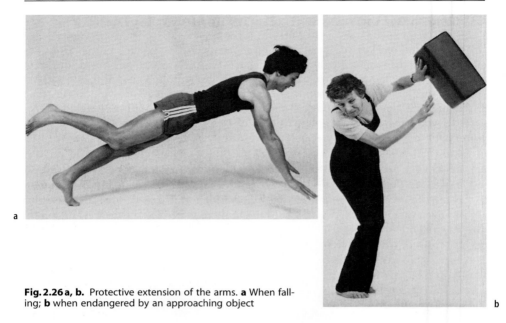

Fig. 2.26 a, b. Protective extension of the arms. **a** When falling; **b** when endangered by an approaching object

Protective Extension of the Arms

If all the reactions have failed to maintain balance and we fall, the outstretched hands spring to our protection, in order to save our head or face from hitting the ground or a fixed object in front of us (**Fig. 2.26 a**). This protective reaction occurs in whatever direction we fall and accounts for the numerous Colles' fractures, particularly among elderly people. We see the same protective reaction when a moving object approaches us rapidly, e. g. when something is thrown at us or falls towards us, or a door slams as we approach it (**Fig. 2.26 b**).

Task-orientated Arm and Hand Movements

The simple task of grasping objects has been studied for centuries by scientists, therapists and engineers who have tried to understand, treat or duplicate the versatility of the human hand. As a result, much has been published on the anatomy and function of the hand, and on factors which enable us, or influence our ability, to perform skilled tasks, just two examples being the 500-page book, *The Grasping Hand* by MacKenzie (1994) and the comprehensive volume titled simply *The Hand*, edited by Tubiana (1981).

When studying the normal movements of the arm and hand in relation to improving activity and function in the upper limb during treatment, some features merit particular consideration:

- Adaptive and dynamic trunk stability is a prerequisite for functional movements of the arm, to ensure balance in postures appropriate for performing the task.
- Mobility and selective control of the scapula, shoulder and elbow are essential for bringing the hand into the right position and maintaining the position for as long as is necessary to complete the task.
- Movements of the arm follow the dictates of the hand, and the movements are task orientated. Results of experiments "support the concept that the CNS programs movements according to endpoint coordinates" (Shumway-Cook and Woollacott 1995). The findings of Morasso (1981) and Abend and co-authors (1982) suggest that "arm trajectory formation is concerned with the motion of the hand rather than with the motion of the joints". "Higher order factors such as the goal, the context (and also probably the knowledge of the result) of the action seem to be able to influence not only duration and velocity, but also the intrinsic kinematic structure of the movements" (Jeannerod 1990).
- The term "motor program" is often used to describe functional movement sequences of the arm and hand, but "the term motor program can be replaced by learned motor routine or motor sequence memory" (Roland 1993). Roland explains that, "once the motor program is released the recruited structures will work together to organize the motor sectors of the brain to execute the motor sequences". "Motor skill thus is the optimal use of programmed movements" (Brooks 1986). Because the time for executing such a movement does not allow for sensory feedback controls and corrections, it occurs all at once "more like a firework exploding," as Morasso so succinctly explains (personal communication).
- The same applies to visual control, which was found to have little effect on either the reaching (transportation phase) or the grasping (manipulation phase) (Jeannerod 1990). Instead, the main role of visual feedback in prehension seems to be to achieve terminal accuracy. It is also not possible, as is often suggested, to use vision as a substitute for kinaesthetic cues, "simply because we never have looked at the movement of our fingers ... but always at the result we are accomplishing. Consequently we have no association between the visual sensation of the moving fingers and the proper impulse to set the muscles into coordinated action" (Woodworth 1899).
- When the hand grasps an object, the shape it adopts is anticipatory and is formed during the reaching movement of the arm, the fingers opening just the right amount, no more and no less than required (Fig. 2.27 a). The size of the maximum grip aperture is proportional to the size of the object (Jeannerod 1990). Furthermore, the adaptation of both reaching and grasping is task dependent. Reaching movements vary according to the goals and constraints of the task, and adaptation of the transportation phase is therefore a prerequisite for effective upper-limb function. "Anticipatory activity is based on prior knowledge about the task itself and the movements that need to be made" (Shumway-Cook and Woollacott 1995). The amount of force that we apply to lift, move or oppose an object depends on our perception of how heavy the object is. "When we estimate how much effort has to be spent on a task, we reach back to previous experience for the answer because our perceptions are rooted in the past" (Brooks 1986). Brooks goes on to explain how the movements

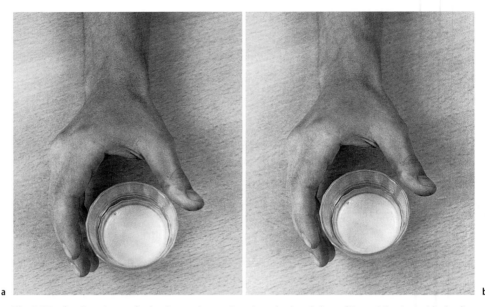

a   b

Fig. 2.27 a, b. Grasping and releasing a glass. **a** Grasping: the hand shaped in anticipation with the fingers opening exactly the right amount; **b** releasing: fingers and thumb do not extend far, but move almost imperceptibly off the surface of the glass

are thus determined centrally until the program is adapted by peripheral feedback to suit the current circumstances.

- It is interesting to note that far fewer studies have been concerned with how the hand releases an object or lets go after holding something. Because of the dearth of information on the subject, many imagine that the fingers extend more than they actually do. In fact the fingers move only millimetre-wise off the surface of the object, the controlled release of their flexor activity playing as important a role as the minute active extension movement. The difference between the shape and activity of the grasping hand and the hand which is letting go of the object is imperceptible without prior knowledge as to which action is being performed at the time (**Fig. 2.27 b**). Even more complex is the coordinated action required to hold the object while releasing the fingers a little to adjust its position in the hand, in order to use it functionally. We perform these skilled movements with our hands and fingers repeatedly in daily life, for example when we pick up and use our knife and fork, a ball-point pen or a nail file. The complexity of such manipulation is clearly illustrated by the example of a highly developed computer-controlled robot which was able not only to play the organ on command, but even to sight-read the music of the piece it was playing with its video eyes. However, only short pieces were possible, because the otherwise skilled robot hand was unable to turn over a page, an action which requires holding while releasing and moving the position of the fingers (von Randow 1991). The author stresses the important role of sensation in the hand, both for appropriate grasping and for skilled activities such as letting something slide through the fingers.

- The ability to hold and manipulate objects with the wrist in palmar flexion while the fingers are flexing is a prerequisite for performing many tasks in our daily lives. There is a common misconception that for precision grip or skilled hand function the wrist must be kept in dorsal extension when the fingers flex, and as a result many therapists strenuously avoid any grasping or holding activities with the patient's wrist flexed. Recovery of functional use of the upper limb will be limited if a patient can only move his arm and grasp and hold objects with some degree of wrist extension. Even with the wrist held constantly in a neutral position by active extension some tasks are rendered difficult or impossible. Careful observation of how we use our hands during activities of daily life reveals that to perform many of them the wrist needs to flex as well as extend, either to pick up an object or to move it in the appropriate way. When we pick up a pen, a knife or even a book, the wrist flexes to bring the grasping fingers into position. The movements involved in wringing out a wet dish cloth, drying the axilla with a towel or putting toothpaste on a toothbrush all include wrist flexion with finger flexion, as do pouring milk into the tea cup or taking a bite of a biscuit **(Fig. 2.28 a, b)** There is anticipatory palmar flexion of the wrist from the very start of many sequences during dressing and undressing, for example to take off a pullover or to pull it down into place when putting it on, and when adjusting the position of the shoulder seam on the same side as the moving hand.

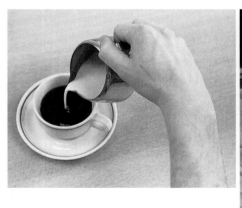
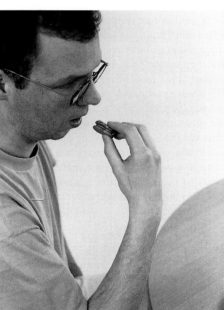

a

b

Fig. 2.28 a, b. Holding or manipulating an object when the wrist is flexed. **a** Pouring milk into a cup; **b** eating a biscuit

Considerations

Normal movements are harmonious, coordinated and always performed with the minimum of effort required for the action or task. When excessive effort relative to the activity is observed it either will indicate a neuromuscular problem or will be the result of a motor skill which is still being learned. The rhythmic fluid nature of normal motion is also disturbed by painful conditions and by stiffness or loss of mobility in some part or parts of the body. Careful analysis is necessary before it can be established exactly which problem is primarily responsible for the disruption of the normal movement characteristics.

Intact balance and saving reactions enable us to go about our daily life without the constant fear of falling. Free righting reactions of the head are a key factor in maintaining balance. Wyke (1985) emphasises the important role of the receptors in the apophyseal joints of the cervical spine in maintaining balance in adults. He reports an increased risk of falling in patients who have no neurological impairment, but who wear a collar as part of the treatment of their cervical spine problems and therefore have limited proprioception information from their neck. The fact that immobilising the cervical spine disturbs balance is particularly significant with regard to the treatment of patients with hemiplegia, because, as a result of hypertonus or overactivity in the muscles in the cervical region, they develop a very stiff neck if it is not mobilised intensively. In a study which seemed to contradict Wyke's findings and indicate that wearing a cervical collar did not affect walking balance (Burl et al. 1992), the test situation was in no way comparable to walking in the varied conditions encountered in real life. There is a vast difference between walking without any distraction along a laboratory walkway, only 6 m long and on one level, and the way we walk during our daily lives, often bombarded by external stimuli. We turn quickly back and forth, avoid objects and other people, negotiate uneven ground and have to concentrate on the task in hand or on finding our way. Balance under such circumstances needs to be anticipatory and adaptive, with the necessary reactions occurring automatically. "Adaptive postural control involves modifying sensory and motor systems in response to changing task and environmental demands. Anticipatory aspects of postural control pretune sensory and motor systems for postural demands based on previous experience and learning" (Shumway-Cook and Woollacott 1995). Every activity in our daily lives is dependent upon adequate balance and equilibrium reactions in a multitude of diverse situations and under everchanging conditions. Even merely lifting one arm requires an adaptation in many other parts of the body. Although balance reactions are automatic they can be modified, altered or suppressed whenever necessary for functional activities. Because each and all of the reactions can be voluntarily inhibited or controlled, they are reactions rather than reflexes in adults.

3 Abnormal Movement Patterns in Hemiplegia

All the balance reactions and smooth, harmonious movement sequences described in Chap. 2 are dependent upon normal postural tone and sensation. The prerequisite for normal tone, sensation and movement is unimpaired nerve impulse conduction in a great variety of postures and activities, which necessitates considerable mobility within the nervous system itself. Any loss of the neurodynamic properties of the system will inevitably alter muscle tone and movement patterns, as explained in Chap. 15. "When a person loses the normal mechanics of the nervous system, certain dynamic and static postural patterns emerge to allow the patient to best cope with the neural movement loss" (Butler 1991). Interestingly, Butler illustrates an abnormal or "antalgic" nervous system posture as an example, which, although that adopted by an orthopaedic patient, reveals many postural abnormalities usually associated with hemiplegia. All active movements occur as the result of muscle contractions, but it should not be forgotten that, "a muscle can only be as efficient as the nerve which supplies it!" (Rolf 1997b). A healthy, mobile nervous system is therefore indispensable for the performance of normal movements. The coordinated movements and variation of posture required for skilled function are also dependent upon the ability to move selectively those parts of the body required for the task, while inhibiting the activity of the other parts. According to Bach-y-Rita and Balliet (1987), "Inhibition is much more important than is generally appreciated; much of what is taught emphasizes excitation while virtually ignoring inhibition". In fact, inhibition of overactivity is one of the most important roles of the central nervous system, and there are more inhibitory than excitatory pathways in the brain stem and spinal cord. Every skilled activity can be said to be surrounded by a "wall of inhibition" (Kottke 1978). When a new skill is being learned, through such inhibition, overactivity decreases proportionally as the performer becomes more skilled.

Learning to drive a motorcar demonstrates clearly this process of increasing inhibition of excess activity as the learner becomes more adept. At first the steering wheel is held in an almost vicelike grasp, and changing gear requires great effort and concentration. The movements of the feet on the accelerator, clutch and brake pedals are abrupt and forceful, so that the car moves somewhat erratically, in fits and starts. Later, the driver manipulates the controls with such appropriate strength, through inhibition, that the changes of gear and speed are smooth and barely perceptible, and he holds the steering wheel lightly.

Normal movements are economical, in that never more energy than that required for the task or activity is expended and the movements are harmonious, flowing and coordinated. If the nervous system is damaged in some way, movements are seen to be too effortful, abrupt or stereotyped as a result of certain problems caused by the loss of central control.

Persistence of Primitive Mass Synergies

Selectivity of normal muscular action is a function of cortical motor control guided by proprioceptive feedback (Perry 1969). Children are born with a high level of anarchy or overactivity in their motor control. As they mature, the overactivity disappears, and it is absent in adults (Basmajian 1981). Reflex patterns are the basis for motion. The repetition of these reflex patterns in infancy teaches the child how to move. However, movement does not become effective unless and until the child learns how to inhibit the undesired components of movements in these reflex patterns at the same time that the desired components are excited (Kottke 1980).

"At birth, the body is under the unopposed control of the lower centres of the central nervous system, which basically generate involuntary reflex movements and postures." "The primitive, postural reflexes primarily involve changes in tone and distribution, which affect posture and movement. These the body responds to automatically and mechanically." "With maturation and integration of the lower centres contributing to the development of the higher centres, with more inhibitory control from the higher centres, the mass movements are integrated and goal-directed movements, which depend on the higher control within the central nervous system, are developed" (Fiorentino 1981).

The primitive but postural reflexes can still be observed in the intact human being, although they have become modified and changed by the activities of the higher centres (B. Bobath 1971). They reappear in an exaggerated form after a lesion to the central nervous system. "Damage to the highest or intermediate centers causes abnormalities in performance by releasing the activity of the undamaged next lower centre from control, rather than by generating a new form of activity originating from the damaged center itself" (Kottke 1980).

When a patient with hemiplegia can move his limbs at all, he does so in a stereotyped way, in total primitive mass synergies which Perry (1969) describes as the primitive pattern responses. These movement synergies should not be confused with the patterns of spasticity which have often been described by B. Bobath, most recently in 1990. The very young baby moves in primitive mass synergies but is in no way spastic. Some hemiplegic patients may have no overt hypertonus, and are nevertheless unable to perform a certain selective or isolated movement, although the therapist, moving the limb passively in the same direction, may encounter no resistance.

Perry differentiates between the two by describing spasticity as "an involuntary response to a sensory stimulus". The primitive pattern response, however, she describes as "a voluntary act, initiated when the hemiplegic patient wishes to perform a task. These synergies are stereotyped because the muscles that participate in patterned motion and the strength of their responses are the same for every effort, regardless of the demand." Naturally, the two overlap to a considerable extent, and one or the other does not appear as an isolated symptom. Thus, it could be said that every patient who moves using primitive mass synergies will also have abnormal tone, and every patient who has abnormal tone due to a lesion of the central nervous system will move without full selection. The movement synergies may not appear exactly as they have been described previously by Brunnstrom (1970), but may differ in some way due to factors such as altered tone, actual weakness or loss of scapula control. When relatively advanced motor control is present in the limb often only the influence of the total synergy on the movement pattern can be observed (see Fig. 3.13)

The Synergies as They Appear in Association with Hemiplegia

In the Upper Limb

The Flexor Synergy (Figs. 3.1 and 3.2)

The flexor synergy is seen when, for example, the patient attempts to lift up his arm, hold it in the air after it has been lifted, reach for an object or bring his hand to his mouth.

Scapula	Elevates and retracts
Shoulder	Abducts and externally rotates (internally rotates)
Elbow	Flexes
Forearm	Supinates (pronates)
Wrist	Flexes
Fingers	Flex and adduct
Thumb	Flexes and adducts

Because of hypertonus the flexion synergy will usually appear with internal rotation of the shoulder and pronation of the forearm.

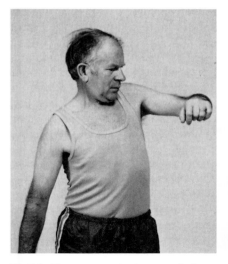

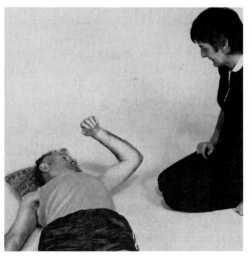

Fig. 3.1. Flexor synergy in the upper limb. The patient is trying to lift his extended arm. Because the shoulder is abducting (flexor component) the elbow flexes as well, instead of extending. In this case pronation rather than supination occurs with mass flexion (left hemiplegia)

Fig. 3.2. While lying, the patient tries to touch his head. The action of flexing the elbow causes the whole flexor synergy with retraction of the scapula and abduction of the arm. In this instance the shoulder rotates externally

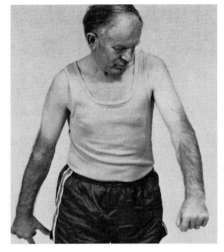
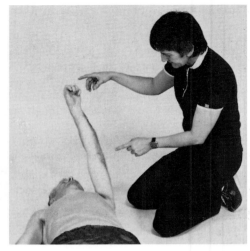

Fig. 3.3. Extensor synergy in the upper limb – the patient is trying to straighten his elbow (left hemiplegia)

Fig. 3.4. While lying, the patient tries to extend his elbow. The shoulder rotates internally and the forearm pronates strongly (left hemiplegia)

The Extensor Synergy (Figs. 3.3 and 3.4)

Scapula	Protracts and pushes downwards
Shoulder	Internally rotates and adducts
Elbow	Extends with pronation
Wrist	Extends somewhat
Fingers	Flex with adduction
Thumb	Adducts in flexion

Because of hypertonicity the wrist will more often be flexed.

In the Lower Limb

The Flexor Synergy

Pelvis	Elevates and retracts
Hip	Abducts and externally rotates
Knee	Flexes
Ankle	Dorsiflexes in supination
Toes	Extend

Because of hypertonicity the toes usually flex. The great toe may be extended.

The Extensor Synergy

Hip	Extends, internally rotates and adducts
Knee	Extends
Ankle	Plantar flexes with inversion
Toes	Plantar flex and adduct

Once again, the great toe may extend.

"The great variety and manifold combinations of movement patterns necessary for skilled activities depend on the ability of any muscle or muscle group to function as part of a great number of patterns and not only as part of one or two total patterns" (B. Bobath 1978). "In damage to the central nervous system, as in stroke, the higher centers containing the complex patterns and the facility for the inhibition of massive gross patterns lose control and the uncontrolled, or partially controlled, stereotyped patterns of the middle and lower centers emerge" (Cailliet 1980). Important for the treatment is that movements in the mass synergies are not encouraged; instead, the patient learns to move his trunk and limbs selectively, because otherwise he will be unable to use recovering motor activity for functional tasks.

Abnormal Muscle Tone

Tone can be described as the resistance felt when a part of the body is moved passively, i.e. lengthening or stretching those muscles which run in the opposite direction to that of the movement.

- Normal tone is felt as an appropriate amount of resistance, allowing the movement to proceed smoothly and without interruption. The opposing or antagonistic muscles adapt instantly to the new amount of stretch, "paying out" appropriately as the part is moved. The amount of resistance felt varies slightly from one normal subject to another, and the therapist needs to experience and become familiar with the possible variations by moving the limbs of many different people.
- Hypotonus is felt as too little or no resistance to the movement, and the limb feels limp and floppy. When released, the part being moved will fall in the direction of the pull of gravity.
- Hypertonus is felt as an increased resistance to passive movement, ranging from a slight delay in the muscles giving way to considerable effort being required before the part can be moved at all. The limb feels heavy and, when released, is pulled in the direction of the hypertonic muscle groups.

The generally accepted and perhaps clearest definition is that formulated by Lance (1980):

"Spasticity is a motor disorder characterized by a velocity-dependent increase in tonic stretch reflexes ('muscle tone') with exaggerated tendon jerks, resulting from hyperexcitability of the stretch reflex, as one component of the upper motor neuron syndrome."

In recent times there has been much discussion as to the use of the words spasticity, hypertonicity, hypertonia, hypertonus or simply increased tension, all of which have much the same meaning and appear to be used interchangeably in the literature. The importance of the words themselves should not be exaggerated because they play only a small part in the actual treatment of patients. They are important, however, with regard to communication and mutual understanding between professionals for purposes of furthering knowledge and improving therapeutic possibilities.

The word tone has been explained as being "the normal degree of vigor and tension", and "tonus, tone or tonicity as the normal state of slight contraction of all skeletal muscles as long as the innervation to the muscle is intact" (*Dorland's Medical Dictionary*), while Duncan and Bradke (1987) explain that, "Muscle tone is a term used to describe the tension attained at any moment between the origin and insertion of a muscle." Any increase in the state of tension could therefore be indicated by adding the prefix "hyper".

Spasticity is not a clearly defined term, and in the current language of stroke rehabilitation, the word "spasticity" is used clinically to signify hyperactive stretch reflexes, increased resistance to passive movement, posturing of the upper extremity in flexion and the lower extremity in extension, excessive cocontraction of antagonistic muscles, clonus and stereotyped movement synergies (Duncan and Bradke 1987; Shumway-Cook and Woollacott 1995). According to these authors, therefore, spasticity does not denote one particular disorder of motor control but describes many abnormal behaviours often seen in patients with a neurological impairment, and a variety of neurophysiological causes are thought to be responsible for its development. It is easy to understand why individual therapists and authors prefer different words to describe the presence of increased muscle tension. Some examples of such preferences as they appear in the literature are: hypertonus and spasticity interchanged freely (Bobath 1990); hypertonicity and spasticity (Duncan and Bradke 1987); hypertonia divided into two types, spasticity or rigidity (Atkinson 1986); spastic hypertonus, spastic hypertonia or spastic hypertonicity (Shumway-Cook and Woollacott 1995), while Ryerson and Levit (1997) use the term hypertonicity exclusively because they believe that, "many hypertonic muscles may not truly fit the scientific definition for spasticity" and that "spasticity is a special type of hypertonicity". Some avoid the conventional terms altogether, postulating that the clinical manifestations usually called spasticity are in fact unnecessary muscular activity which has become habitual, certain muscles whose mechanical advantage is greatest and which can be activated most easily contracting persistently to the disadvantage of others (Carr and Shepherd 1996, 1982).

At present, the pathophysiology of spasticity appears to be as controversial as its definitions, and hypotheses range from increased motor neuron excitability resulting in an enhanced response, to stretch evoked input, to the reduced influence of descending inhibitory systems (Katz and Rymer 1989). Whatever the underlying mechanism for the abnormal stretch reflex response, and regardless of which term is preferred, hypertonus or spasticity manifests itself in typical stereotyped patterns of either flexion or extension. The condition is never isolated to one muscle group but is always part of a total flexion or total extension synergy (Atkinson 1986). So stereotyped are the patterns that they allow a patient to be identified instantly as having a hemiplegia.

With explanations of hypertonus and its pathophysiology being so controversial, it must also be taken into account that all human beings will have increased muscle tone under certain circumstances, and similar causative factors will likewise precipitate hypertonicity in patients with central nervous system lesions. In the case of the patients, the increase in tone is far more obvious because of the disturbed inhibitory mechanisms resulting from the lesion (Davies 1994). Factors which normally cause such increased tone include learning a new motor skill, painful stimuli, loss of balance or fear of falling, rushing to complete a task, confusing sensory information, loss of sensation, a sudden unexpected noise or loud voice and coping with unfamiliar technical appliances or an unknown environment (Lipp 1996). Even meeting new people or being interviewed can cause an increase in muscle tension. These additional factors are important considerations, for preventing the development of hypertonicity in the overall care and treatment of patients as well as for reducing existing spasticity.

Although the patient may demonstrate hypertonicity or exaggerated reflex activity in all muscle groups following stroke, the recognised patterns would seem to be the result of the pull of the strongest muscle groups, and the influence of the tonic reflexes. K. Bobath has often described the strongest muscles as being the phylogenetically antigravity muscles – those in the upper limb which would be involved in pulling the body weight up into a tree, and those in the lower limb which support the body weight in standing.

Typical Patterns of Spasticity or Hypertonicity

When considering spasticity, care must be taken to differentiate between the position in which the joints may find themselves and the resistance encountered when the limb is moved passively. For example, although the hip joint may be seen to be in some degree of flexion when the patient is standing, there will nevertheless be a resistance when passive flexion of the hip and knee is attempted in the presence of extensor spasticity.

The most common patterns, according to Bobath (1974, 1978, 1990), are:

Head	The head is flexed laterally toward the hemiplegic side and rotated so that the face is toward the sound side.
Upper limb (flexion pattern)	The scapula is retracted and the shoulder girdle depressed.
	The shoulder is adducted and internally rotated.
	The elbow is flexed with pronation of the forearm (in some cases supination dominates).
	The wrist is flexed with some ulnar deviation.
	The fingers are flexed and adducted
	The thumb is flexed and adducted.
Lower limb (extension pattern)	The pelvis is rotated backwards on the hemiplegic side and pulled upwards.
	The hip is extended, adducted and internally rotated.

Due to the rotation backwards (of the pelvis) the leg usually shows a pattern of external rotation in spite of extensor spasticity which, in cases with bilateral spasticity, is combined with internal rotation. A change of this pattern of external rotation can be observed if one moves the pelvis forward on the affected side, when internal rotation occurs (B. Bobath 1978).

The knee is extended.
The foot is plantar flexed and inverted.

(The term "supination" is often used to describe the turning inward of the foot. Supination, however, is the movement which occurs when the foot is dorsiflexed and the unopposed pull of the m. tibialis anterior is clearly seen. In the extension pattern, the foot is plantar-flexed and the m. tibialis anterior is not active. The term "inversion" or "plantar inversion" should be used to differentiate between the two positions. Inversion is caused by the uninhibited activity of the m. tibialis posterior.)

> The toes are flexed and adducted. (Occasionally the great toe extends in the presence of a marked positive Babinski sign.)

Although extensor spasticity usually predominates in the lower limb, in certain situations flexor spasticity may be more apparent. For example, patients who remain in the wheelchair for many months in a position of flexion will tend to have flexor spasticity in the lower limb. Any painful stimulus to the foot or leg will result in a flexor withdrawal response, with flexor spasticity being manifested. Any flexion contracture of the lower limb will tend to elicit a flexion pattern, due to the stretch reflex in the flexor muscle groups being stimulated earlier, each time the leg moves towards extension. The flexor pattern of spasticity is the same as the pattern of the mass movement synergy which has already been described.

The difficulties caused by both the mass synergies and hypertonus can be felt and observed by the therapist when she tries to place the head, trunk or limbs in different positions as part of her assessment.

Placing

The normal limb, head or trunk responds instantly and actively to being moved by another person, without a verbal command being required. For example, if someone's hand is lifted into the air, it feels light because the subject immediately takes the weight of his own arm actively. The arm remains for a short time in the position in which it is placed before returning to a relaxed position once again. The arm can be placed in an enormous variety of positions and combinations of positions. The automatic response is dependent upon normal tone and reciprocal innervation, as well as on an intact superficial or tactile sensation, and forms the basis of our ability to use our hands functionally and automatically.

The placing reaction of any part of the body can be tested during assessment and also used as a treatment procedure. Placing is difficult if not impossible for most patients because of the problems of abnormal tone and loss of selective movement (reciprocal innervation) as well as that of inadequate superficial sensation. In the case of the upper limb, for instance, if a patient cannot feel in which direction the examiner's hand is moving his, he will not be able to follow correctly or leave his arm in position when she releases his hand. Careful analysis is required to ascertain which of the difficulties is primarily responsible for the altered reaction or its loss. Typical difficulties are revealed by comparing normal subjects with hemiplegic patients.

When he is lying supine, the normal subject's head feels light and reacts at once to the therapist's touch indicating a movement direction. The model lifts her head without

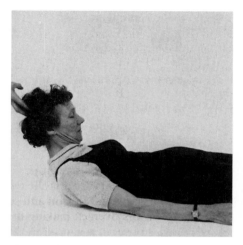

Fig. 3.5. Placing the head, normal subject. The arms remain relaxed at her side

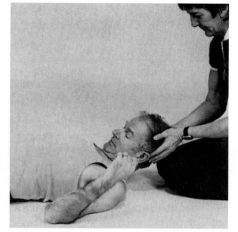

Fig. 3.6. Placing the head, patient with left hemiplegia. As the head is lifted, the arm pulls strongly into flexion

effort and it remains in any position (**Fig. 3.5**). The patient's head pushes back and feels heavy. It requires effort for the patient to maintain the position, and the therapist needs to assist the lifting movement before he can take over the activity. A verbal command is often necessary before activity occurs. As the neck flexes the patient's arm may pull up into flexion (**Fig. 3.6**).

In standing, the normal model's trunk moves forwards without any resistance, and rotates easily in response to the slight pressure of the therapist's hand on one shoulder (**Fig. 3.7**). The model is able to hold any position which the therapist's hands indicate. The patient attempts to react to the therapist's hands, but there is considerable resistance to trunk and hip flexion. Because activity in the extensor muscle groups is required to support the patient against gravity, the whole extensor synergy is elicited with no selective activity. The foot pushes down against the floor in plantar flexion, and so the patient's hip is also shifted backwards. The hip extensors overact, making the movement forwards impossible. No trunk rotation takes place in response to the therapist's hand on the left shoulder; instead, the scapula pushes back, and the arm flexes. The patient extends his neck strongly, which increases the extension in the lower limb (**Fig. 3.8**).

In lying, the normal model's leg can be placed in any position or combination of positions. For example, the therapist can place the leg in a position where the hip is flexed; the knee must hold with active extensor activity while the foot remains dorsiflexed (**Fig. 3.9**). The patient's leg, when placed in the same position, pulls into total flexion, as he cannot extend the knee actively while holding his hip in flexion (**Fig. 3.10a**). If he attempts to straighten his knee the total extension pattern is evoked, and the hip moves more into extension, the knee extends and the foot pushes into plantar flexion (**Fig. 3.10b**).

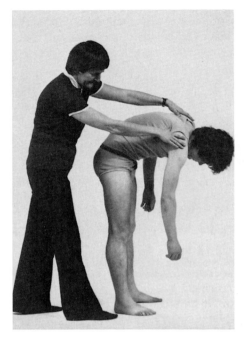

Fig. 3.7. Placing the trunk in a standing position, normal subject

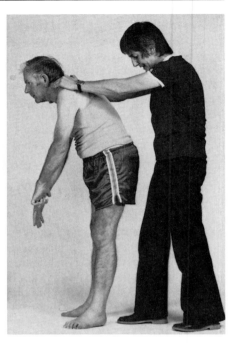

Fig. 3.8. Attempting to place the trunk, patient with a left hemiplegia. A resistance is encountered by the therapist, and she is not able to move the trunk into the various positions

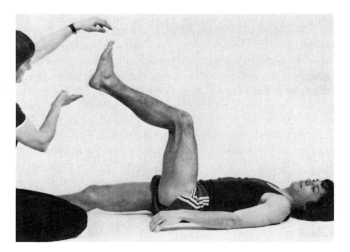

Fig. 3.9. Placing the leg, normal subject. The position requires selective hip flexion, knee extension and dorsiflexion of the foot

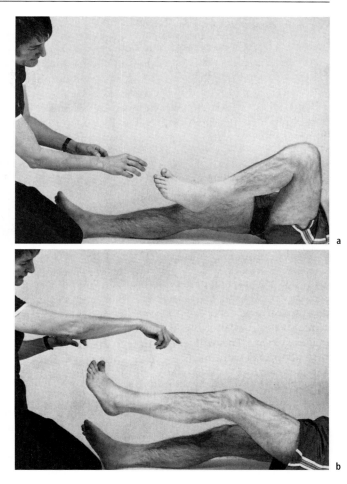

Fig. 3.10 a, b. Placing the leg, patient with a left hemiplegia. **a** The leg pulls into the total flexion pattern without the knee extension component being possible while the hip is flexed. **b** The patient tries to extend his knee as required, and the whole limb extends in the total pattern. He is unable to keep the hip flexed as a result, and the knee extends further than it should

If the model is seated and his arm is placed forward, it remains in exactly the same position when the therapist removes her hands. Without any effort he keeps his shoulder in active flexion, holds the elbow in position with active extension and is able to keep the wrist and fingers in active extension **(Fig. 3.11)**. When the patient's arm is placed in a similar position he attempts to hold it there but requires tremendous effort to do so. He elevates the shoulder girdle, has difficulty in stabilising the scapula and, because he is maintaining flexion of the shoulder, is unable to extend his elbow. Despite the activity in the elbow extensors, the elbow pulls into further flexion. The fingers flex and the thumb flexes and adducts **(Fig. 3.12)**.

The difficulties that the patient demonstrates when the limb cannot be placed in selected combinations are also seen clearly whenever he moves actively. The degree of difficulty varies considerably, but the effect of the mass synergies can still be observed

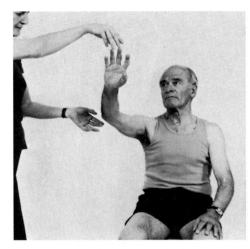 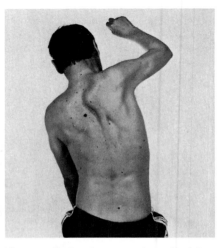

Fig. 3.11. Placing the arm, normal subject

Fig. 3.12. Placing the arm, patient with right hemiplegia. Because the arm is being lifted, flexor hypertonus increases and the total pattern of flexion makes the desired movement unattainable. The patient is unable to extend his fingers at all

even when the patient has regained a significant amount of voluntary function in the hemiplegic limbs. For example, he will not be able to extend his arm in front of him with the palm turned upwards. The activity requires a combination of movement patterns: holding the arm in the air is a flexor activity and the scapula therefore elevates and retracts. Straightening the elbow is an extensor activity and the forearm pronates as a result, with the wrist flexing and the fingers adducting with flexion (**Fig. 3.13 a**).

The same difficulty can be observed when the patient tries to clap his hands together above his head. The activity requires flexion of the shoulder and extension of the elbow, but with supination of the forearm and extension of the wrist and fingers (**Fig. 3.13 b**).

Holding the extended arm horizontally abducted and outwardly rotated also requires very selective activity. The elbow is difficult to extend, because holding the abducted arm in the air requires flexor activity at the shoulder. As the patient tries to extend the elbow, the shoulder rotates inwardly and the forearm pronates as part of the extensor synergy (**Fig. 3.13 c**).

The inability to move the leg selectively can be observed, for example, during the swing phase of gait. The patient brings the hemiplegic leg forwards but is unable to extend the knee for the last part of the swing phase. Because he is flexing his hip, the knee is also flexed and the foot is in supination (**Fig. 3.14**). The patient who extends his knee before placing the foot on the floor in front of him has difficulty in dorsiflexing his foot for heel strike because the ankle is plantar flexing in the extensor synergy (**Fig. 3.15**).

These abnormal movement patterns arising in association with hemiplegia result from the combination of abnormal tone, the re-emergence of primitive mass synergies, a disturbed feedback system and other factors, such as loss of selective trunk muscle ac-

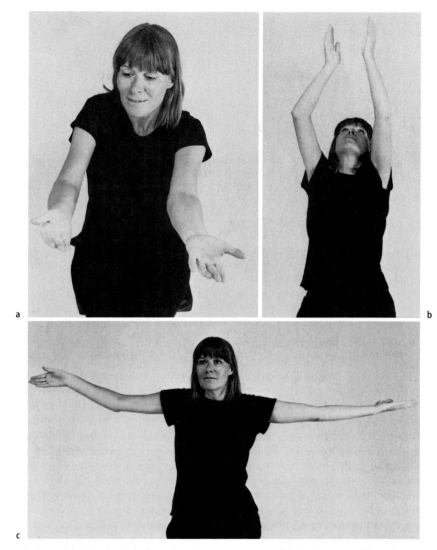

a

b

c

Fig. 3.13 a–c. Patient with right hemiplegia and active movement possible in the arm. **a** When she attempts to stretch both arms out in front of her with the palms facing upwards, the component of the flexor synergy can be seen. **b** When clapping her hands above her head the patient has difficulty in extending her elbow with the forearm supinated and the shoulder externally rotated. **c** When holding the arms in abduction, the patient cannot extend her elbow or turn the palm to face upwards

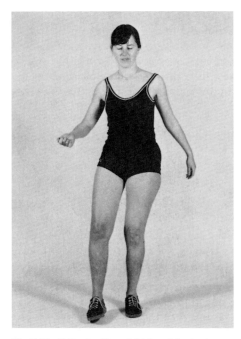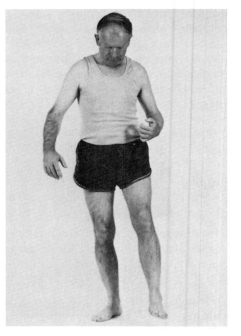

Fig. 3.14. Patient with a right hemiplegia steps forward with her hemiplegic leg using the total pattern of flexion

Fig. 3.15. Patient with a left hemiplegia brings his extended leg forwards and is unable to dorsiflex the foot with the knee extended

tivity, particularly that of the abdominal muscles (Davies 1990). Some variations may occur due to the patient using his abnormal movement patterns repeatedly for functional activities. "This will lead in time to the development of secondary or compensatory abnormal patterns of a greater variety" (K. Bobath 1971). It has also been suggested that, "If some degree of recovery is possible, however, it seems likely that frequent repetition of adaptive motor patterns may generate stronger neural connections, these patterns, rather than more effective and efficient patterns, becoming 'learned' or more stable" (Carr and Shepherd 1996). An important consideration for treatment is therefore that, "If unchecked, improper motor control can become a highly reinforced program" (Bach-y-Rita and Balliet 1987)

Many reflex mechanisms unleashed from the necessary inhibition also play a role in causing increases in postural tone and for the reappearance of primitive movement synergies. "In essence, there are no pathological reflexes but merely normal stereotyped lower spinal and middle supraspinal reflexes that are no longer activated, modified or inhibited" (Cailliet 1980).

Reappearance of Tonic Reflex Activity

Certain reflexes would appear to be particularly relevant to the movement problems commonly encountered. Understanding their influence will help the therapist in her treatment, which aims at inhibiting abnormal tonic reflex activity and facilitating normal movement sequences, including the higher integrated righting and equilibrium reactions. Abnormal postural reflexes can be observed only in patients with lesions of the central nervous system, where their release has led to their re-appearance in an exaggerated form. But even then it is difficult to isolate the various postural reactions, as the picture is usually complicated by the simultaneous action of a number of reflexes and by the patient's volitional efforts (B. Bobath 1971). Fiorentino (1981) describes the role of the postural reflexes in the normal development of movement in babies, and illustrates most clearly the results of their persistence in cerebral palsy as a typical neurological disability.

Tonic Labyrinthine Reflex

The tonic labyrinthine reflex is evoked by changes in the position of the head in space. It originates in the otolithic organs of the labyrinths and is believed to be integrated at brain-stem levels (K. Bobath 1974; Fiorentino 1981). In supine, extensor tone increases throughout the body. The head pushes back as the spine extends, the shoulders retract and the limbs extend in the pattern of extension. In prone lying, flexor tone increases throughout the body, although it may appear only as a reduction of extensor tone if the patient has severe spasticity, particularly in the lower limb. Because the reflex is stimulated by the relative position of the head in space, its effect can also be noticed in standing and sitting positions. For example, if the patient extends his neck and holds his chin in the air, extensor tone in the leg is increased.

The following are some effects of the reflex which may appear pathologically in hemiplegia:

- When the patient is lying supine, the extensor hypertonicity in the leg increases. The head pushes back against the supporting surface, and the whole affected side is seen to be retracted. There is a resistance to protraction of the scapula.
- Patients who are nursed continually in the supine position show marked increase in the extensor tone in the lower limb, and in the upper limb, particularly in the retraction of the scapula.
- When the patient attempts to roll over he extends his head, and the movement is prevented by the increased extensor tone. Rotation is made difficult or impossible because he is unable to bring either his shoulder or his lower limb forwards to initiate turning over. If he flexes his head when rolling, the increased flexion prevents him from turning into the prone position. The lower limb and the arm remain flexed and block the movement, as does the trunk flexion.
- When the patient sits for long periods in his wheelchair, the trunk is flexed and the neck must of necessity be extended to enable him to see. Extensor tone increases in the lower limb, and the resulting hip extension causes his seat to slide forwards in the chair. The knee extends and the foot is pushed forwards off the footplate, so

that eventually he may slip right out of the chair, or be left in a half-lying asymmetrical position in the chair.
- When the patient attempts to stand up without sufficient preparation or adequate tone, he struggles to do so by extending his neck. The total extension pattern occurring in his leg as a result pushes him backwards, as does the retraction of the shoulder. The extending knee is unable to move forwards over his foot, and the necessary dorsal flexion of the ankle is prevented by the simultaneous thrust of the plantar flexors.
  The same difficulty is experienced if he sits down with the head held in extension. Should he flex his head as he sits down, he collapses suddenly onto the chair as the total pattern of flexion is activated. The patient who can maintain sufficient extension of his trunk and leg in standing only by lifting his head will have difficulty in taking a step forwards with the affected leg when he walks. The increased extensor tone prevents the relaxation of the hip and knee at the initiation of the swing phase to allow sufficient flexion for the leg to swing forwards reactively.
- When the patient attempts to extend his elbow while lifting his arm, he reinforces the extension by pushing his head back. The movement is effortful and compromises functional use.

Symmetrical Tonic Neck Reflex

The symmetrical tonic neck reflex is a proprioceptive reflex, elicited by the stretching of the muscles and joints of the neck. Interacting with the labyrinthine reflexes, the symmetrical tonic reflex enables the baby to achieve the crawling position in normal development. In adults the reflexes interact to provide balance and equilibrium and orientate the head. When the neck extends, extensor tone in the arms and flexor tone in the legs increase. With the neck flexed, the extensor tone in the lower limbs increases, with more flexor tone in the arms.

The influence of the reflex seen in hemiplegia is as follows:
- The patient who is nursed in bed in the half-lying position, with the head and trunk flexed by the supporting pillows, shows increased tone in the extensors of the affected leg and the flexors of the arm. Sitting with his head down while in the wheelchair produces the same pattern of spasticity.
- The patient has difficulty when moving from lying to sitting because he must lift his head to initiate the movement, and the resulting increase in extensor tone at the hip resists the movement. Often, the whole leg will show marked extensor spasticity as he struggles to sit up, particularly if he attempts to do so symmetrically.
- The patient who holds his neck flexed when walking and fixes his eyes on the ground has increased extensor tone in the leg. The knee hyperextends, the foot plantar flexes against the floor and the hip is pushed backwards during the stance phase. The patient has difficulty in relaxing the extensor activity to permit the necessary flexion of the hip and knee for the swing phase (Fig. 3.16). During walking the arm pulls strongly into flexion, the associated reaction reinforced by the position of the head.
- When the patient attempts to transfer from his bed to the wheelchair he extends his head and his arms, and the affected leg may show increased flexor tone, either sliding under the bed or lifting off the floor. He is unable to take weight on the leg.

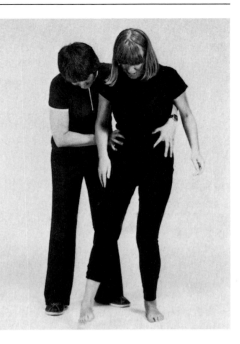

Fig. 3.16. Patient with a right hemiplegia flexes her neck to look at the ground when she walks. She is unable to release the hip and knee when taking a step and the position of the foot in the extensor pattern makes it difficult for her to place it correctly on the floor to initiate the stance phase

- When the patient attempts to kneel as he goes down onto the floor or stands up from the floor, he lifts his head and the affected leg collapses in total flexion.

Asymmetrical Tonic Neck Reflex

The asymmetrical tonic neck reflex is elicited as a proprioceptive response from the muscles and joints of the neck. When the head is turned, extensor tone increases in the limbs on the side towards which the face is turned. The limbs on the occiput side show an increase in flexor tone. In the normal baby, the reflex is fundamental to visual fixation, with the hand reaching out for objects. It also prepares the way for rolling over to prone with rotation at about 4–5 months in normal children.

Effects of the reflex seen pathologically in hemiplegia are as follows:

- The patient's head is usually turned away from the affected side in lying and sitting, and flexor tone increases in the hemiplegic arm as a result. Patients who remain in the wheelchair for many months, when standing and walking are delayed, often show an increase in flexor tone in the hemiplegic leg as well. The leg shows flexor spasticity when the patient is helped to stand up. Even when the patient is lying supine, a resistance may be felt when passive extension of the leg is attempted. A flexion contracture of the knee may develop.
- When attempting to straighten his hemiplegic arm, the patient turns his head strongly to the affected side to reinforce the extension at the elbow. He may be unable to extend the arm without turning his head.

- Although flexor spasticity predominates in the arm and it assumes a flexed position, the patient is unable to flex his hand to touch his head or face when his head is turned towards it. The therapist feels a resistance to flexion when she attempts to assist the correct movement.
- The patient with hypotonus in the lower limb will often turn his head towards the affected side when he is attempting to stand with help. He fixes his head in a position of rotation to the hemiplegic side, to reinforce extension in the leg. (The attitude is often misinterpreted as compensation for an existing hemianopsia, but when the patient is sitting the head does not adopt the same posture.) The fixed head position should be discouraged, as it interferes with normal balance reactions.

Positive Supporting Reaction

The positive supporting reflex is more a reaction following an exteroceptive stimulus to the skin of the toe pads and the ball of the foot, often elicited as these touch the ground. A proprioceptive stimulus follows, due to the stretching of the interosseous muscles of the foot caused by the pressure on the ball of the foot. Extensor tone throughout the limb is increased, together with a simultaneous contraction of the opposing muscles to stabilise the joints for weightbearing. In normal development the reflex is a precursor to standing and walking.

The effects of the reflex seen pathologically in hemiplegia are as follows:

- If the ball of the hemiplegic foot makes contact with the ground first, as it will do with premature plantar flexion of the ankle, the exaggerated reflex causes an immediate increase in extensor tone throughout the limb in a total pattern. The leg becomes a rigid pillar, with the knee hyperextended, and the patient has difficulty in keeping his heel on the floor during weightbearing, or in releasing the hip and knee for the swing phase during walking. He also has difficulty in transferring weight over the hemiplegic leg at the start of the stance phase, as the plantar flexors push against the direction of the movement.
- Attempts at maintaining dorsal flexion at the ankle by traditional passive movements fail, because the therapist's hands on the ball of the foot increase the hypertonus in the plantar flexors and the full range of motion is impossible.

Crossed Extensor Reflex

The crossed extensor reflex is believed to be a spinal reflex, causing an increase in extensor tone in one leg when the other leg is flexed. In normal development it is a precursor to amphibian-type movement in preparation for crawling and walking (Fiorentino 1981).

B. Bobath (1971) discusses the animal experiments of Magnus and Sherrington, who described the reflex as appearing when a painful stimulus is applied to one limb, causing a flexor withdrawal reaction. Extensor tone increases in the other leg(s) in order to support the additional body weight.

The effects of the reflex seen pathologically in hemiplegia are as follows:

- When lying supine, the patient is able to lift his buttocks off the bed, the weight being supported by both his legs. If he lifts the sound leg off the bed in flexion, the affected leg is pushed into total extension pattern, and the "bridge" collapses.
- When the patient stands from sitting with the weight only on the sound leg, the hemiplegic leg will often flex as the other leg extends actively. The patient has difficulty in transferring his weight over the affected leg in order to initiate walking.
- A patient may be able to stand on his hemiplegic leg alone in the exercise situation. The leg remains mobile, and he can even flex and extend the hemiplegic knee during weightbearing without the toes flexing. However, during walking, when the sound leg is flexing forward to take a step, the hemiplegic leg pushes into the total extension pattern, making balance difficult and the subsequent step forwards with the affected leg stiff and effortful.

The Grasp Reflex

The grasp reflex is elicited by tactile and proprioceptive stimuli in the palm of the hand and palmar aspect of the fingers, causing a grasp response with the fingers flexing and adducting. The reflex is present at birth in normal babies and disappears gradually as voluntary grasp develops. The reflex consists of an initial catching phase, elicited by a distally moving object in the palm of the hand in contact with the skin. The subsequent holding phase of the reflex results from a pull on the already contracting flexor muscles. "The stimulus for the proprioceptive phase is undoubtedly stretch, an increment of passive tension, acting on a centre already facilitated by deep cutaneous pressure" (Seyffarth and Denny-Brown 1948). The authors differentiate between the grasp reflex and the instinctive grasp reaction, which is a "deliberate progressive closure of the whole hand made in a series of small movements, upon a stationary contact within the palm. This movement terminates in a final complete grip."

The effects of the reflex seen pathologically in hemiplegia are as follows:

- An object placed in the patient's hand may increase flexor tone in the flexors of the wrist and fingers and cause flexion of the elbow, which is affected by the proximal insertion of the muscles involved. Patients with flexor spasticity in the hand are frequently treated by placing a firm roll in the hand to prevent flexion, or by applying a firm resting splint which includes the fingers. Both of these procedures will tend to increase the spasticity by eliciting the grasp reflex and reaction.
- The patient who shows some return of activity in the hand should not be encouraged to squeeze a rubber ball, as flexor tone will be stimulated and release of the grasp become increasingly difficult.
- The patient may have difficulty in clasping his hands together in order to carry out his self-assisted arm exercises. As he attempts to interlace his fingers, the grasp reflex is stimulated by the fingers of the sound hand moving distally on the palmar aspect of his other hand. The fingers flex and adduct and resist the attempt.
- A patient who has active extension of the fingers may still have an active grasp reflex which prevents him from releasing objects during functional activities. The inability to release or prevent the grasp is not necessarily related to weakness of finger extension.

- Some patients have difficulty in preventing involuntary, inappropriate grasping. The affected hand, even when not involved in an activity, may hold tightly to an object, e.g. the leg of the trousers, when walking. The patient may even grab hold of the therapist and not be able to let go, which is embarrassing for him, particularly if the grasp is so forceful as to be painful for her.

Clinical observation has shown that patients who demonstrate reflex grasping will always have diminished or disturbed sensation in their hemiplegic hand. If the therapist avoids placing anything in the patient's hand because she is afraid of eliciting the reflex and does not guide his hands during the manipulation of objects, then the situation becomes self-reinforcing. The less tactile input the hand experiences, the more impoverished the sensation becomes and thus the stronger the grasping tendency. Hard objects are more easily felt and released than flimsy, pliable ones, and the patient should therefore be helped to hold and release those which offer a definite resistance at first, such as a wooden pole, a cucumber or a chair, and only later progress to manipulating softer materials. As sensation improves the reflex gradually disappears.

Associated Reactions and Associated Movements

Associated reactions in hemiplegia are abnormal reflex movements of the affected side, and they duplicate the stereotyped spastic patterns of the arm and leg (**Fig. 3.17**). Walshe (1923) described associated reactions as "released postural reactions deprived of voluntary control". Riddoch and Buzzard (1921) defined associated reactions as "automatic activities which fix or alter the posture of a part or parts when some other part of the body is brought into action by either voluntary effort or reflex stimulation". The reactions are seen when the patient moves with effort, is trying to maintain his balance, or is afraid of falling. Mulley (1982) reports associated reactions in the hemiplegic arm in 80 % of a group of patients, occurring in conjunction with yawning, coughing and sneezing. During functional activities, such as putting on shoes using the sound hand, associated reactions are prevalent in both the arm and the leg if attention is not given to inhibitory positions and the way in which the task is performed.

Associated movements are normal automatic postural adjustments which accompany voluntary movements. They occur in normal subjects, to reinforce precise movements of other parts of the body, or when an activity requires a great deal of strength or concentration. Associated movements can be observed in the unaffected limbs of the hemiplegic patient when he is trying to move his affected limbs. They should not be confused with associated reactions, which are pathological, and they can be differentiated by the ability of the patient to alter or relax them. Associated reactions are stereotyped and occur even when no active movement is present in the limb. The patient is unable to relax them at will. The limb returns to its previous position only after the stimulus has ceased, and then often only gradually.

The detrimental effects of associated reactions are as follows:

- The abnormal flexed position of the hemiplegic arm is cosmetically unacceptable for the patient. It draws immediate attention to his disability.

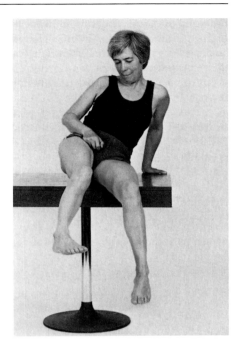

Fig. 3.17. Patient with a right hemiplegia shows typical associated reactions in the arm and leg when moving incorrectly and pulling herself back with her sound arm to sit on a table

- The affected limbs in the fixed spastic positions of associated reactions make functional activities more difficult. For example, putting on a shoe, with the leg in extension and the foot plantar flexed and inverted, becomes almost impossible. As the patient struggles to perform the activity, the extensor spasticity is further increased. Washing the hemiplegic hand and putting on a coat become equally difficult if the arm is pulling strongly into flexion.
- If the arm is constantly pulled up in flexion, there is a danger of contracture, particularly of the elbow and the fingers.
- The continuously flexed position makes functional use of the affected arm impossible, and return of activity may even be prevented altogether.
- Recovery of active control of the elbow extensors and the foot dorsiflexors is negatively influenced by the reciprocal inhibition of antagonists when they are constantly hyperactive.
- Balance reactions in both the arm and leg are prevented by the associated reactions, making the maintenance of equilibrium difficult.
- Hypertonicity may be increased throughout the affected side, making movements effortful and less adaptable to the demands of the environment and the task.

Because of their many adverse effects, every attempt should be made to avoid such hypertonic reactions from being elicited in the course of the patient's daily routine. During treatment, associated reactions should act as a barometer for the therapist, informing her whether the activity is too difficult, whether she is giving too little support, whether balance is inadequate, or whether the patient is trying too hard or is not receiving enough sensory information. She will need to analyse which of these needs to be adjusted, the reduction in the hypertonus guiding her to the correct solution.

Abnormal Tension in the Nervous System

Prolonged abnormal postures such as those caused by associated reactions can easily lead to reduced mobility in the nervous system (Rolf 1997b). In turn, such increased tension may further add to the strength of the associated reactions, so that a self-reinforcing situation occurs. If the nervous system is unable to lengthen adaptively then body movements will be altered as a result. The effects of the loss of the normal neurodynamics on movement are described in Chap. 15, together with ways in which mobility can be regained.

Disturbed Sensation

All skilled movements require a refined feedback system to provide exact information as to the correctness of the activity being performed, feedback normally being used to adjust programmed movements. "Feedback brings the program commands up to date with how their execution is coming along" (Brooks 1986). Maintenance of balance is also dependent upon sensations throughout the body.

It is difficult, if not impossible, to know exactly what the hemiplegic patient feels and what information he receives when he moves. Although conventional testing of sensation can provide only a guideline, the results can be recorded, allowing changes to be noted at a later date. What is recorded states only that the patient at a specific time, in a given situation, gave the examiner information about what he was feeling. Even if all the answers he gave were correct as to the position of his limbs, the direction of their movements and the pressure or light touch he was able to perceive, an hour later he might be observed sitting with his hand trapped in the wheel of his wheelchair while attempting to move it forwards. The phenomenon of tactile suppression has been described, whereby the patient correctly identifies which hand is touched by the examiner but when both are touched simultaneously, he feels only the touching of the sound hand. It seems that the stimulus of the sound side suppresses that of the affected side (Isaacs 1977).

Observation of the way in which the patient moves during the performance of different activities can be a reliable guide as to how accurately he feels. Video films of his movements can be taken and studied to reveal any difficulties. Observations such as the patient using too much effort, holding parts of his body too tensely or pressing too hard against the supporting surfaces are all indications that his sensation is impaired. No patient feels exactly as he did before the hemiplegia; it is just that all presently available methods of sensory testing are too gross to detect fine differences in feedback.

Patterns of spasticity and mass movement synergies are closely related to sensation, either as cause or effect. The patient can move only in an abnormal way, and so the feedback he receives is of an abnormal movement. He moves in abnormal patterns because the sensation is inaccurate and inadequate. With so much tension in the muscles there is little chance of his being able to feel objects accurately. When sensation is disturbed, the patient will tend to increase the tension in his muscles to provide him with more information as to where his body is in space, and with increased tone his ability to interact more appropriately with his environment is further reduced.

One difficulty encountered by the patient with disturbed sensation is the inability to plan the required movements in anticipation of the performance, in the normal manner. "The term 'motor set' indicates that the CNS (central nervous system) is ready to carry out a planned motor action, that plans have been made to implement the intention" (Brooks 1986). The anticipatory nature of motor activity is also a feature of balance, in that "postural supports have to be coordinated early to steady the body, head and limbs for the expected movements". Likewise, "During reach and grasp, the shaping of the hand for grasping occurs during the transportation component of the reach" (Shumway-Cook and Woollacott 1995). The anticipatory shaping of the hand is dependent upon the characteristics of the object which is to be grasped, and the size of the maxi-

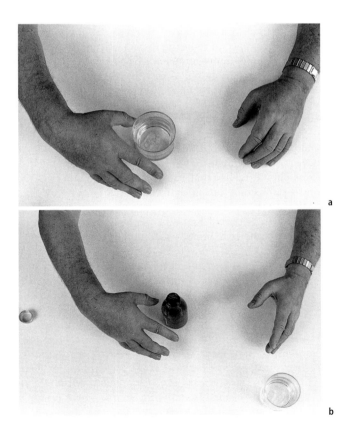

a

Fig. 3.18a, b. No anticipatory shaping of the hand (right hemiplegia). **a** Hand and fingers have not assumed the form of the glass. **b** When the bottle is being released the grip aperture is disproportionately wide, with the fingers too extended

b

mum grip aperture is proportional to the size of the object (Jeannerod 1990). A patient may be able to flex and extend his wrist and fingers voluntarily, but if he cannot plan the timing and the agonist and antagonist muscle activity before the movement then functional use of the upper limb will be hampered. There is characteristically no anticipatory shaping of the patient's hand, and the fingers extend too much (**Fig. 3.18 a**). The same applies when the patient is letting go of an object and opens his hand as widely as possible instead of the fractional amount of activity normally used to remove the fingers from the object (**Fig. 3.18 b**; compare with **Fig. 2.27 a, b**). The therapist should therefore avoid instructing the patient to open his fingers wide, a command which is often used if the finger flexors are hypertonic, because by doing so she would be encouraging an incorrect grasping or releasing action.

Considerations

Although normal muscle tone is considered to be a prerequisite for economical and harmonious movement in normal patterns, the role of hypertonicity or spasticity should not be overestimated with regard to the movement difficulties experienced by the patient with hemiplegia. An overemphasis of its importance for successful stroke rehabilitation has led to a number of research studies concentrating too specifically on treatment forms aimed at reducing hypertonus by physiotherapy techniques, antispasmodics or injections of botulinum toxin. The results have proved disappointing in the long term, although the initial effects may have seemed promising (Hesse et al. 1994). Improvements which have been noted have tended to be subjective as reported by the patients rather than reflecting true functional gains, possibly because the distal symptoms and not the underlying cause of the problem were influenced. In fact, real improvement of independent motor behaviour or performance has not been demonstrated after tonic and phasic stretch reflexes have been decreased or reflex contractions weakened by CNS depressants (Landau 1980). For successful treatment it is therefore logical that, "Clinicians should realize that in stroke rehabilitation it is more appropriate to concentrate on reestablishing normal active motor control rather than reducing the hypersensitivity of the stretch reflex in response to passive movement" (Duncan and Bradke 1987). Despite having devoted much of her professional life to discovering ways to normalise tone, Betha Bobath, in her wisdom, nevertheless reminded therapists:

> It cannot be expected that a reduction of spasticity and the activation of certain muscle groups during treatment, i.e. when the patient is lying supine or prone, or while rolling, or sitting, or kneeling, will lead directly to more normal use of arm and hand or to an improved gait. Even if the muscles can function well in such 'developmental exercises', it will be impossible for the patient to carry over the obtained movement patterns into the activities of daily life, or to use the newly acquired but not established movements in different functional situations. Everything done in treatment, therefore, should serve as a direct preparation for specific functional use. The sequences of movement chosen for such preparation should be as similar as possible to those movements needed in daily life. In this way a bridge can be built between treatment and functional use" (Bobath 1977).

Recent research indicates that other factors, such as inadequate recruitment of agonist motor neurons, may be more disabling than simply hypertonicity (Shumway-Cook and Woollacott 1995).

Movements are learned through repetition and become more skilled as inhibition of unwanted activity increases. However, the repetition must be "repetition without repetition" in a great variety of situations, because "Motor skill is not a movement formula and certainly not a formula of permanent muscle forces imprinted in some motor center. Motor skill is an ability to solve one or other type of motor problem" (Bernstein 1996b). To be successful the practised movements must also be correct, because, as Bernstein emphasises, if only the existing clumsy or unskilled movements are repeated, the exercise does not result in any improvement. The therapist must therefore use her hands to enable the patient to move correctly and not, as is sometimes advocated, leave him to struggle on his own to solve the problem in the only way possible for him at the time. If the patient moves in stereotyped mass movement synergies, he will learn only these, to the exclusion of more defined, selective and thus effective movements. Right from the beginning, the treatment should aim at helping him to move in the most normal and economical way possible, to avoid abnormal movement patterns from becoming habituated through their constant repetition. "Just as repetition of good programs leads to good results, repetition of bad programs leads to bad results and the need to 'unlearn' them" (Brooks 1986).

4 Practical Assessment – A Continuing Process

To assess the patient's abilities and difficulties fully and accurately, the therapist requires exact observation, ready hands, analytical thinking and the time to listen to what the patient says. She needs to understand fully how people normally move and react in different situations and perform certain tasks, so that she can notice at once if the patient acts or reacts differently.

No scientific system of measurement is as yet available for the therapist when assessing a patient with a hemiplegia. A purely functional chart which can be ticked off briskly, such as the still widely used Barthel Index, provides only quantitative information, stating what the patient can or cannot do (Mahoney and Barthel 1965). However, the recording of the patient's functional abilities alone is not sufficient for adequate treatment planning. For example, the statement "Patient cannot transfer from wheelchair to bed" does not answer the question "Why?" It states only that he is unable to perform the activity. In order to treat his particular difficulty, it is necessary to know whether his legs were too weak or his balance too poor, whether he was too spastic, or even whether he was too obese to lift his body from the seat of the chair.

Similarly, a patient might be described as having an adequate functional gait, even able to use public transport. However, because of extensor hypertonus, he may be unable to flex his knee while the hip is extended. In order to bring his foot forwards, he therefore circumducts his leg as he takes a step, and this would be the information needed for treatment aimed at improving his walking.

The lack of such qualitative information also characterises the many other evaluation forms presently being used for comparing treatment outcomes, for providing prognostic indicators, or even for deciding which patients should receive intensive treatment. Such scales may well be useful for research, in that they provide statistical data for computerised analysis, but as yet no trials have taken into account that the skill and experience of the therapists can be important in obtaining a satisfactory rehabilitation outcome following stroke (Ashburn et al. 1993).

For providing informed and appropriate treatment a qualitative rather than a quantitative assessment is essential.

The Aims of Assessment

Assessment is aimed at:
- Establishing what the patient is able to do independently, how he does so and what he cannot as yet do

- Eliciting what is preventing the patient from performing some activity or from moving in a normal way, in order to plan the treatment
- Making frequent reviews possible so that the treatment can be altered whenever necessary
- Providing sufficient information to enable another therapist to step in at short notice and treat the patient effectively
- Recording the patient's condition accurately for future therapeutic or statistical purposes

Recommendations for Accurate Assessment

In order to ascertain what the patient can do and what difficulties he has at the present time, he must be observed while he is moving actively. Assessment involves far more than merely asking the patient to move his limbs while lying on a bed or plinth. The actual problems really come to light only when the patient is moving at the very limit of his present ability, and not when he is being helped to perform an activity which is easy for him. The therapist needs to observe and note when exactly an activity cannot be performed at all or only in an abnormal or alternative way. There will, of course, be a great difference in the level of performance possible for individual patients, according to what stage of rehabilitation or recovery they have reached. In the acute phase a patient may be able only to turn his head or roll over in bed, while at a more advanced stage the therapist will need to search diligently to observe subtle deviations in the way he moves. Sometimes it may even be necessary to observe the patient jogging or clapping his hands behind his back before a problem is revealed.

The therapist should watch the patient as he arrives for his first treatment; from this valuable moment onwards assessment is a continuous process, involving important variables which will come to light over a longer period.

A full evaluation cannot be made on one particular day. Even a sleepless night or constipation can adversely affect the patient's performance.

Assessment is always carried out in conjunction with treatment. The therapist is trying to discover where the patient's main problem lies and if she can change some factor. If she inhibits hypertonicity, can he then move in a more normal pattern? What can he do if she helps him a little or supports him in a certain way? Assessment is therefore an integral part of the treatment itself and not a separate entity.

The therapist is constantly assessing and reassessing during treatment to see if she has reduced hypertonus, stimulated activity or enabled the patient to move in a more normal way during a certain activity.

The therapist should take the trouble to put the patient at ease and speak in such a way that he understands what is required of him. Many assessments may be inaccurate simply because the patient is confused as to what activity the therapist wishes him to perform.

The patient should always undress sufficiently and wear appropriate clothing for the assessment and all subsequent treatment sessions. Many significant problems may otherwise be overlooked. During treatment, adequate stimulation and observation are not possible if the patient remains fully dressed. A bathing costume or shorts and a sleeveless undershirt are most suitable for assessment and treatment. How the patient undresses and dresses himself again and the amount of support or assistance he requires when doing so is an important observation in the assessment. For example, with even a comparatively slight hemiplegia the patient may reveal balance problems in his inability to step out of his trousers. Through observation, the therapist can be building up a composite picture long before she handles the limbs or tests functions specifically.

Specific Aspects of Assessment

Immediate Observation

The therapist should note how the patient enters, whether he is escorted, held or supported. If he is in a wheelchair, she notes how he pushes it or assists, how he is sitting, whether he looks alert or uninterested. The same applies whether he is seen in bed, on the ward or in his home.

The therapist observes the patient carefully as he approaches and while he is greeting and talking to her, irrespective of whether he is lying, sitting or standing. How the patient behaves in the situation will provide information about possible perceptual disturbances, through comparing his behaviour with that which would normally be expected under similar circumstances. Failure to respond to the introduction and greeting in the

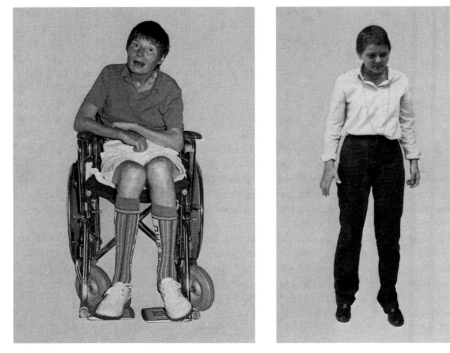

Fig. 4.1. Patient with bilateral hemiplegia following a thrombosis in both internal carotid arteries

Fig. 4.2. Patient with ataxia

usual way, talking excessively or laughing inappropriately are typical symptoms and
are most likely symptomatic of the lesion rather than being of a purely psychological
nature.

Figures 4.1–4.3 illustrate patients as they might appear when arriving for their assessment and treatment. The following points can be observed that could prove valuable
later for treatment purposes.

In Fig. 4.1 the absence of facial expression is inappropriate to the situation, where the
patient is greeting the therapist. The mask-like face and very wide-open eyes suggest a
hypertonus of the facial muscles, as does the withdrawn upper lip on the left side. Her
eyes are turned towards the therapist but her head remains turned to the right and
side-flexed to the left, and the hyperactivity apparent in the left sternomastoid muscle
could account for the position.

She appears to have difficulty in lifting her head against the pull of the flexor spasticity in neck and trunk. She will certainly have problems with balance if her head is not
free to move. The open mouth indicates that she will have problems with eating and
drinking. Is it because of weakness in the jaw-closing muscles, or is she unable to close
her mouth due to hypertonus in the antagonistic muscle group?

The upper trunk is markedly flexed, particularly on the left side, and her weight is
over the right side. The left side is probably more affected than the right. Her arms are
in the pattern of flexor spasticity. Is it just spasticity, or are there contractures or painful

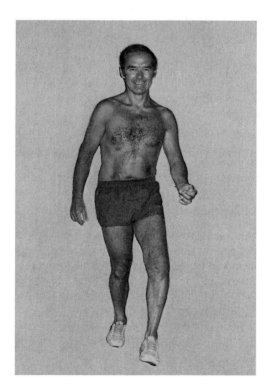

Fig. 4.3. Patient with a left hemiplegia

limitation of range? Can she use her arms at all? The patient's right arm is pressing heavily on the arm of the wheelchair. Is she unable to maintain the upright position without the help of her arm? Her legs are in adduction. Is this due to her position in the chair, or is there a resistance to abducting them, caused by spasticity?

Her left foot is plantar flexed with the heel off the footrest. Is the Achilles tendon only spastic, or is there shortening of the muscle as well?

In **Fig. 4.2**, as the patient walks towards the physiotherapist, she does not look up to greet her but fixes her eyes on the floor with much concentration. From the position of the head, shoulders and arms it would seem that she has difficulty in stabilising and balancing. She takes only a short step, more to the side than forwards. The right foot has remained in contact with the floor until her weight is on the left leg. She has transferred her weight sideways rather than forwards as in normal walking.

In **Fig. 4.3** the patient walks confidently towards the therapist with an appropriate and symmetrical facial expression and normal eye contact. His balance is obviously good, as he shows no fear of falling. The sensation in his left leg appears adequate, as he does not need to look at it in order to step forwards. His pelvis shows a marked lateral shift to the right with his right knee remaining in flexion. Although he is stepping forwards with his left leg, his left arm is moving forwards as well, instead of his right arm swinging reactively forward. His pelvis is retracted and hitched upwards as he brings the leg forwards in the flexion synergy, with abduction and outward rotation at the hip and the foot pulled into supination by the strong activity of the anterior tibial muscle. The muscle bulk in his whole leg shows that weakness is not the problem, but rather that hypertonus is restricting selective movement.

With the effort of bringing his left leg forwards, his arm shows an associated reaction in flexion, particularly marked distally, with his fingers flexing strongly and his thumb adducted and flexed. The forearm is supinated and not pronated as would be expected in the flexion pattern.

A Subjective History

A short history is taken from the patient, and while he talks the therapist observes him carefully and gains an impression of the following:

1. Voice: (a) Does he speak clearly and with sufficient volume? (b) Are his sentences very short because his breath control is inadequate? (c) Is his voice hoarse or monotonous?
2. Facial expression: (a) Is it appropriate and does it change it all? (b) Does he look at her and make normal eye contact?

If he is unable to speak at all, some other person who knows him well, for example his wife, should be present to provide the necessary information. The whole history should not be taken at the start of the treatment session, as many patients find it distressing to sit and talk about what has happened to them. The therapist observes the patient's abilities first, then uses her hands to facilitate certain movements and between activities gradually builds up a composite picture of the problems.

While listening to him, the therapist learns whether he understands his disorder and has a clear picture of the prognosis. She discovers what his attitude is to home and work, and whether he is prepared to accept a new way of life now that he is disabled.

She hears from the patient what he thinks his main problem is, and why he has sought help. His subjective opinion of what he considers to be his main problem and what he hopes to achieve through the treatment is an important clue to how realistically he sees his disability.

It is also important for the therapist to compare her goals with those of the patient, because they must somehow be brought together to form a realistic aim. Failure to have a common goal will lead to disappointment and frustration for the patient or the therapist, or both. For example, where the therapist's aim is that the patient should learn to walk again, while his is to have a new wheelchair, success is possible only if they come to a mutual agreement. Similarly, if the therapist is concentrating on enabling the patient to walk without a walking-stick and his main wish is to be able to use his hemiplegic hand again, the treatment sessions will be disappointing.

Muscle Tone

While the patient is moving either to sit on the plinth or to stand up from his chair, the therapist can be gaining an impression of his muscle tone on a more automatic level, before he is conscious of being tested. She is looking and feeling all the time as he moves or is being assisted to move.

Muscle tone is usually defined as being the amount of resistance to passive movement of the part, in other words, to stretch or elongation. Observation alone can be very deceptive, so the therapist needs to feel the resistances.

The muscle with normal tone responds to being moved by taking the weight of the part it affects and allowing the limb, head or trunk to be guided without resistance into a position which is spontaneously maintained with ease. In the presence of normal tone the part moved can be described as having a feeling of lightness, with those muscles responsible for movement in the opposite direction playing out smoothly to allow unimpeded motion. If placed in a certain position, the part will stay there for a time before returning slowly to a resting posture.

Hypertonicity makes the limb or trunk heavy and difficult to move because it resists movement to a greater or lesser degree. When released, the part is pulled in the direction of the muscles which have increased tone.

Hypotonicity allows the movements with less than normal resistance, causing the part to feel floppy and lifeless. The weight of the limb is not taken and it will fall in the direction of the pull of gravity (see Chapter 3).

Joint Range

Although there is often interobserver variability in the measurement of joint range, the measurement provides an important record of the patient's state at the time and will influence the planning of the treatment. Care must be taken, however, to differentiate between hypertonicity impeding motion and actual structural limitation of range, and also between soft tissue shortening and bony changes, because the information will be necessary for planning the treatment approach. Any contracture will affect the pattern of movement and may even prevent the return of functional activity. When testing, it is effort-saving to examine all parts of the body first in one position and then in another, but when the facts are recorded it is helpful to have both muscle tone and joint range measurement grouped under the heading pertaining to the particular part of the body. For example, it is far easier to refer to the section on upper limbs to see whether the elbow was contracted at the time of the last assessment than to have to search for a chart kept on a separate page.

A photograph or a diagrammatic sketch of the movement possibility is often clearer than a recorded number of degrees. Actual measurement of a contracture can be noted by measuring the distance between two definite points; e.g. for a flexion contracture of the elbow the patient lies supine and his shoulder is held flat on the supporting surface. The distance between the dorsal aspect of his wrist and the plinth is measured and re-corded.

Muscle Charts

A specific muscle-testing chart is not included in the assessment. In the presence of hypertonicity, which is a varying force, it is not possible to estimate accurately the strength of a muscle acting against it. The manual muscle test and its corresponding evaluation scale were originally designed for patients with lower motor dysfunction where individual muscles were affected. The manual muscle test is unsuitable for patients with upper motor neurone lesions because of the large numbers of muscles involved in the paralysis, the abnormalities of tone and the influence of manual contact on both (Michels 1959; La Vigue 1974) Posture and the position of the limb also influence or alter the activity of different muscle groups, so that the results of testing do not reflect functional use. For example, a patient with possible grade-5 dorsiflexors may be unable to dorsiflex his foot against the hypertonus of the calf muscles, particularly when the leg is extended. Muscle strength may be adequate in certain positions, but if the patient can move only in synergistic, nonselective patterns he cannot use the limb or part functionally. The hemiplegic patient is often able to extend his elbow against gravity when lying supine with his arm above his head and the flexor spasticity inhibited. In this position the therapist may be unable to overcome the extensor activity, which would then be classified as a grade 5 in triceps (**Fig. 4.4 a**). When the patient is standing or sitting, however, he is unable to extend his elbow, even though gravity is assisting the movement (**Fig. 4.4 b**).

Increased Tension in the Nervous System

Because the patient will invariably have abnormally increased tension in his nervous system as a result of the lesion, the presence and amount of tension should be tested and recorded. The loss of normal neurodynamics has a marked influence on posture, muscle tone, voluntary muscle activity, the patterns of active movement, joint range and sensation (Rolf 1997). The tension tests described by Butler (1991) are an integral part of the overall assessment because of their importance for future treatment, as described in Chap. 15.

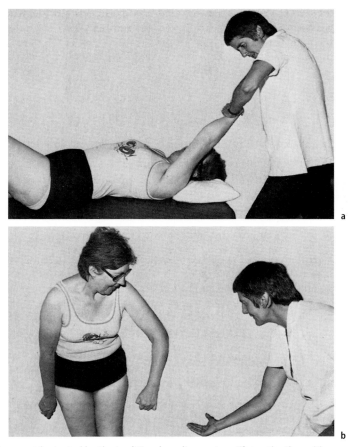

Fig. 4.4 a, b. Muscle strength cannot be tested by the traditional grading system. The patient's position and the variable tone in the antagonists give results which are not applicable to function. **a** A patient lying supine is able to hold her elbow extended against gravity despite considerable resistance from the therapist. **b** Even with gravity assisting the movement, in standing the patient is unable to extend her elbow (left hemiplegia)

Recording the Assessment

There is no short cut to recording the assessment, no chart that would suit all patients and all therapists. The information should be clearly headed and neatly written or printed so that important facts are not overlooked. A recent, carefully prepared assessment form for hemiplegic patients made no mention of abnormal tone, so omitting one of the most relevant factors.

To make recording easier it is possible to have printed sheets giving headings and space, to ensure that each aspect is examined. Any difficulty observed in one part of the body will influence the posture or movement of the other parts. The following headings are suggested:

The head	Walking
The trunk	Comprehension
The upper limbs	The face, speaking and eating
The lower limbs	Sensation
Sitting	Functional abilities
Standing	Leisure activities and hobbies
Weight transference and balance	
reactions	

Obviously, should there be other outstanding features in individual cases, they can then be recorded under an appropriate heading.

Not all the suggested tests and activities will be suitable or possible for every patient, depending upon the degree of disability or stage in rehabilitation. For example, the patient in the acute stage cannot be turned to lie prone, and in all probability will not yet be able to walk. The therapist will need to select those activities which are feasible at the time of the assessment.

The Comprehensive Evaluation

The Head

Under this heading and those that follow it is not necessary to answer all the questions separately, only to record when something of significance is noted.

■ **In Supine.** Does the head lie centrally at rest or does it incline or rotate to one side? Does it remain flexed? Does it push back onto the plinth? Can the patient correct its position and turn it freely? Can he raise it as if to look at his feet? When the therapist moves the head passively is there resistance in any direction, and does the patient support its weight automatically himself? Is there structural loss of range of motion in the cervical region?

■ **In Sitting.** The position which the head assumes is observed and then tested to see if it is freely movable. Is there resistance to passive movement, and can the patient move it actively?

■ **In Standing.** The same tests should be made with the patient in a standing position.

The Trunk

■ **In Supine.** Does the body lie symmetrically or is it shortened on one side? Is the umbilicus right in the middle? Is the pelvis rotated? Has the lumbar spine a fixed lordosis, and if so, can it be corrected passively by flexing the hips and tilting the pelvis? Is passive rotation of the upper and lower trunk fully mobile? Can the patient roll over to both sides? Can he roll from supine to prone and back again over either side? How does he do so? Can he sit up from lying without using his arms?

■ **In Sitting.** Can the patient hold his trunk erect, or does he sit with a kyphosed posture? Is his trunk symmetrical? Can he rotate his trunk actively to either side? Is there a resistance to passive rotation in either direction? Is lateral flexion of the lower trunk possible?

■ **In Standing.** What position does the trunk assume? Can the patient move his trunk selectively, e.g. tilt his pelvis forwards and back without moving his thoracic spine? Can he rotate his pelvis without moving his upper trunk?

The Upper Limbs

■ **In Supine.** What position do the arms assume at rest? Can the patient move them voluntarily in a normal manner? If not, state the pattern of movement. Is there resistance to passive movement in any direction? Do the arms move involuntarily on effort or when the patient yawns or coughs? If so, in what pattern of movement?

Does the tone in the arms change according to which way the head is turned? Is contracture present at any joint even after release of spasticity? Is there pain on movement in any direction?

■ **In Prone Lying.** Can the patient bring his arms forwards, or is there too much flexion in this position? Is full elevation of the shoulders with extension of the elbows possible in this position? Can he support his weight on his elbows? Can he support his weight on extended arms?

■ **In Sitting and Standing.** The tests carried out in supine and prone lying should also be done with the patient sitting and standing. Many patients have comparatively good movement when lying fully supported, and the problems may be obvious only when they have to hold themselves upright against gravity and maintain their balance at the same time.

It is even more important to know how the patient actually uses his hands. Testing the different movements in a free exercise situation will not provide the information as to what happens when he performs a task. For example, the patient should be asked to carry out an everyday activity which normally requires the use of both hands, such as opening a bottle, pouring himself a drink and then drinking it. He could also be asked to cut a slice of bread, spread it with butter and then eat it. The therapist observes whether he performs the activity in any way differently from other people. Even how hard he has to concentrate to perform such relatively simple tasks will indicate whether he has problems in using his hands.

The Lower Limbs

■ **In Supine.** Active and passive movements are tested in a way similar to that used for the upper limbs. In addition, the following are observed with the patient lying prone.

■ **In Prone Lying.** Can the patient flex his knees actively without flexing his hips as well? Is there resistance to flexing the knees passively, and do the hips flex if this is done? Do the knees remain flexed if left in this position?

■ **In Sitting.** The patient moves his leg actively in different directions, e.g. crossing one leg over the other one. The therapist also moves the leg passively to note any resistance or limitation of range.

■ **In Standing.** The patient lifts his leg in different directions and can be observed while he takes a step or kicks a football with the hemiplegic foot. The therapist should also feel the resistance when she moves his leg passively.

Sitting

Can the patient come to a sitting position from lying unaided, and how does he do so? Does he sit with the trunk flexed, or does he push or fall backwards? Does he lean more to one side than to the other?

Does he bear weight equally through each buttock? Is the trunk rotated, for example is one shoulder or one side of the pelvis drawn backwards? Is one shoulder lower than the other?

Do the legs hang in a normally flexed position over the side of the bed or couch, or do the knees extend, showing hypertonus? How is his balance in this position? Can he move his head, arms and legs, or have them moved passively, without falling over? Can he save himself from falling?

Standing

How does the patient stand up from sitting? Does he push backwards in his effort to assume the upright position? Does he come up more over one side than the other?

Once upright, does he bear weight equally on both legs? Does his posture deteriorate as he comes upright against gravity? For example, what posture does he assume? Does the pelvis tilt in an anterior or posterior direction or shift laterally? Does he show associated reactions in the rest of the body due to his efforts to maintain the upright position? Is there overactivity in the sound side as the patient tries to maintain the upright position?

Does he require an ankle support or brace for standing, and if so, how does he manage without it? Is he able to put it on without assistance?

Weight Transference and Balance Reactions

■ **In Sitting.** Can he shift weight to either side without the support of his arms and lift or free the opposite leg for movement? Does his leg lift reactively and automatically? When his weight moves over to the side does the head right freely and adequately to the vertical position? Does the trunk lengthen and shorten adequately when the weight is transferred to either side?

■ **In Standing.** Can he move his weight over one leg, and is the supporting leg hyperextended or flexed to permit this? Can he stand on one leg and move the other leg? In step position, can he transfer weight easily from the front leg to the one behind? Can he take steps to regain his balance sideways, forwards and backwards? When the therapist steers the patient in different directions, with her hands placed lightly on his shoulders as he walks, does he follow quickly and easily by taking automatic rhythmic steps in all directions?

Walking

It is difficult to give an accurate description of walking, but it is probably best done by describing variations from the normal. The walking pattern is recorded as vividly as possible, describing also the ease with which the patient walks, the speed, rhythm and length of stride. Stride width should be noted as well and the position of his feet on the floor. Whether the patient hyperextends his knee when bearing weight or hitches up his pelvis or fails to flex his knee during the swing phase are key factors for the gait pattern analysis. The description of the walking pattern is far clearer when the weight-bearing phase and then the step forwards are described separately.

The arm swing gives a good indication as to how freely he walks and whether rotation takes place. Do the arms assume a fixed position during walking, either due to associated reactions or in the patient's attempt to maintain his balance? Can the patient move his head freely while walking, and is he able to talk and walk at the same time? Can he walk freely out of doors, even on uneven surfaces? Is he able to walk in the street when there is traffic, and can he negotiate the pavement without hesitation?

Approximately how far does he walk without becoming unduly tired? (It is useful to record how long it takes the patient to walk a certain distance for comparison at a later date.)

Does the patient require support when he walks, manual support from another person, a cane or a crutch and does he wear a calliper or ankle brace? (It is also important to describe what happens when he walks without these aids if it is possible for him to do so.) Can he walk barefoot?

■ **Negotiating Stairs.** Can the patient go up and down stairs? Does he do so in a normal manner, i.e. with one foot on each step? Is he able to manage without holding on to the bannister?

■ **Getting Up from the Floor.** Can the patient get down onto the floor unaided? How does he do so? Is he able to come from lying through kneeling to standing again? What support does he require, if any?

Comprehension

Does the patient understand verbal instructions, or is he merely imitating or anticipating what is required in the familiar situation rather than actually understanding the words? His ability to understand simple verbal commands can be tested by showing him two objects, for example a cup and a spoon. Without the therapist giving him any nonverbal cues she can ask him to look at either the cup or the spoon. If he follows correctly she can give him a two-part instruction by asking him to do something unusual with the spoon, e. g. "Take the spoon and tap it against the side of the cup before replacing it." His response will give an idea of his ability to follow a command during therapy. Often, as the therapist reaches out a hand expectantly while saying, "Give me your hand", the patient responds correctly, and she may think he has full comprehension when he is, in fact, responding to nonverbal cues in a known situation. The patient's ability to comprehend language is frequently overestimated because he is adept at interpreting nonverbal signals. Many therapists believe that their patients understand everything just because they follow so well in therapy sessions. Language entails far more than following simple commands in a familiar environment. Davenport and Hall (1981) describe how many patients fitted into a category labelled "High-Level Language Disorder", which involved not just spoken and written language but a deficit in reasoning as well. "Their language, both oral and written, often seemed impressive at first, though inclined to be pedantic, but on closer examination there was considerable evidence of circumlocution, inappropriate use of words and phrased and dogmatic repetition." It should always be remembered that aphasia refers to all aspects of language communication, namely, speaking, understanding, writing and reading and not, as is sometimes erroneously thought, to only one or two of these difficulties. Just as with learning a new language, it is always far easier to read and understand than it is to produce the language by speaking or writing. Any patient who has language difficulties should receive speech therapy from a qualified speech therapist. A patient who can write or type correct, full sentences but is unable to speak clearly is most probably suffering from dysarthria, a sensory/motor disorder with diverse causative factors, which can indeed be helped by informed physiotherapy. It is therefore important to distinguish between the existing problems.

The Face, Speaking and Eating

While listening to the patient giving his subjective history, the therapist will already have formed an opinion as to the patient's ability to speak and to vary his facial expression appropriately. In addition:
- Does the patient sound different when the therapist assists breathing, indicating that poor breathing is handicapping his speech?
- Does his position influence voice production because abnormal tone is affecting speech, making it sound effortful and/or monotonous? Is neuromuscular dysfunction slurring his speech and rendering him incapable of producing certain sounds? For example, are labials impossible for him due to the facial paresis? He can be asked to whistle or blow out his cheeks and move the air from one cheek to the other.

Can he move his tongue from side to side equally? Can he move his tongue up and down outside his mouth? If he cannot, the chances are he cannot do it inside his mouth. Is he able to put his tongue in his cheek and move it rapidly up and down or to put its tip behind his upper front teeth?

Can he eat and drink without difficulty? Often, moving the food around in the mouth to prepare it for swallowing is the problem, and not the actual swallow itself. It is extremely important for the therapist to question the patient's relatives about any difficulties, because often the patient will reply that he has no trouble with eating merely because he has enough to eat and drink each day. The therapist should therefore observe the patient while he is actually partaking of food so that she can assess exactly how he manages and record her observations.

Are his teeth and mouth clean, or are pieces of food left stuck anywhere? A quick and easy way for the therapist to check whether the independent patient is eating safely and to assess his ability to move his tongue adequately is for her to offer him a dry biscuit and eat one herself at the same time. As soon as she has finished her biscuit and feels that her mouth is completely clean again, she examines the patient's mouth and determines whether he, too, has finished and if there are any crumbs or pieces of biscuit still left in his mouth or throat.

Can he pronounce easily and rapidly the consonants "t", "g" and "k"? The first requires that he be able to place the tip of his tongue up behind his front teeth and the latter two require that he raise its posterior portion. These movements are necessary not only for articulating clearly when speaking, but also for transporting the prepared food back for swallowing.

Many patients with hemiplegia have inadequate or inappropriate facial expression, which can be a most distressing handicap. They may be misjudged as a result and thought to be depressed, unmotivated, or unfriendly. The patient and his relatives are very sensitive to facial abnormalities, particularly should dribbling occur or pieces of food remain unnoticed on his lips or chin. Activities to improve the movement, tone and sensation of the face and mouth should be included in the treatment if any difficulties exist, no matter how slight they may seem to be. (see Chap. 13).

Sensation

Testing of sensation is often totally omitted by the therapist, although it may well hold the key to the problem being treated. All tests for sensation must be done without the patient being able to see at all. A towel should be held in front of him, as he may otherwise obtain clues by seeing movement if the eye closure is not complete (Fig. 4.5). If the patient is unable to speak, he should be shown how to respond nonverbally, by signalling or indicating with his sound hand or foot.

Without going into too much detail, the therapist should test the following:

1. Light touch, deep pressure, and differentiation between hot and cold. It is not sufficient for her merely to touch various parts of the patient's body with her hand, saying, "Can you feel me touching you here?" The patient should not only acknowledge each time she touches him, but also inform her as to exactly where she is touching or pressing.
2. Position sense. The patient should be able to describe the direction in which the joint is being moved or the position in which it is placed. The therapist moves the hemi-

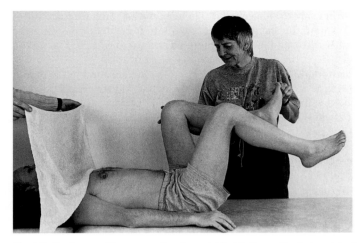

Fig. 4.5. Testing position sense: the therapist holds the patient's hemiplegic leg in a certain position and he tries to copy the movement and position exactly with his sound leg (left hemiplegia)

plegic limb into certain positions and the patient then places his sound limb in exactly the same positions (**Fig. 4.5**). The test is performed in two ways:
- The patient moves his sound limb simultaneously as the therapist places his affected limb in a position.
- The therapist selects a position and then, after an interval, asks the patient to imitate it with his other arm or leg.
3. Stereognosis. Can he identify a familiar object placed in his hand, for example a key? If he has speech problems, he can indicate a duplicate object near at hand. Where there is inability to manipulate the object the therapist can move the patient's hand for him to simulate his own grasp.

The testing of sensation is always a complex performance, and the hemiplegic patient may therefore fail due to reasons other than his poor sensation. Testing first with visual control until it is clear that he understands what is required will ensure that he is able to perform the task as such. Then his vision can be excluded and the actual test for sensation carried out.

It must not be forgotten, however, that there are no tests available which can really test sensation accurately with all its manifold refinements, as Brodal (1973), from personal experience of stroke, points out. Even if a patient responds successfully during all forms of formal testing, the way in which he moves and handles objects will demonstrate to a careful observer that he is not able to differentiate and adapt as finely as he did before the stroke.

All patients will perceive objects differently and receive altered feedback from the way they did before, so that there is in fact no pure motor stroke, only different degrees of impaired sensation.

Functional Abilities

The therapist must record the patient's ability to carry out the routine activities of daily living. It is one of the few objective measurements of his progress and capability that she has. She should assess thoroughly the activities concerned with personal hygiene, dressing and eating, and note how long each activity takes him. The patient should be observed while he performs these tasks, to avoid any discrepancies. Careful discussion with nursing staff, or with those people nearest to him if he is already living at home, may bring other difficulties to light, which is particularly important if the therapist is unable to assess the patient in his own environment. How he carries out the activities should also be noted, so that even small qualitative improvements can be appreciated in future assessments.

Recording the patient's profession and age gives the therapist some idea of his life before the hemiplegia and what sort of stimulus might be of help to him in the treatment. The information will also be a guide to his life style and his expectations of the rehabilitation.

Leisure Activities and Hobbies

There is a tendency in this day and age to associate a positive outcome of rehabilitation with a return to gainful employment. However, quality of life depends on more than merely going to work each day, particularly for stroke patients, who are often in the older age-group. Even with the younger age-group, Evans (1981) found of the unemployed or unemployable that, "quite a few have made new lives for themselves, taken up new skills and interests, and appear to observers to be leading satisfying lives." It therefore behoves the therapist to ascertain what interests the patient had before suffering a hemiplegia so that she can advise him and help him to find new leisure activities that he can enjoy in the future, depending on his personal tastes and abilities. Experience has shown that most patients prefer to take up a new form of sport or hobby, one which they had not experienced before becoming disabled, in order to avoid the inevitably negative comparison (F. M. Mueller 1997, personal communication).

Considerations

The assessment which has been described is a very full one and is not necessarily carried out during the first treatment session. If the patient is seen during the acute phase of his illness, many of the tests will not be applicable. In the same way, a patient who has not had adequate treatment and has a painful shoulder or is afraid of moving will not be tested in the prone position or asked to kneel down on the floor. The therapist estimates which of the tests are feasible at the time.

When a patient comes for treatment at a later stage in his progress, the whole assessment may be necessary to discover exactly where his difficulties lie. It should also be noted how much treatment he has already had, and what type.

Although the assessment may seem long, time is actually saved by accurate assessment, and without it comprehensive rehabilitation and further improvement are impossible. Even if the information is not fully recorded, the therapist nevertheless needs to consider all the points that have been mentioned.

A "scribe" writing down the observations during the assessment can be a great help. Alternatively, a small tape recorder could be of assistance and the actual writing be done afterwards. Perhaps one of the greatest aids to recording movement is video film. A short video of a patient performing an activity will describe the action far more vividly than words and can be used for comparison later. Even a photograph, as shown earlier, can be a clear record of some aspects of the patient's ability or disability.

Compensatory or "trick" movements can allow a degree of independence, but once they become established they are difficult to change and may even inhibit the return of normal activity. Care should be taken to assess whether the trick movement is really necessary, or if it has become a habit which could possibly be changed and so allow a more normal and economical movement sequence.

A detailed neurological assessment separate from a purely functional assessment is recommended, because it is the only way in which the therapist can treat the condition itself, rather than merely pushing for rapid independence, possibly at the expense of the patient's chances of regaining more normal function and recovery of activity in the affected parts.

When the results of the assessment show a marked discrepancy from the patient's ability to perform independently the activities of daily life, the problem will almost certainly be a perceptual one (see Chap. 1). For example, where the therapist has recorded that the patient can move his arms and legs and maintain his balance in a sitting position, he may be unjustly labelled "unmotivated" when he fails to put on his shoes and socks unaided. It is important to understand the complex requirements for carrying out such tasks and why the patient is unable to manage them on his own. For the patient there is a huge step between the recognition level, for example putting on the shoe handed to him by the therapist, and producing the whole sequence independently when he dresses in the morning. The same applies when any person is learning something new. He recognises what is required or is correct long before he can reproduce what has been taught without any cues being provided.

5 The Acute Phase – Positioning and Moving in Bed and in the Chair

Successful rehabilitation depends not only on the various therapy sessions but also very much on what happens to the patient during the remaining hours of the day and night. Even the position in which he sleeps can make a remarkable difference to the end result. No matter how good the therapy, if during the rest of the time the patient moves with effort in abnormal patterns of movement, spasticity will increase and functional gains achieved during therapy will be lost and not carried over into his daily life. Likewise, if he lies and sits in grossly abnormal postures for prolonged periods, not only will tone increase; range of motion will almost certainly be lost as well. Rehabilitation should therefore be regarded as a 24-hour management or way of life for each and every patient.

It is more satisfactory and easier for all concerned if such a concept is adopted from the very beginning, immediately following the stroke. However, even if a patient comes for treatment at a later stage, some months after the stroke, the same principles apply, and he too must be helped to achieve what he has missed. It will merely require more time because he will have established other habits, some of which may be difficult for him to change. The following positions and ways of moving him, or helping him to move, are recommended whether the patient is being nursed in an intensive care unit, in a general ward, in a rehabilitation centre or at home.

The Arrangement of the Patient's Room

How the patient's bed and chair are placed in relation to his surroundings can play an important role, particularly in the early stages of the illness when his ability to move about on his own is restricted. It is well worth going to considerable trouble to change the arrangement of the room if it is not ideal. Because of the lesion, the hemiplegic patient's head turns away from the affected side and he tends to neglect not only that half of his body but also the space on that side. Often the sensory modalities of feeling, hearing and seeing are reduced on the hemiplegic side. Intensive stimulation is necessary to counteract the resultant sensory deprivation. The room must be so arranged that the hemiplegic side automatically receives as much stimulation as possible during the day.

If the bed is so placed that the patient's affected side is towards a wall or where little activity will take place, the sensory deprivation will be reinforced. All nursing duties will be carried out from the unaffected side, and doctors and visitors will approach from that side too. When he starts sitting out of bed, he will transfer towards the sound side, look to that side and neglect his hemiplegic side still further.

Merely by altering the position of the bed so that all activity and interesting events take place on the patient's hemiplegic side, the situation can be changed remarkably. The nurse will approach from his affected side, to wash him, to help him with brushing his teeth, or when she brings him his food and assists him with eating, to mention but a few instances. The doctor, likewise, will sound his chest, take his blood pressure and carry out other regular examinations and observations from the hemiplegic side. If the patient has difficulty in turning his head at first, all who work with him can assist him to do so by placing a hand flat on the side of his face, and then holding the head in the corrected position until they feel the resistance subside.

With the room arranged in this way, the patient is constantly encouraged to turn his head toward his hemiplegic side to look at the people attending to him. The hemiplegic side will be required to react and will have input throughout the day. The bedside table should be placed on his affected side so that he will need to turn his head to look at objects on the table and must move his arm across the midline to reach for anything he requires. If necessary, the table can at first be so placed that it is almost in front of him and then gradually moved further and further to his affected side, as his condition improves and he is better able to turn his head and reach over to that side. Transferring to the chair next to his bed will also be a movement towards the affected side.

Many patients enjoy watching television, as they may be unable to read at first. The television set should also be placed so that the patient turns his head to the affected side when watching it. Relatives and friends can be of great assistance if carefully instructed. They should sit next to the patient on his hemiplegic side, or in front of him but more to that side. The patient will then spontaneously turn his head in their direction when they are talking to him, and the visitors can encourage him to move his eyes and look directly at them during the conversation. In addition, close relatives or friends can hold the patient's hemiplegic hand while talking with him, providing further stimulation (**Fig. 5.1**).

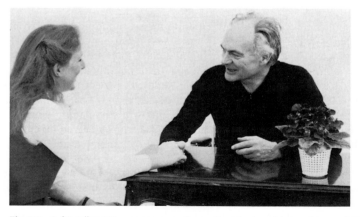

Fig. 5.1. A friendly visitor encourages the patient to turn his head toward the hemiplegic side (right hemiplegia)

Normal eye contact with other people and fixation of objects will often continue to cause difficulties if these steps are not taken, with the eyes being pulled constantly towards the sound side by the overactivity of the unopposed muscles on that side. Frequently, a supposed visual field defect is in fact the patient's inability to turn his head or move his eyes to the affected side. Through the improved rearrangement of the room not only will the patient's neck be more mobile but the eye muscles will be activated on that side as well. If a hemianopsia is present, then the patient's ability to turn his head freely will enable him to compensate for the loss of visual field more easily.

Positioning the Patient in Bed

In the very early stages, the patient will spend most of his time in bed, and how he lies will therefore be of great importance. As soon as possible, he should sit out of bed, and in fact there are very few circumstances which would necessitate his staying in bed for more than a few days. Experience has shown that the longer the patient is left lying or half-lying in bed, the more spasticity increases and the greater is his fear of moving in upright positions when he eventually starts to sit and stand again. Other serious complications can arise as a result of prolonged immobilisation in bed, particularly for older patients: thrombosis, pressure sores and hypostatic pneumonia, to name but a few. Even patients who are out of bed during the day will still be spending 8 hours or more in bed at night, and they too will need to be positioned correctly, if secondary complications of hypertonus and loss of range are to be avoided.

If an infusion is necessary, it is not a contraindication to turning the patient and positioning him correctly in bed or when he is sitting in a chair.

The patient's position must be changed at regular intervals, particularly during the acute phase, for the same reasons as when nursing any paralysed or unconscious patient. At first he should be turned every 2 or 3 hours, but later, when he is able to turn over and move himself in bed, the time can be extended until he resumes a normal routine of changing his position when he wakes and feels uncomfortable.

Lying on the Hemiplegic Side

Lying on the affected side is the most important position of all and should be introduced right from the beginning. In fact, most patients seem to prefer it, possibly because the side which feels more normally is uppermost. Hypertonicity is reduced by the elongation of the whole side, and the awareness of the affected side is increased because the patient's weight presses it firmly against the surface of the bed. Another obvious advantage is that the patient's more skilled hand is free to carry out tasks such as pulling up the bedcovers, arranging the pillow or holding the telephone receiver.

In the *ideal position* (**Fig. 5.2**), the head is well supported so that it lies slightly higher than the thorax. If the head lies comfortably, the patient is far more likely to remain in the correct position and sleep. The head should be flexed in the upper cervical region and not pushed back into extension. The trunk is rotated somewhat backwards and supported from behind by a pillow tucked firmly in behind the patient.

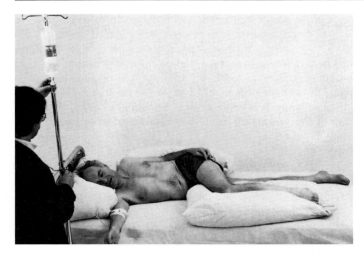

Fig. 5.2. Lying on the hemiplegic side in the correct position. The intravenous drip does not prevent the patient from lying on his side (right hemiplegia)

The hemiplegic arm is drawn forwards until it lies at an angle of not less than 90° to the body. The forearm is supinated and the wrist lies in passive dorsiflexion. The assistant, working from the front, places one hand under the patient's shoulder and scapula and brings the latter forwards into protraction. The patient's body weight maintains the protraction, and when the shoulder-blade is protracted flexor spasticity in the entire arm and hand is reduced, enabling the correct position to be maintained. To check that the scapula is indeed protracted, the assistant should always feel across the back of the thorax. When the patient is correctly positioned the medial border of the scapula does not protrude at all, but lies flat against the chest wall. Without sufficient protraction, the patient will often complain of shoulder pain or discomfort after a short time, as he is lying on the point of his shoulder.

The patient's other arm rests on his body or on the pillow behind him. If the sound arm lies in front of the patient, it brings the whole trunk forwards, which automatically results in retraction of the hemiplegic scapula.

The legs lie in a step position, with the sound leg flexed at the hip and knee and supported on a pillow. Both hip and knee should not be flexed fully but should lie comfortably at an angle of not more than about 80°. The large pillow beneath the limb also helps to maintain the position of the hemiplegic leg, which is extended at the hip and slightly flexed at the knee.

Lying on the Unaffected Side

Achieving a comfortable position on the sound side may cause some difficulty, because with the affected side uppermost the patient feels more helpless and the flaccid arm needs to be particularly well supported for it to remain in place without the shoulder becoming painful. Because the patient has to be turned regularly and lying supine has so many disadvantages, it is essential, however, that he be helped to lie correctly on his other side as well.

In the *ideal position* (**Fig. 5.3**), the head is again well supported on a pillow, to ensure that the patient feels comfortable and to maintain side flexion of the cervical spine to the other side as well. The trunk is at right angles to the surface of the bed; i.e. the patient is not pulled forward into a semi-prone position.

The hemiplegic arm is supported on a pillow in front of the patient in approximately 90° elevation with the scapula well protracted. To ensure a comfortable position, care must be taken that the shoulder girdle does not fall into elevation as it will tend to do during the flaccid stage, with the point of the shoulder almost touching the patient's ear. The large, supporting pillow needs to be placed well against the patient's chest and beneath the whole length of the upper arm right up to the axilla. If the shoulder rotates medially and the forearm pronates, then the elbow should be slightly flexed to avoid the persistent extension pattern.

The other arm lies wherever it is most comfortable for the patient. Sometimes it is flexed with the hand underneath the head pillow, or it lies across his chest or abdomen; some patients prefer to let it lie straight down along the front of their body.

The hemiplegic leg is brought forwards and fully supported on a pillow with some degree of flexion at the hip and knee, placed carefully to ensure that the foot does not hang in supination over the edge of the pillow. The other leg remains flat on the bed in some extension of the hip with slight flexion of the knee, and the large pillow prevents the limb from being drawn forwards as it tends to do in the early stages.

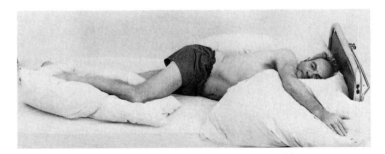

Fig. 5.3. Lying on the unaffected side. The hemiplegic arm is well supported by the pillow (right hemiplegia)

Lying Supine

The supine position should be used as little as possible, because in this position abnormal reflex activity is at its highest due to the influence of the tonic neck and labyrinthine reflexes. For hemiplegic patients it also involves the highest risk of pressure sores developing on the sacrum and, even more commonly, over the outside of the heel and on the lateral malleolus. The pelvis is rotated backwards on the hemiplegic side and pulls the hemiplegic leg with it into outward rotation, causing pressure on the two sites mentioned.

However, it may be necessary to use the position as an alternative, during specific nursing procedures or for those patients who have been nursed for a long time only on their backs and find it difficult to tolerate side-lying at first. In such cases, the supine position will need to be used, but only for as short a period as possible before the patient is turned onto his side again.

In the *ideal position* (**Fig. 5.4**), the head is well supported on pillows, with the upper cervical spine in flexion. Care must be taken that the thoracic spine does not flex as well.

A pillow is placed beneath the hemiplegic buttock and thigh to bring the side of the pelvis forward and thus prevent the leg from pulling into outward rotation. It is contraindicated to hold the limb mechanically in place by putting sandbags or other hard objects against the lower leg itself, because the position of the leg is in fact secondary to the backward rotation of the pelvis on that side. If the posture of the pelvis is not corrected, the leg will therefore continue to press against any form of fixation, and pressure sores or damage to the nerves in that area could easily be caused.

A pillow placed beneath the hemiplegic scapula maintains protraction and allows the arm to lie in a corrected, raised position, i.e. extended at the elbow, with the wrist in dorsiflexion and the fingers extended.

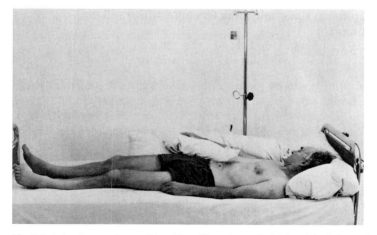

Fig. 5.4. Lying in a supine position. The pillows beneath the hemiplegic buttock and scapula keep the whole side forwards and correct the position of the limbs. The head is turned to the affected side (right hemiplegia)

The legs lie extended. Supporting pillows underneath the knee or calf should be avoided because the former tends to lead to too much flexion at the knee, and the latter could cause hyperextension of the knee or unwanted pressure over the vulnerable veins of the lower leg.

General Points to Note When Positioning the Patient

- The bed should be kept flat and the head end should not be raised at all. The half-lying position should be avoided at all times, as it reinforces unwanted flexion of the trunk with extension of the legs (**Fig. 5.5**). In addition, the increased pressure over the sacrum and coccyx can easily lead to the development of decubitus over the bony area. In the preferable side-lying positions the patient tends to slide down the bed if the head of the bed is raised.
- Nothing should be placed in the hand in an attempt to counteract flexor spasticity. The effect will be just the opposite, as the influence of the grasp reflex causes the hand to close on an object placed in the palm. In a study comparing electromyographic (EMG) activity in the finger flexors of the hemiplegic hand when using a volar splint, a foam-rubber finger spreader and no device at all, Mathiowetz et al. (1983) write that "... the effects of positioning devices over time generally show that no device evokes the least amount of EMG activity." In fact, the volar splint actually demonstrated increased EMG activity while it was being put on and during the period when the patients were grasping something with their sound hand. The correct positioning proximally will allow the hand to remain open, particularly as the patient is at rest and not exerting himself against gravity.
- Many patients have difficulty in aligning their body in relation to other objects in their vicinity. It is helpful to position the patient in bed so that he lies parallel to the sides of the bed, and not diagonally across it, as so often happens when he is left to his own devices.

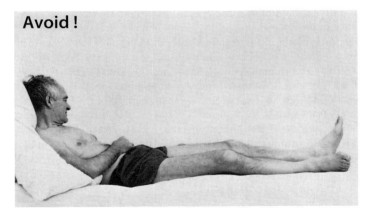

Fig. 5.5. The half-lying position should be avoided, at all times. It reinforces the patterns of spasticity (right hemiplegia)

- Pillows vary considerably in size and consistency in different countries. Ideally, they should be large and well-filled with a soft material, e.g. down, which will mould to support and maintain the part of the body in the desired position. Most positions require about three to four continental pillows or five to six English/American pillows. It is confusing for staff and for patients and their relatives to have pillows of various sizes and shapes to use for different parts of the body.
- Nothing should be placed against the balls of the feet in an attempt to avoid a plantar flexion deformity, because firm pressure against the ball of the foot actually increases unwanted reflex activity in the extension pattern. The hemiplegic patient will shift himself away from the uncomfortable fixation in any case. Heavy or tightly tucked-in bedclothes should be avoided, and a bed-cradle should be used to support their weight, if necessary.

Sitting in Bed

It is difficult for the patient to sit in bed with a good upright posture, and the position should therefore be avoided whenever possible. Flexion of the trunk is encouraged and the hips remain in some degree of extension. Remaining in such a sitting or in fact half-lying position for any length of time will almost inevitably cause a decubitus between the buttocks directly over the coccyx, a wound which can be extremely troublesome to heal. However, in the acute phase it is usually not feasible for the nursing staff to transfer the patient to an upright chair as often as would be necessary during the day. The patient needs to sit up every time he eats or drinks (Chap. 13), a minimum of five times a day. He has to sit when he brushes his teeth or needs to empty his bladder or bowels. If sitting in bed cannot be avoided, the position should be made as optimal as possible.

In the *ideal position*, the hips should be flexed in as near to a right angle as is feasible and the spine extended. Sufficient pillows placed appropriately behind the patient help to achieve the erect position, and the head should be left unsupported so that he starts to hold it actively. An adjustable table placed across the bed, beneath the patient's arms, will help to counteract the pull into trunk flexion. If the downward pull is strong, a pillow should be placed beneath his elbows to avoid pressure over the vulnerable tissues in the area.

Some modern hospital beds have an adjustable back rest that can be brought almost to a vertical position. A pillow behind the patient's back will provide trunk extension, and the recommended upright sitting posture is achieved (**Fig. 5.6 a**). If, however, the back rest can be adjusted only to slope upwards, it should be left flat and the patient moved so that he is supported against the head of the bed with sufficient pillows behind him (**Fig. 5.6 b**).

In both these ways, the detrimental half-reclining position is avoided, but even so, the patient should not be left for long in the sitting position because he will soon slide down the bed and assume very undesirable postures for prolonged periods.

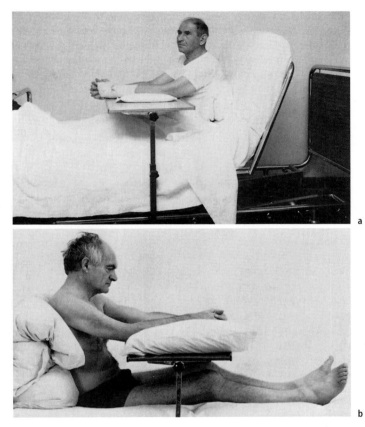

Fig. 5.6 a, b. Sitting upright in bed (right hemiplegia). **a** Easily achieved in a modern hospital bed with a fully adjustable back rest. **b** If the head end is not sufficiently adjustable, the bed is left flat and the patient is moved up the bed and supported by pillows

Sitting in a Chair

In a suitable chair a far more upright posture can be achieved and maintained, and it is therefore advisable to transfer the patient out of bed as soon as his general condition allows. If the patient is unable to stand and walk at all even with assistance, a wheelchair is the best answer. He can then be easily transported to therapy sessions or to X-ray or other investigations, and can also enjoy the change of scene, particularly when he learns how to propel the chair himself. If the back rest of the wheelchair encourages too much flexion of the trunk, a padded board should be placed in the chair to help the patient to maintain an upright position. The board should be adjustable so that it can be tilted forwards when the patient is sitting at a table. Whenever he is not moving from place to place he is positioned with his arms on a table in front of him, spine extended and hips flexed **(Fig. 5.7 a, b)**. If a more stable table without wheels is used the patient will feel more secure and a correct sitting posture will be easier to achieve **(Fig. 5.7 c)**. When positioned in this way, there is far less tendency for him to slide his seat forwards and half lie in his chair, which is such a common problem in the beginning **(Fig. 5.8)**. In the corrected position he can stay erect far longer, watching television, talking to visi-

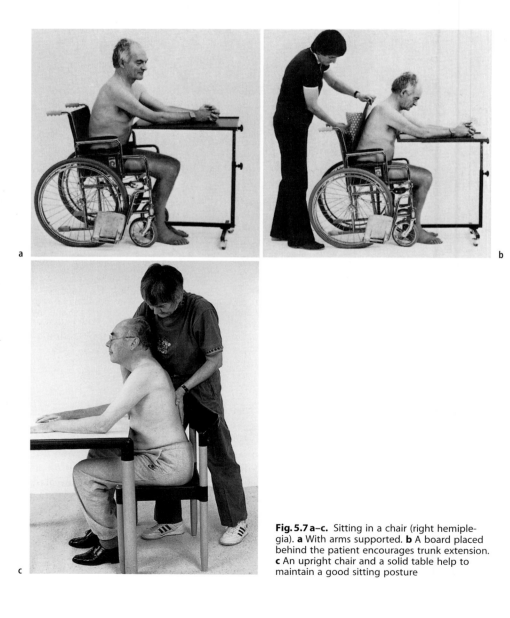

a

b

c

Fig. 5.7 a–c. Sitting in a chair (right hemiplegia). **a** With arms supported. **b** A board placed behind the patient encourages trunk extension. **c** An upright chair and a solid table help to maintain a good sitting posture

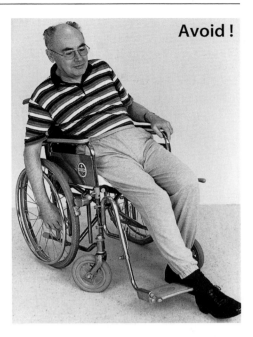

Fig. 5.8. Typical undesirable sitting posture. Without a table in front of him the patient often slides down in the wheelchair and is in danger of falling

tors or other patients, or even reading and writing. However, it must be realised that in the early days following a stroke the patient will tire quickly, particularly if left on his own, and it will be necessary to let him rest in bed frequently. It is better to sit him up again for short periods than to let him sleep uncomfortably in the chair in a position which emphasises abnormal tone and posture.

Gradually, the time which the patient spends out of bed can be increased, and the more stimulation he receives the longer he will be able to tolerate sitting up. He should not be left to his own devices but should be kept occupied with appropriate activity in the company of others.

Re-adjusting the Patient's Position in the Wheelchair

If the patient has slipped down in his chair he should always be helped to correct his posture at once, to avoid his falling to the floor or injuring his arm or hand.

■ **Single-handed.** The therapist, nurse or whoever may be helping him, immediately places both his feet flat on the floor with his knees well flexed. Standing in front of him, she presses her knees firmly against his knees to prevent him from sliding still further down in the chair and helps him to clasp his hands together (**Fig. 5.9 a**). The helper asks the patient to lean forwards as far as he can and guides his hands to one side of her legs (**Fig. 5.9 b**). Because he will tend to fall towards his hemiplegic side, it is usually advisable that his arms are moved towards his unaffected side. Once his trunk is sufficiently

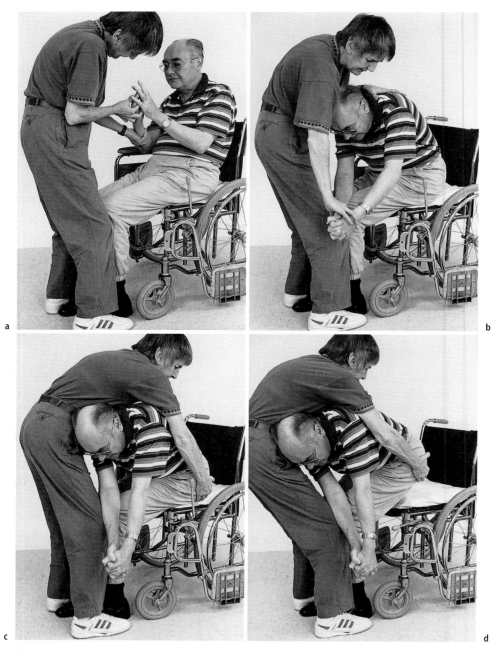

Fig. 5.9 a–e. Helping the patient to sit upright again after he has slipped down in the chair (right hemi-plegia). **a** Clasping his hands together with further sliding prevented. **b** Bringing his trunk and hands well forwards. **c** Shifting weight sideways to place a hand beneath each trochanter. **d** Lifting his but-tocks into the air

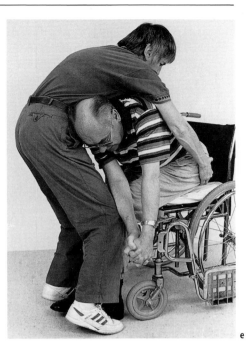

Fig. 5.9 e. Placing his seat well back in the chair   e

far forward, the helper shifts his weight to one side and then the other to enable her to place one hand beneath each of his trochanters (**Fig. 5.9 c**). She lifts his buttocks into the air by leaning backwards and at the same time pressing her knees against his knees (**Fig. 5.9 d**). The patient's seat can then be placed right back in the chair (**Fig. 5.9 e**). Because the helper is using her body weight to lift the patient, her own back is protected. The patient learns to help more actively until eventually he is able to correct his sitting position on his own in the same way (**Fig. 5.10**). The method is also a useful preparation for standing up from sitting, as it teaches him to lean well forwards and take weight over his feet while lifting his buttocks.

■ **With an Assistant.** When adjusting the position of a very disabled or heavy patient, the therapist may require the help of a second person (**Fig. 5.11 a**). She proceeds in the same way as before, but with an assistant standing behind the patient's chair to help lift his seat from the chair at the right moment (**Fig. 5.11 b**). Together they lift his bottom into the air and place it right back against the back rest (**Fig. 5.11 c,d**). The patient is able to sit upright once again, and a wheelchair table, together with a strategically placed cushion, can help him to maintain the corrected position (**Fig. 5.11 e**).

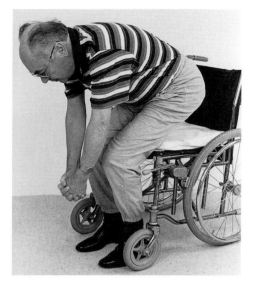

Fig. 5.10. The patient learns to place his seat well back in the chair unaided

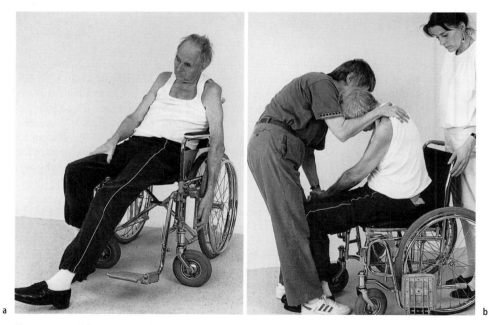

a

b

Fig. 5.11 a–e. When two people are needed to adjust the position of a very disabled patient (left hemiplegia). **a** Sliding out of the chair. **b** Bringing weight forwards with knees stabilised and hands clasped

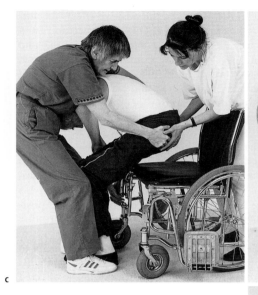

c

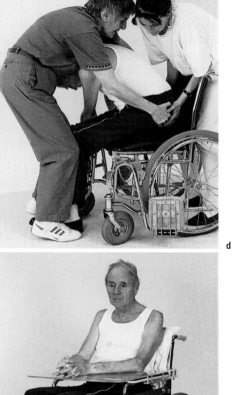

d

Fig. 5.11 c–e. **c** An assistant behind the chair helps to lift the patient's seat. **d** Placing his seat right back in the chair. **e** Able to sit upright again; a wheelchair table helps to maintain the corrected position

e

Learning to Propel the Wheelchair Independently

For the patient, the ability to propel the wheelchair on his own and move about independently is a very positive experience. Some therapists are reluctant to allow the patient to do so because they fear that the one-sided activity may cause associated reac-

tions with increased tone in the hemiplegic limbs. However, the positive effects far out-
weigh the negative, and if the method of propulsion is carefully taught, hypertonicity in
the hemiplegic side will not increase. In fact, the active movement of the trunk and
limbs is most beneficial both physically and psychologically. It may be some weeks or
even months before the patient is able to walk safely on his own, particularly as most
hospitals have very long corridors. Not only is having to sit and wait for someone to
push him wherever he wants to go frustrating; it can lead to pronounced passivity and
lack of initiative. Two ways in which a normal wheelchair can be propelled have proved
most satisfactory for most patients.

1. The patient uses his sound hand on the wheel of the chair and at the same time
   makes a stepping action with his sound foot on the ground. The footrest on his
   sound side must be removed to allow his foot to push against the floor unencum-
   bered. He must be encouraged to keep his bottom well back in the chair with his
   trunk moving forwards instead of lying back against the back rest in a flexed position (Fig. 5.12 a). The patient keeps his hemiplegic arm forward with the hand resting
   on his thigh.
2. To avoid retraction of the hemiplegic side, right from the start the patient is taught to
   place his clasped hands over his hemiplegic knee and push the chair using only his
   sound leg (Fig. 5.12 b). In this way, the danger of associated reactions in the affected
   arm is eliminated and, should the limb already be spastic, any increase in hypertonus
   is avoided. In fact, the sustained position of the upper limb combined with the movement of the trunk proximally has an inhibitory effect.

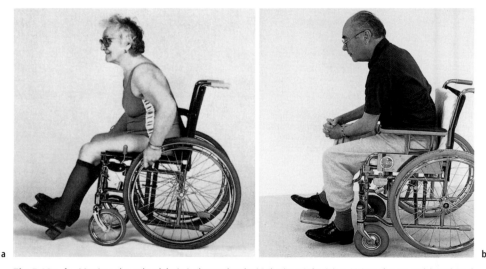

a   b

Fig. 5.12 a, b. Moving the wheelchair independently (right hemiplegia). **a** Using the sound hand and
foot. **b** Clasped hands placed over one knee prevent associated reactions while the patient is propelling
the chair with the sound leg

Self-assisted Arm Activity with Clasped Hands

From a very early stage the patient is taught how to release the spasticity in his arm, in his hand and around the scapula, and how to maintain full passive elevation of his shoulder (**Fig. 5.13 a**). Due to its special construction, allowing for functional mobility in daily life, the shoulder is a vulnerable joint and reacts badly to immobilisation. Following a stroke it is therefore important to keep it moving, passively if need be. The hands are clasped together, fingers interlaced with the hemiplegic thumb uppermost in some abduction (**Fig. 5.13 b**). Whether lying, sitting or standing, the patient is taught to start the movement by pushing his clasped hands well forwards, assuring protraction of his scapula, before he attempts to lift the arm. With the elbows extended and the balls of his hands always together, he then raises his arms above his head. The activity is practised many times during the day and can be encouraged by all members of the team and by relatives and other patients. Even if the patient is on an intravenous drip he should continue to lift his hemiplegic hand carefully during the day to maintain full pain-free range of motion (**Fig. 5.14**). It is important that the activity be carefully taught and carried out correctly, as otherwise the patient may traumatise his shoulder, cause himself pain and be discouraged from moving his arm. The balls of both hands must be kept symmetrically and firmly against each other with the fingers interlaced ade-

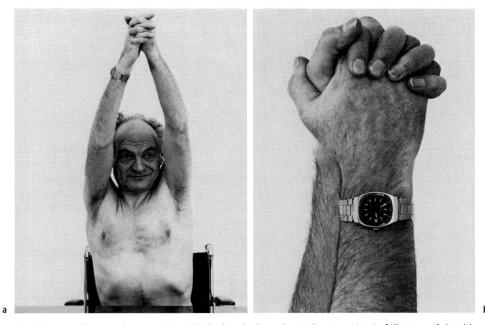

a   b

Fig. 5.13. a Self-assisted arm activity with the hands clasped together to maintain full range of shoulder movement. **b** With the fingers interlaced, spasticity is inhibited (right hemiplegia)

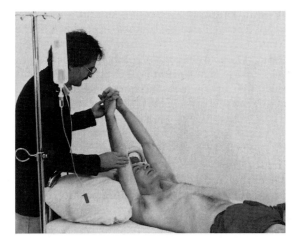

Fig. 5.14. Even the doctor can encourage the patient to move his arm after adjusting the infusion (right hemiplegia)

quately; this will prevent any possible trauma to the joints of the hand. Because the activity has proved to be so beneficial, many have recommended that it be used during therapy or when the patient is being helped to move into different positions and certainly as part of his home exercise programme (Biewald 1989; Bobath 1990; Geisseler 1993; Kamal 1987; Todd and Davies 1986).

Clasping the hands together with the fingers interlaced is important for the following reasons:

▶ The hemiplegic hand and shoulder are protected while the patient moves himself in bed, is being transferred from bed to a chair or particularly when he is sitting down from standing.

▶ Because the fingers of the sound hand abduct the fingers of the hemiplegic hand, the flexor spasticity in the whole arm is reduced.

▶ The hands are brought together in the midline, and sensation and awareness are improved by the act of interlacing the fingers.

▶ Sitting with clasped hands looks natural and, if adopted whenever the patient is sitting for any length of time, will reduce hypertonicity quite amazingly or even prevent its development in the first place. During the day the patient can sit with his legs crossed and his clasped hands over his knee to help him to maintain a correct posture while travelling in a car or train, while watching television or simply when he is enjoying the company of other people (**Fig. 5.15**).

▶ With the hands held forward, the retraction of the scapula and in fact of the whole side is prevented, making certain movement sequences such as coming to standing easier and less effortful for the patient.

▶ When the patient is moving, associated reactions in the arm are prevented. Because the patient is using his sound hand to hold the other hand, he is not able to pull or push with it as he moves. He therefore uses other parts of the body more normally, and trunk activity is stimulated and symmetrical movement and weightbearing are improved.

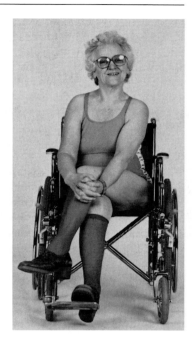

Fig. 5.15. Patient sitting with her hands clasped over one knee. The hemiplegic arm is prevented from pulling into flexion and the weight is over the affected side (right hemiplegia)

▶ Perhaps most important of all, a stiff, contracted hand can be prevented altogether if the simple manoeuvre is used in conjunction with appropriate treatment of the upper limb. Loss of range of motion due to joint stiffness, tendon shortening and loss of tissue mobility such as described by Ryerson and Levit (1997) and Kamal (1987) may otherwise develop, limiting the return of voluntary activity and compromising normal movement patterns.

▶ At home, if the patient is able to interlace his fingers easily, he will be able to perform an essential exercise on his own, one which prevents shortening of his finger and wrist flexors by inhibiting and maintaining the full mobility of the hypertonic muscles. In fact, if he cannot fold his hands together, there is almost no way in which a patient can maintain the full length of his finger flexors himself, once he has been discharged from treatment. Patients who have not been taught to clasp their hands together in this way are in very real danger of developing a contracted, unsightly hand which is not only cosmetically embarrassing for them but will also be difficult to keep fresh and clean and will create problems with nail care **(Fig. 5.16)**.

Merely holding the hands together in some other way with the fingers left free in flexion instead of interlaced will not have all these advantages, so that it is well worth teaching the patient the right way from the very beginning. Should a patient already have developed marked hypertonus or even some degree of shortening and be unable to fold his hands, the therapist must work to overcome the problem with intensive treatment until he too can achieve the inhibitory position on his own without difficulty.

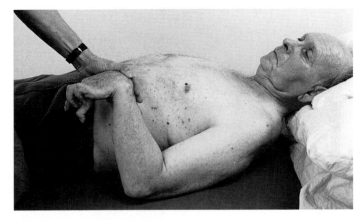

Fig. 5.16. Patient with distressing contractures of elbow, wrist and fingers, which could have been prevented had he been taught how to clasp his hands and move his arm from the beginning (left hemiplegia)

Moving in Bed

If the patient is unconscious or is still unable to participate actively, he must be turned onto his side by an assistant. The turn is easier if both legs are flexed with the feet remaining on the bed and the knees then turned to one side. The shoulders and trunk follow. The assistant places one hand behind and the other in front of his axilla to lift and turn the patient away from her.

Two helpers using a recommended lifting method can also move him passively into an upright sitting position. For the Australian lift the assistants stand on either side of the patient, facing in the opposite direction to him. The hands nearest to the patient are placed beneath his thighs and the assistants grasp and hold each other's wrist. Placing their shoulders under his shoulders and leaning towards each other, the assistants straighten their knees to lift the patient off the bed (**Fig. 5.17 a**). With their free hands the assistants can support themselves on the bed to avoid straining their backs, or they can adjust the bedclothes or pillows (**Fig. 5.17 b**).

This method of passive lifting is recommended because it is comfortable and safe for the patient and will not traumatise his shoulder. It can also be used to lift the patient back into bed if the height of the bed is not adjustable. Very soon, however, the patient is able to assist, and activity should be encouraged, but always with sufficient facilitation to allow the movement to take place in a normal pattern, without his having to struggle. Because the aim is to re-establish normal movement patterns, a monkey chain should never be used. If it is there attached to the bed, the patient will naturally reach for it and try to pull himself into position with his sound hand. Immediately, an abnormal, one-sided response follows, leading to increased tone on the hemiplegic side.

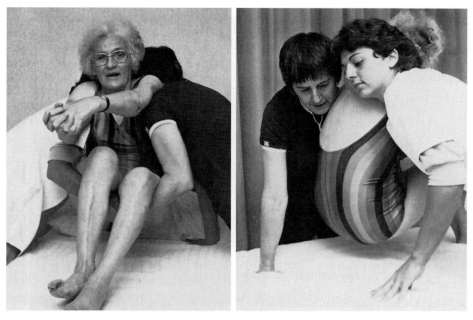

a   b

Fig. 5.17 a, b. Moving the patient passively in bed (left hemiplegia). **a** The Australian lift is safe and comfortable. **b** The assistants can support themselves with their free hand to protect their backs

Moving Sideways

With his legs flexed and his feet on the bed, the patient raises his buttocks off the bed and moves them to the side. The assistant facilitates the movement by pressing down on his hemiplegic knee, drawing the knee forwards over his foot as she does so (**Fig. 5.18**). The patient then moves his shoulders into line, help being given to prevent the scapula from retracting. The same assistance can be given when the patient needs to move up or down the bed.

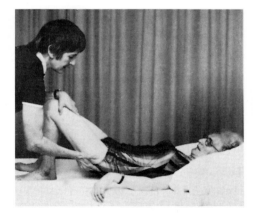

Fig. 5.18. Bridging used to move in bed (left hemiplegia); see also Figs. 6.5, 6.6

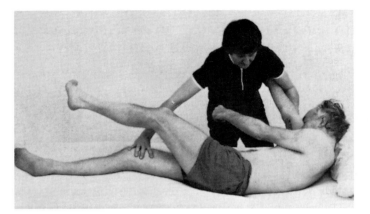

Fig. 5.19. Turning over onto the hemiplegic side. The therapist protects the hemiplegic shoulder from injury (right hemiplegia)

Rolling Over Onto the Hemiplegic Side

Rolling is most therapeutic, as it stimulates reactions and activity throughout the body. How it can be used during therapy is described in Chap. 11. When the patient is turning towards the affected side, it is important that the assistant protect his hemiplegic shoulder while the he rolls over. She does so by cradling his arm against her side, using one hand beneath his upper arm to rotate the joint laterally and maintain the position of the humeral head in the glenoid fossa. The patient lifts his sound leg off the bed and swings it forwards, without pushing off with his foot on the bed behind him **(Fig. 5.19)**. He brings his sound arm forward actively and must also be discouraged from grasping the edge of the mattress to pull himself over. The assistant facilitates the lateral rotation and extension of the hemiplegic leg with her hand placed over his knee.

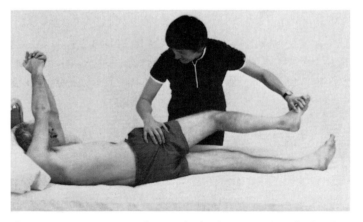

Fig. 5.20. Turning over onto the sound side. The patient clasps his hands to protect his shoulder while the therapist facilitates the correct leg movement (right hemiplegia)

Rolling Over Onto the Unaffected Side

The patient clasps his hands together, so that the hemiplegic arm is supported. The assistant facilitates the correct movement of the hemiplegic leg, helping him to bring it forward over the sound leg, which plays no active part in the movement (**Fig. 5.20**).

Moving Forwards and Backwards While Sitting in Bed

With help, the patient moves up the bed by transferring his weight first over one buttock and then over the other. The opposite side, when relieved of weight, is moved backwards each time, as if the patient were walking on his buttocks. The assistant stands on his hemiplegic side and holds his trochanters; using her body to keep his trunk forward and to help him to transfer his weight, she facilitates the walking action (**Fig. 5.21**).

The patient can use the same movement pattern when moving himself to the edge of the bed before transferring into a chair, or later, before standing up from the bed. In this case, help is given from the front. The assistant places one hand under his trochanter and the other over the contralateral shoulder, to prevent his falling backwards. She helps the patient to transfer his weight over to one side and then brings the hip on the freed side forward (**Fig. 5.22 a**). She then changes her hands, to facilitate the step with the buttock on the other side. When the patient is returning to his bed from the wheelchair, she uses the same facilitation to help him move back onto the bed, moving the freed buttock backwards instead of forwards.

The patient soon learns to move himself in this way unaided, and by so doing avoids the extensor spasticity in his hemiplegic leg, which is strongly increased in an associ-

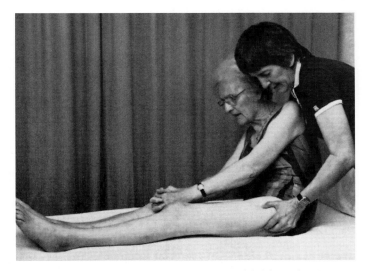

Fig. 5.21. The patient "walks" on her buttocks to move up and down the bed (left hemiplegia)

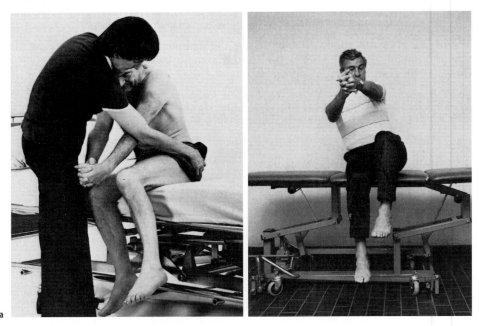

a   b

Fig. 5.22 a, b. Moving to the edge of the bed or back again (right hemiplegia). **a** The therapist facilitates "walking" on the buttocks. **b** Patient moving back on a plinth, unaided

ated reaction if he pulls himself with his sound hand to move to the edge of the bed. The same sequence is used later when he moves to sit further back on the plinth in the physiotherapy department (**Fig. 5.22 b**). Not only is the activity functional; it can also be used therapeutically, as it stimulates automatic weight transference and active trunk movement with rotation and balance reactions similar to those required for walking.

Sitting Up Over the Side of the Bed

Sitting up over the hemiplegic side is stressed because of the therapeutic effect. When we sit up over one side normally, that side is forward when we reach the upright position. For the patient this will mean that his hemiplegic side is forward instead of in its usual retracted position. The sequence starts with the patient lying on his back. He brings his hemiplegic leg over the side of the bed keeping the knee flexed, with the assistant facilitating the movement at first. He then brings the sound hand forwards across his body to push on the bed on the hemiplegic side, rotating the trunk in order to do so. He pushes himself up to the sitting position, swinging his sound leg out simultaneously to aid the movement by its counterweight (**Fig. 5.23 a**). The head rights to the vertical and the hemiplegic side elongates during the movement, and the weightbearing through the side is beneficial.

Fig. 5.23 a–c. Sitting up over the side of the bed. **a** Coming up over the hemiplegic side with the sound hand pushing down on the bed (right hemiplegia). **b** Supporting the trunk to help a more disabled patient (left hemiplegia). **c** The therapist leans sideways and presses down over his iliac crest

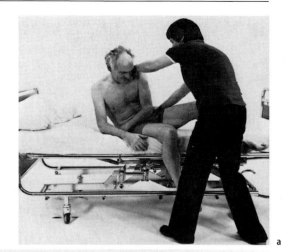

a

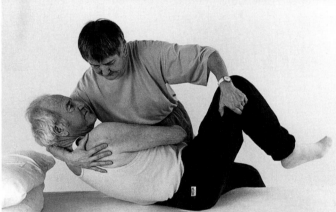

b

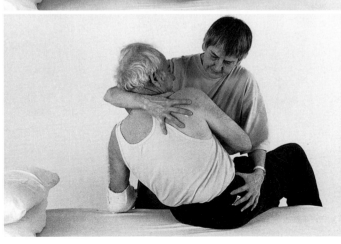

c

The assistant facilitates the movement by placing one hand on the sound shoulder, which she presses down firmly, and the other hand on the iliac crest, doing the same. Should the patient require more help, she can encircle his head and hemiplegic shoulder with one arm and lean her body weight sideways to bring him to the upright position (**Fig. 5.23 b, c**).

Lying Down from Sitting Over the Side of the Bed

To lie down in bed again the patient uses the same movement sequence in reverse. The assistant facilitates the movement by guiding his sound shoulder backward with one hand and supporting his weight as much as is necessary with her other arm placed round behind his trunk (**Fig. 5.24 a**). Once he is safely lying down, she facilitates the movement of the affected leg to lift it into bed without effort (**see Fig. 6.5**). As the patient's ability improves the assistant reduces the amount of support and uses only her hands to draw his hemiplegic shoulder forwards and guide the other one back as he lies down (**Fig. 5.24 b**).

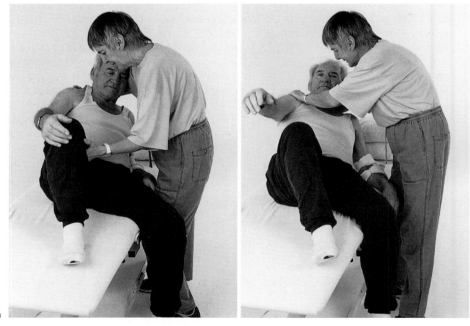

a   b

Fig. 5.24 a, b. Lying down in bed. **a** The therapist's arm behind the patient supports the weight of his trunk and helps him to lift his leg. **b** Guiding only the hemiplegic shoulder forwards and the other one back when motor control improves

Transferring from Bed to Chair and Back Again

Transferring correctly and without undue effort will later enable the patient to stand up easily, and will assist in achieving weightbearing through the hemiplegic leg without using the total pattern of extension. If transferring is easy for the patient and nursing staff alike, the problem of incontinence will be far easier to overcome.

Transferring is easier and safer when the patient is nursed in a bed of adjustable height, which can be lowered until it is approximately the same height as the chair. At home, the bed is usually low enough, but in a hospital where the beds cannot be lowered both patient and staff are at risk of being injured. The therapist will need all her ingenuity to find a safe and easy method of transfer if the bed is too high, particularly when she is helping the patient back into bed again. A possible solution is to support his hemiplegic leg in the way shown in **Fig. 6.30**, and then help him to lift his sound buttock on to the high bed. Once that buttock is on the bed, the therapist places an arm round over his sound shoulder and uses her free hand to bring his other buttock up as well.

The Passive Transfer

When the patient is unable to help actively, the following methods can be used to transfer him into his chair:

1. The assistant moves him to the edge of the bed until both his feet are flat on the floor. With her feet beside his feet, she supports his knees with her knees, from the front, and at the same time prevents his knees from falling into abduction. She rests his forearms on her shoulders and places her hands over his scapulae, gripping their medial borders to keep them forward. She splints the patient's arms with her extended arms. She then brings his weight forwards over his feet and presses downward on his scapulae until his seat lifts off the bed. Weightbearing through his legs is assisted if he lifts his head. The assistant pivots the patient round and lowers his seat far back into the chair (**Fig. 5.25**). The patient should not clasp his hands round the helper's neck because he would pull too hard and come to the upright position with total extension of his leg. The chair should be so placed that the patient transfers towards his hemiplegic side. On moving back into bed, the same procedure is followed.

2. For the patient who is very heavy and unable to participate actively when being transferred to or from his bed, a slidingboard should be used as his shoulder might otherwise be traumatised, or the assistant's back injured. The same applies for a patient whose shoulder has unfortunately been traumatised in some way and is already acutely painful.

The therapist leans the patient towards his sound side, her arm around his shoulder to prevent his falling. She places the end of a wooden slidingboard under the buttock on his hemiplegic side, which is no longer taking any weight (**Fig. 5.26a**). With the board spanning the gap between bed and chair, the therapist moves the patient gradually along it until she can ease him gently on to the chair seat, or the bed (**Fig. 5.26b**). Throughout the transfer, the therapist keeps the patient's trunk forward with her hand behind his thorax, and her knees against his keep him safely on the board. With her other hand she helps the patient to move slowly along the board.

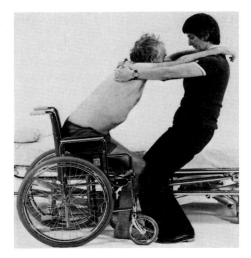

Fig. 5.25. The passive transfer (right hemiplegia). The therapist guides the patient's trunk forwards and downwards while pressing his knees back with hers

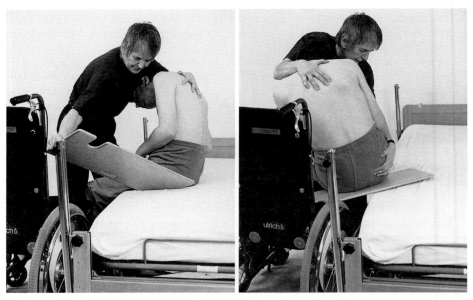

a

b

Fig. 5.26a, b. Using a sliding board (left hemiplegia). **a** Leaning the patient sideways to place the end of the board under one of his buttocks. **b** Sliding him across into the wheelchair with his weight fully supported

The More Active Transfer

As soon as the patient is able to understand what is required of him and participate actively, the transfer becomes more active. A stool or chair is placed in front of him, on which he supports his clasped hands. The stool should be sufficiently far away so that when his hands rest on it, his head is over his feet. The assistant grasps his trochanters, and two separate movements follow to facilitate the transfer. The patient first lifts his seat from the bed and then turns to sit in the chair (**Fig. 5.27**). The assistant gives only as much help as the patient requires to carry out the movement easily and smoothly.

The Active Transfer

When the patient can transfer with the help of a stool in front of him, he can learn to do the same movement, only now with his clasped hands held actively in the air. The assistant facilitates by placing her hands lightly on his scapulae, helping him to keep his trunk well forward and then to turn and place his seat in the chair (**Fig. 5.28**). Some patients may require help to keep the hemiplegic foot flat on the floor. The assistant then places one hand on his knee, presses down on it and draws the knee forwards over the foot as he transfers.

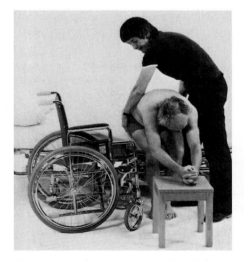

Fig. 5.27. Transferring more actively with the patient's clasped hands supported on a stool in front of him (right hemiplegia)

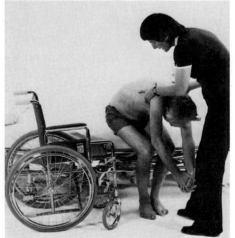

Fig. 5.28. The active transfer (right hemiplegia). The therapist's hands rest lightly on the patient's scapulae and guide the right side forwards and the left one back to facilitate his turning towards the chair

Incontinence

In the acute phase of the disease some patients may have difficulty in controlling both urine and faeces. Once the patient is more mobile and able to help himself the difficulties usually disappear, so that they are seldom a problem after the first 3 months. Persisting difficulties are associated with perceptual problems or pre-existing urological conditions.

The patient with severe perceptual difficulties is unable to plan sufficiently to be continent. The incontinence is not an isolated problem, but will appear in conjunction with failure to perform tasks of a similar complexity (see Chap. 1). The patient will also be unable to dress himself or carry out other activities of daily living independently. The uncontrolled bladder can be likened to that of an infant who has not yet learned to inhibit its emptying appropriately, rather than being regarded as pathologically neurogenic.

Because many patients who suffer a hemiplegia are in the older age-group they may already have been experiencing difficulties with micturition, e.g. due to prostate enlargement or sphincter weakness. Under normal circumstances, before the onset of hemiplegia, careful planning and anticipation assured continence, as did the ability to move easily and independently within a known environment. With loss of mobility following stroke, and in the unfamiliar hospital routine, the patient becomes incontinent or may have retention. Once the patient is able to walk and arrange his own clothing once again, he usually regains continence by re-establishing his former routine.

Whichever of the problems is causing the patient to be incontinent before he is sufficiently able to manage on his own, those who are looking after him should assist him at regular, timed intervals so that the humiliation of incontinence is avoided. When an indwelling catheter has been used in the acute phase, it should be removed as soon as possible, i.e. when the patient has progressed in his ability to move and care for himself. If necessary, specific problems such as urinary tract infection or persisting prostatic difficulties will need to be treated accordingly.

Constipation

Constipation is invariably a problem in the early stages of hemiplegia and, if no adequate steps are taken, may well continue to be a problem at later stages of rehabilitation as well. The patient is immobile in bed, his diet is restricted due to eating difficulties, his fluid intake is reduced as he has difficulty swallowing liquids and he is inhibited psychologically by the presence of the person who is required to assist him. His usual timing is altered by the hospital routine, and he misses the dietary or medicinal aids he used at home. Even when he is no longer confined to bed, he will not be moving as much as he did before.

Constipation is distressing for the patient and may affect him in other ways:
- He has difficulty in concentrating on his rehabilitation and may become depressed.
- He may have apparent diarrhoea, because he is unable to empty his bowels completely.

- The pressure from the loaded bowel may interfere with urination or catheter drainage.
- If severe, the constipation may lead to obstruction or to difficulties with breathing.

Continence of faeces is easily re-established if constipation is avoided right from the beginning by using appropriate doses of a laxative. The correct dose is estimated by taking into account the patient's previous history, obtained either from him or from his close relatives, and then by observing the results. The laxative is given in the evening, and after breakfast the patient is transferred onto the toilet or a commode next to his bed, as it is extremely difficult to "perform" in bed. He is encouraged to breathe deeply and press down gently. Should he be unable to pass a soft-formed stool, a suppository is used to enable him to empty his bowels or, if necessary, an enema is given to ensure emptying. The dose given that evening is then increased as required to ensure success the next day. If, on the other hand, the initial dose was too great and the patient suffered diarrhoea the following day, it will need to be decreased appropriately.

Considerations

If the patient is taught to move in normal movement patterns right from the beginning his whole rehabilitation will be easier and quicker. Sometimes it is advisable to wait a bit longer before pushing for independence if the patient can manage only with a great struggle and in a way detrimental to the return of active movement. If an incorrect movement pattern has been established it will be more difficult for the patient to change the habit later because it involves re-learning. When assistance is given in the ways described in this chapter, the patient will not be afraid to move and his shoulder will have been protected from trauma. Each position and way of moving is a preparation for independent movement later. Although it is not possible to prevent hypertonicity altogether, the correct positioning and handling of the patient in the acute phase will reduce its development considerably.

The positions in which the patient lies in bed are those which he should use even when he is at home and independent. He will then no longer require all the supporting pillows, but the basic side-lying positions remain the same and serve to inhibit hypertonus. During his rehabilitation he is taught to turn himself in bed and achieve the correct position without the help of another person.

Time spent in the acute phase is time well spent because it will certainly decrease the period of intensive inpatient treatment required and will enhance the possibility of achieving a more successful rehabilitation outcome.

6 Normalising Postural Tone and Teaching the Patient to Move Selectively and Without Excessive Effort

Perhaps the most important and difficult task for the therapist is to normalise muscle tone and teach the patient how to move easily in a normal pattern. When the tone is too low, the patient will be unable to support himself or parts of his body against gravity. Where tone is too high and spasticity is a problem, the patient will be able to move only with great effort in stereotyped mass patterns against the resistance of the hypertonic antagonists. One or other of these problems may be predominant, but very often there is a mixture of the two, or a state of muscle tone which fluctuates between the two. How the patient moves or is positioned throughout the day will influence the tone considerably (Chaps. 5 and 10). Striving to move unaided in whatever way he can in the presence of hyper- or hypotonus will in turn lead to further tone abnormalities. From the beginning he should therefore learn to move selectively and be assisted sufficiently so that the mass movement synergies do not become habituated, with tone increasing further as a result. It has even been postulated that, "what is usually called spasticity is in most cases following stroke unnecessary muscular activity which has become habitual, certain muscles, those whose mechanical advantage is greatest, contracting persistently to the disadvantage of others" (Carr and Shepherd 1982). Not only does repeated use of abnormal movement increase hypertonicity, but the habitual patterns are difficult to change later and may even prevent the return of useful functional activity for patients for whom such recovery might otherwise be possible. "It seems likely that frequent repetition of adaptive motor patterns may generate stronger neural connections, these patterns, rather than more effective patterns, becoming "learned" or more stable" (Carr and Shepherd 1996). During treatment the principles of facilitation should be followed, after tone has become as normal as possible. The treatment is not a series of isolated exercises but a sequence of activities to achieve a specific aim. When a therapeutic activity has normalised tone, a selective movement is practised and then used in a functional way. Although one part of the body cannot be treated in isolation, as each part influences the others, this chapter deals more specifically with trunk and lower limb activity and Chap. 8 with the trunk and upper limbs.

The activities which follow are a preparation for walking, and the selective movements are necessary for a correct stance phase and swing phase during walking. They can also change and improve the way in which a patient walks even if he has already been using an abnormal pattern of walking. While working for control of the leg it is important that the arm should not pull into flexion, and should remain instead at the patient's side (see Fig. 6.2). The therapist may have to inhibit the hypertonicity first, and then ask the patient to try and leave his arm at his side, consciously inhibiting its tendency to flex. He should perform the activities in such a way that associated reactions do not occur, because by so doing he will be learning to inhibit the associated reactions which can often be a problem during walking or when performing other functional tasks.

Such intrinsic inhibition of spasticity is preferable to having him clasp his hands together and maintain the arms in extension above his head or stretched out in front of him while practising lower limb activities. The patient's arm should, in fact, serve as a barometer for the therapist, informing her at once if something is going wrong. Should the arm pull up in flexion she will need to decide whether the activity is too advanced for the patient, whether he is using too much effort, whether her support is inadequate or her verbal stimulation too great. Using the sound hand to hold the hemiplegic arm forcibly in an extended position while learning to move selectively has several additional disadvantages:

- Considerable effort is required and the sound shoulder may suffer as a result of the prolonged holding. A supraspinatus tendinitis is not uncommon.
- The effort increases the tone in the lower limb which the patient is concentrating on moving selectively and without overexertion.
- The fixed position of the arms prevents normal reactions and movement patterns from occurring spontaneously in the rest of his body.
- In standing, holding the hands clasped in front of him increases flexion of the trunk and hips while he is trying to extend them.
- The position cannot be carried over into functional activities, because the patient will need his sound hand to perform more skilled tasks.
- Later, when he is able to walk outside on his own, he will not be able to hold his hands above his head all the time, but should have learned to let his arm remain relaxed in a normal position at his side.

Important Activities for the Trunk and Lower Limbs in Lying

Inhibiting Extensor Spasticity in the Leg

The patient lies with both legs flexed and encircles his knees with his clasped hands. Lifting his head from the pillow, he rocks gently into more flexion and then less **(Fig. 6.1)**. The movement reduces the extensor spasticity in his leg and simultaneously brings the scapula into protraction, which inhibits flexor spasticity in the arm. Lifting his clasped hands, he tries to hold the legs in flexion, and then to flex them actively as he replaces his hands over his knees. The same activity can be performed holding the hemiplegic leg alone while the other lies flat on the plinth.

Retraining Selective Abdominal Muscle Activity

For the patient to be able to walk safely with a more normal gait pattern, selective abdominal muscle control is essential. In hemiplegia there is a loss of both voluntary and reflex activity in the abdominals, with far-reaching effects on tone and motor control (Davies 1990). From the beginning, the activity in the abdominal muscles must be retrained selectively, that is, with the thoracic spine remaining extended despite the flexor activity of the abdominal muscle group. After tone and overactivity in the extensors of

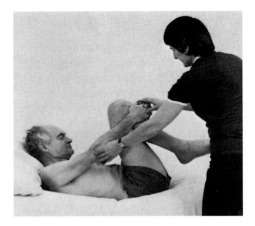

Fig. 6.1. Inhibiting extensor hypertonicity in the leg. Later the patient learns to carry out the activity on his own (right hemiplegia)

the lumbar spine and lower limbs have been inhibited, the therapist places the patient's feet on the plinth or bed, close to one another and in line with his trunk. She helps him to cross one leg over the other and facilitates abduction and adduction of his hips by moving his knees rhythmically from side to side. With her other hand she stabilises the patient's chest, pressing lightly down on his sternum (**Fig. 6.2 a**). The patient is asked to assist actively with the movement back and forth and then changes, so that his other foot is supported on the plinth (**Fig. 6.2 b**). As soon as the movement is taking place smoothly and without effort, the therapist reduces the amount of help she is giving, taking her hand slightly away from his knee, but is always ready to help again if necessary. Should the movement falter or become effortful and its rhythm lost, she at once resumes her facilitation. Finally, when the activity is possible without his affected arm showing an increase in tone, the patient lifts his sound arm and holds it in outward rotation with 90° of shoulder flexion (**Fig. 6.2 c**).

Control of the Leg Through Range

With the patient's leg flexed at the hip and knee, the therapist holds his foot in dorsiflexion and pronation with one hand while using her other to keep his hip in position (**Fig. 6.3 a**). She guides his leg down towards extension, and the patient holds the weight of his leg actively, avoiding the influence of the mass movement synergies. He tries to maintain the position of the leg in flexion without abduction and external rotation at the hip, and as the leg is moved toward the plinth he tries to prevent it from pushing into adduction with internal rotation as it extends (**Fig. 6.3 b**). If the therapist feels that the leg is pushing into extension she quickly asks him to lift it again a little before proceeding, taking some of its weight with her hand beneath his knee The activity is practised until the patient can eventually control the movement with eccentric muscle activity all the way down until his leg is lying flat on the plinth.

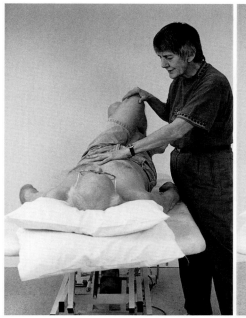
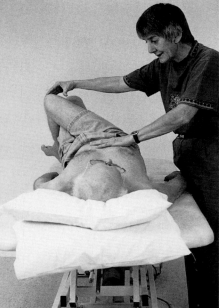

a

b

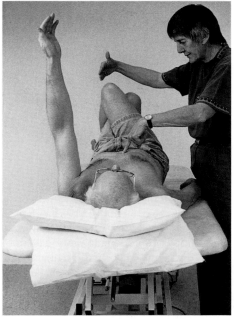

Fig. 6.2 a–c. Regaining selective abdominal muscle control (right hemiplegia) (**a**) with one leg crossed over the other and moving the knees from side to side. **b** The therapist helps to stabilise his thorax and maintain the rhythm. **c** With his sound arm raised the patient stabilises his chest actively with less help from the therapist

c

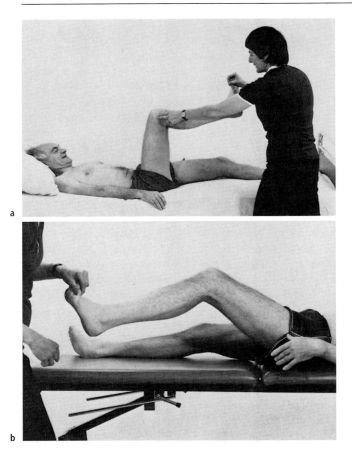

Fig. 6.3 a, b. Learning to control the leg actively. **a** At first it is easier for the patient to hold his leg in a flexed position (right hemiplegia). **b** Later he must learn to maintain control in increasing degrees of extension (left hemiplegia)

Placing the Leg in Different Positions

The therapist places the leg in various positions and the patient maintains the exact position after she has removed her hands. At first only full flexion of hip and knee may be possible, and positions where the foot is supported on the plinth. As control improves, the positions can be made more demanding. Flexion of the hip with internal rotation and adduction is important for function, as is hip flexion with various degrees of knee extension, i.e. selective knee extension (see Fig. 3.9).

Inhibition of Knee Extension with the Hip in Extension

The patient's hemiplegic leg is brought to lie over the side of the bed or plinth. The therapist inhibits plantar flexion fully by lifting his foot and toes into full dorsiflexion with her fingers and giving counterpressure with her thumbs over the tarsal area

(Fig. 6.4). At the same time, she eases the knee into flexion until all resistance to the movement disappears. The patient then brings his foot actively onto the plinth, the therapist having released one of her hands to assist at the knee if necessary (Fig. 6.5). He then lowers his foot over the side of the bed again, maintaining the knee in flexion as he does so. The ability to flex the knee while the hip is extended is essential for the initiation of the swing phase in walking. The activity also enables the patient to bring his leg out of bed before sitting up over the side.

Active Control at the Hip

Lying with his feet supported on the plinth and his knees flexed, the patient brings the hemiplegic knee away from the other knee, which is kept stationary. He learns to do so smoothly and to stop the movement at given points, instead of letting the leg fall into abduction. He can also practise keeping the affected knee still while moving the other knee.

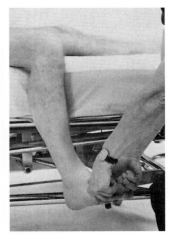 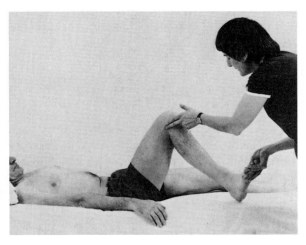

Fig. 6.4. Inhibition of knee extension with the hip extended. The therapist also inhibits plantar flexion of the ankle. She avoids touching the ball of the foot, as this could stimulate extensor spasticity (right hemiplegia)

Fig. 6.5. After inhibition, selective flexion to bring the leg back onto the bed. The arm remains at the patient's side without pulling into flexion (right hemiplegia)

Selective Hip Extension (Bridging)

From the same starting position, the patient lifts his buttocks from the plinth, with his pelvis held level. The therapist facilitates the movement by placing one hand on the patient's thigh on the hemiplegic side and pressing down over his knee with her forearm as she draws the femoral condyles forwards over his foot (**Fig. 6.6**). With the extended fingers of her other hand she helps him to extend his affected hip by tapping lightly to stimulate activity in the gluteal region. The patient is then asked to lift his sound foot a little way off the plinth, so that all weight is on the hemiplegic side (**Fig. 6.7**). He must still maintain the pelvis on one level, not allowing it to rotate back on the sound side. The therapist reduces her help, and the patient controls the movement without letting his knee push into extension or fall to the side. The patient repeats the movement, lifting and replacing his foot in approximately the rhythm of normal walking. He should

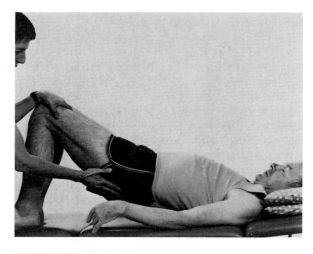

Fig. 6.6. Bridging with facilitation (left hemiplegia)

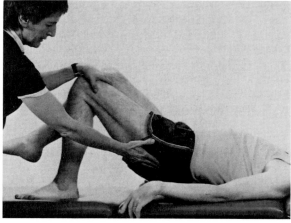

Fig. 6.7. Bridging, and keeping the pelvis level when the sound foot is lifted off the plinth (left hemiplegia)

place his whole foot flat down on the surface each time and not just tap up and down with his toes first. As control improves, the patient can raise and lower his buttocks with the weight only on the hemiplegic leg. When the patient can perform the activity easily, he will be better able to prevent his knee from locking in hyperextension when walking. The further away the feet are placed during bridging activities, the greater is the amount of selective activity required to maintain knee flexion as the patient extends his hips.

Isolated Knee Extension

Lying with his foot and toes held in full dorsiflexion by the therapist's body and with his heel resting on the plinth, the patient extends his knee isometrically, with a static iso-metric contraction of the extensor muscles (**Fig. 6.8**). In order to ensure really full dorsi-flexion of his foot, the therapist may first have to flex his knee somewhat to enable her to achieve the passive range and then, while maintaining the position firmly by leaning forwards against the sole of his foot, slowly straighten his knee. The therapist stimulates the desired activity in his knee extensors and asks the patient not to push against her body with his foot or toes as he tenses his thigh. It usually helps the patient if he per-forms the activity correctly first with his unaffected knee. It may also be helpful for the therapist to flex his knee slightly before the attempt at extension, but once he can do this, the isometric contraction should be practised with no movement of the knee at all. Apart from enabling the patient to stand without the foot pushing into plantar flexion, the activity also inhibits spasticity in the calf muscles and can be used before stimulat-ing active dorsiflexion of the foot.

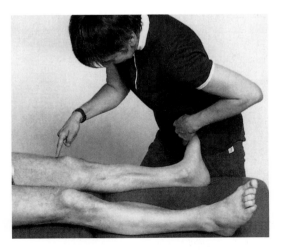

Fig. 6.8. Selective knee extension, with the foot held in full dorsiflexion. With her finger the therapist indicates to the patient exactly where the activity should occur (left hemiplegia)

Stimulating Active Dorsiflexion of the Foot and Toes

The movement of dorsiflexion is most easily stimulated when the patient is lying with his leg flexed and the foot supported on the bed. In lying, extensor spasticity in the leg is reduced, as he is not required to hold himself upright against gravity. The patient should not try desperately to pull his foot up, but should just lift the toes up lightly and let them relax again immediately. If he struggles to perform the movement the tone in the antagonists will increase, making the desired movement impossible, or causing the foot to pull into supination. Showing the patient exactly what is required on his sound foot helps him to move correctly. To inhibit the hypertonus in the antagonists before attempting the movement, the therapist holds the whole foot in front of the ankle firmly down on the plinth, and then moves the patient's leg over it from adduction into abduction; i.e. the foot is pronated by the movement of the leg proximally. The movement releases the pull into supination and relaxes the small muscles of the foot. She then pushes down through the ankle with the web between her extended thumb and index finger, while with her other hand she lifts the toes and foot into full dorsiflexion with pronation (**Fig.6.9**). When the foot offers no resistance to the passive movement, the therapist stimulates dorsiflexion with the active participation of the patient. The therapist seeks a stimulus which will elicit dorsiflexion in a normal pattern without supination, asking the patient to lift his toes simultaneously. The following are useful; in fact they almost always elicit the desired response:
- Stroking the tips of the toes briskly with a chunk of ice, or even pushing the ice between the two most lateral toes (**Fig.6.10**)
- Stroking the lateral border of the foot with the ice
- Brushing the tips or dorsum of the toes with a bottlebrush
- Tapping the dorsum of the foot laterally with the bottlebrush

Sometimes the whole foot needs to be immersed in melting ice before the bottlebrush is effective. Some patients may need less stimulation, and merely tickling the toes or flicking the lateral toes upwards will evoke a response. Whichever stimulus is effective, the

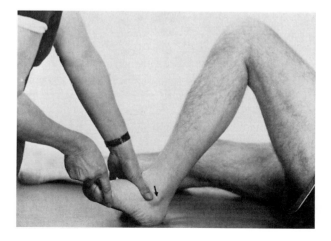

Fig.6.9. Inhibiting plantar flexion of the foot. The toes are held in full dorsiflexion (left hemiplegia)

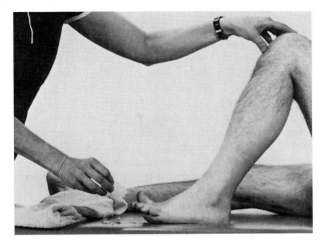

Fig. 6.10. Stimulating active dorsiflexion with ice after inhibition of the antagonists. The towel is not placed under the patient's foot, as it tends to stimulate plantar flexion (left hemiplegia)

patient must learn to reproduce the movement actively on his own. He feels the movement or gets feedback from the therapist informing him when the movement is correct. She then reduces the intensity of the stimulus and asks him to perform the movement again until eventually only her verbal stimulus is required. Once the movement is established, she stimulates the activity in the same way with the patient in a sitting position, after inhibition, and ultimately when he is standing upright. The ability to dorsiflex the foot actively without supination means that the patient will not have to wear a calliper at all times, so it is a very important aspect of the treatment.

Rolling Over

Rolling is a very effective way not only to inhibit hypertonicity throughout the body, particularly when rotation of the trunk is emphasised, but also to regain active control once tone has been normalised. The patient can move freely and confidently without having to maintain his balance against gravity, and movement without effort can be facilitated. Head-righting reactions are also stimulated. The active movements of the legs and trunk which are used when rolling over onto the side are similar to those necessary for walking. Facilitating rolling in a normal pattern is therefore a useful and effective way of preparing the patient for learning to walk again. Therapeutic rolling should be practised only on a wide supporting surface such as a bed, a mat on the floor, a high mat or two plinths pushed together. If the patient is asked to roll on a narrow plinth, he will be afraid of falling off it and will not move freely and normally. The facilitation of rolling is described in Chaps. 5 and 11.

Activities in Sitting

Correcting the Sitting Posture

Patients at all stages of their rehabilitation nearly always sit with their hips too extended and their spine in flexion to compensate (**Fig. 6.11**). As a result, many functional activities are impeded or can be performed only in an abnormal way and the all-important abdominal muscles are unable to work efficiently. Balance reactions in sitting cannot be regained with the trunk flexed, and possible recovery of voluntary activity in the arm is severely hampered if the thorax cannot provide a stable origin for the muscles controlling the scapula and shoulder. When standing up from sitting, the patient has to round his back in order to bring his weight forwards. Sitting for long periods with extended hips leads to an increase in extensor tone in the whole leg, making function more difficult. Regaining the ability to sit upright with the hips sufficiently flexed is therefore of prime importance in the treatment. It is of little use for the therapist to tell the patient to sit up straight, as he will pull his shoulders back obediently but will be able to maintain the apparent correction for only a very short time. The posture needs to be corrected from its base, by adjusting the position of the patient's hips and pelvis The therapist stands or kneels in front of the patient, and with one hand on his lumbar spine she draws it forwards until his hips are sufficiently flexed and his trunk vertically over his pelvis (**Fig. 6.12**). With her other hand she helps him to extend his thoracic spine without leaning backwards. The earlier the patient is taught how to correct his sitting posture, the easier it will be for him to do so automatically later and also to maintain the position.

    Patients in the acute phase and patients who have not had such early training may have great difficulty in bringing their trunk sufficiently far forwards if they are sitting

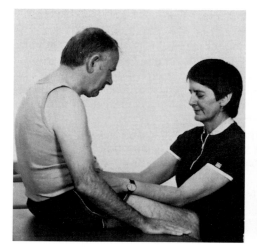

Fig. 6.11. The typical sitting posture, with insufficient flexion of the hips, needs to be corrected from its base (left hemiplegia)

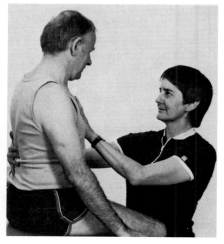

Fig. 6.12. Correcting the patient's sitting posture (left hemiplegia)

unsupported on a plinth or bed. The same applies to those with severe perceptual disorders, because they will be afraid to move their trunk forwards if there is only an empty space in front of them.

Careful progression will be required for all such patients, starting with a table placed in front of them and their arms supported on it while flexing and extending their trunk. To facilitate the movement and posture, the therapist stands behind the patient but slightly more to his hemiplegic side. She puts one arm right around the patient's lower ribs and helps him to round his whole back completely until he touches the backrest of the chair (**Fig. 6.13 a**). With her other hand over his scapula, she eases his shoulder girdle forward on that side and helps him to flex his thoracic spine as well. The patient is then asked to move away from the backrest and bring his lower chest forwards to touch the edge of the table. The therapist places one hand over his lower thoracic spine in the region of the typical kyphosis and presses it firmly into extension. With her other hand on his sternum in front, she guides his chest upwards and backwards to extend his trunk (**Fig. 6.13 b**). The patient continues to flex and extend his trunk, the chairback behind and the table in front providing him with points of reference each time. Once he can perform the movement freely and rhythmically, he stays in the extended position with his lower ribs in contact with the table. Without moving away from the table at all, he can try to lift his sound arm off its surface while still maintaining the trunk extension. Once he has learned to sit upright with the table in front of him, he can be encouraged to adopt the posture frequently during the day, for instance when watching television, talking to visitors or having his meals.

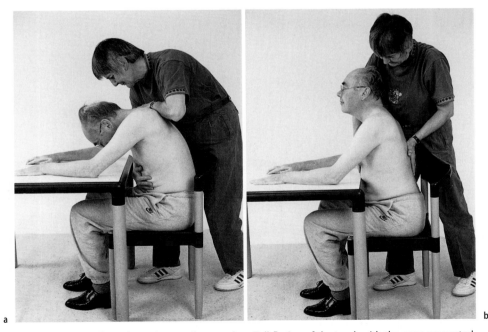

a   b

Fig. 6.13 a, b. Teaching the patient to sit correctly. **a** Full flexion of the trunk with the arms supported. **b** Extending the trunk with his hips flexed (right hemiplegia)

Selective Flexion and Extension of the Lumbar Spine

When the patient has practised flexing and extending his trunk as a whole with his neck moving as well, the activity should become more and more selective until he can localise the movement to his lumbar spine without his upper trunk, shoulders or neck moving at all. He learns to localise the movement more easily while still sitting with his arms supported on the table. The therapist helps him to stabilise his chest wall by placing her arm round in front of his lower ribs and holding them firmly together and asking him to move only the lumbar area.

Once the patient has the feel of the small localised flexion and extension movement, the activity can be attempted without the table supporting his arms. At first it will be easier for him to move his lumbar spine selectively if he sits on a raised plinth with his feet unsupported, because when his feet are on the floor, he will usually push down against it with his sound foot, thus impeding the free movement of his pelvic girdle.

Once the patient can perform the selective movement freely, he must also learn to do so when he is seated on a chair with his feet flat on the floor. The therapist kneels in front of him and places one hand on the front of his chest to indicate that it should remain motionless, while with her other hand she shows him exactly where the movement should take place and helps him to extend his lower back for a correct starting position (**Fig. 6.14 a**). With one hand on the side of his pelvis, she facilitates its movement back and forth rhythmically in order to flex and extend the lumbar spine selectively (**Fig. 6.14 b**). If the patient's legs are usually in abduction, then the therapist holds his knees nearer together while he moves proximally. If, on the other hand, his hemiplegic leg adducts and medially rotates, she keeps his legs apart during the activity. The move-

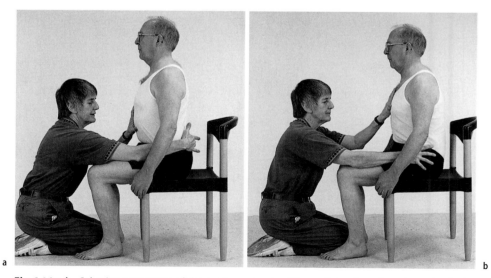

a
b

Fig. 6.14 a, b. Selective movement of the lumbar spine in sitting. **a** Extension of the lower back; the therapist indicates where the movement should take place. **b** Maintaining extension of the thorax when the lumbar spine flexes (left hemiplegia)

ment of his trunk against the lower limbs reduces extensor spasticity around the hips and knees remarkably. When the patient can extend his spine with his hips in flexion, standing up from sitting will be far easier for him and will be possible in a normal way because he will be able to bring his weight sufficiently far forwards over his feet.

Selective movements of the lumbar spine will later be performed in standing and are of inestimable value for improving the patient's walking pattern.

Placing the Hemiplegic Leg and Facilitating Crossing It Over the Other Leg

The therapist holds the patient's foot in dorsiflexion with one hand beneath his toes, while with her other hand she helps him to lift his leg without any external rotation or abduction. The patient takes the weight of his leg actively as he lowers his foot slowly to the floor **(Fig. 6.15)**. He tries to maintain his upright sitting posture while doing so, without leaning back or allowing the hemiplegic side to retract. The therapist facilitates the action of crossing the leg over the sound leg **(Fig. 6.16)**, a movement he will need in order to put on his trousers, shoes and socks (see Chap. 10). He must learn to cross and uncross the leg without pulling it with his unaffected hand and without pushing the heel of the sound foot off the floor.

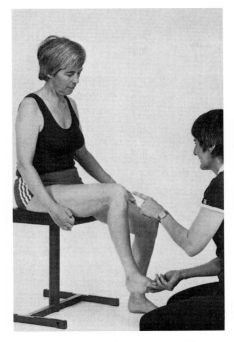

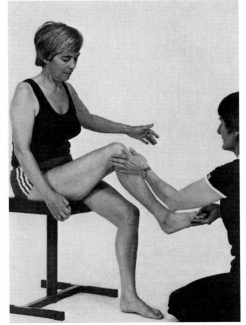

Fig. 6.15. The patient learns to control her hemiplegic leg in sitting (right hemiplegia)

Fig. 6.16. Learning to cross the hemiplegic leg actively over the other one without pulling it with the sound hand (right hemiplegia)

Stamping the Heel on the Floor

When the patient's heel is banged on the floor, tone in his knee extensors is built up and activity is often elicited automatically. Active dorsiflexion of the foot is stimulated at the same time. He also becomes more aware of his heel on the ground, and the activity is therefore a very good preparation for standing up and bearing weight on the affected leg, whether the problem is due to hypotonicity, poor sensation or too little active control. The therapist kneels down in front of the patient and holds his foot and toes in full dorsiflexion with one hand; her other hand is placed over his knee from above. She lifts his leg from the foot, and then pushes down on his knee to bang the heel on the floor. The ankle must remain firmly dorsiflexed so that the ball of the foot does not make contact with the ground (**Fig. 6.17**). In order to support the weight of the patient's leg sufficiently with the knee and foot held in position, the therapist props her forearm on her thigh and, by so doing, needs only to flex her elbow and let it extend again. The patient can also try to participate actively with the stamping movement, as it facilitates selective hip extension, with the knee and foot flexed.

If the patient does not feel his heel on the ground, the therapist can rub it against the floor backwards and forwards. She maintains full dorsiflexion of the foot with the web between her extended thumb and index finger pushing down through his ankle, while her other hand holds his toes in extension (**Fig. 6.18**).

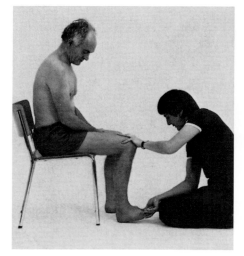 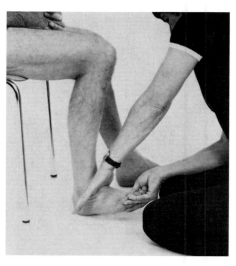

Fig. 6.17. Banging the heel on the floor to stimulate tone and activity in a hypotonic leg before standing. Active dorsiflexion is also stimulated (right hemiplegia)

Fig. 6.18. Rubbing the patient's heel firmly on the ground to improve sensation (right hemiplegia)

Coming From Sitting to Standing

Weightbearing with Selective Extension of the Leg

Once the patient's lower extremity has been carefully prepared for weightbearing, he should practise coming up to a standing position using the normal pattern of movement. Most patients, if not trained correctly, push themselves up with the unaffected hand, most of their weight over the sound side, while the hemiplegic leg thrusts into the total extension pattern. The weight is therefore too far back, the activity is effortful and the resulting posture is asymmetrical and the spastic pattern of extension emphasised.

Sitting with his feet flat on the floor, the patient places his clasped hands on a stool in front of him. The stool should be so positioned that when his hands rest on it with the elbows extended, his head is further forward than his feet, as it is in the normal pattern of standing up. The therapist guides him as he lifts his hips off the chair or low plinth, drawing his affected knee forwards over his foot with one hand, and helping him to lift his weight with her other hand over his trochanter on the opposite side. With her shoulder against his scapula she prevents him from pushing back with his trunk (**Fig. 6.19**). He learns to maintain this position when she withdraws her support, and practises moving his hips from side to side and then back onto the chair or plinth.

When the patient can perform the activity easily, his hands can be placed separately flat on the stool, and he lifts his hips while the hemiplegic hand remains in place, without his arm pulling into flexion (**Fig. 6.20**). Finally, the patient practises the movement without folding his hands together and without the stool in front of him, but with both arms swinging lightly forward in a more normal way (**Fig. 6.21**).

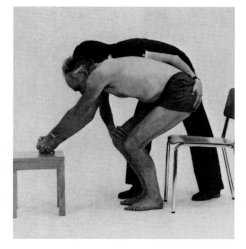

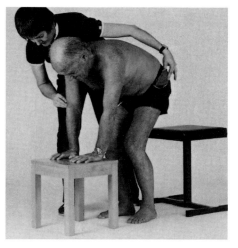

Fig. 6.19. Teaching the patient how to stand up from sitting using the normal pattern of movement. The stool is so placed that his head is in front of his feet. The therapist assists the forward movement of the hemiplegic knee (right hemiplegia)

Fig. 6.20. Preparation for coming to standing. The patient lifts his hips while his hands remain in place on the stool (right hemiplegia)

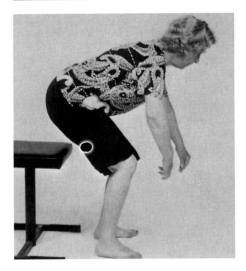

Fig. 6.21. Standing up with the arms swinging freely (right hemiplegia)

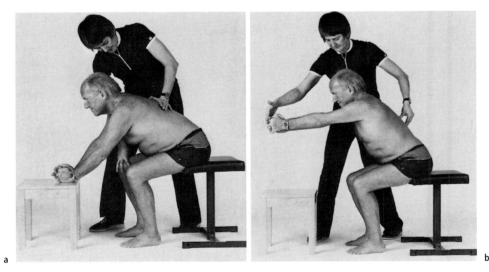

a

b

Fig. 6.22 a, b. In sitting the patient learns to extend his back while his hips are flexed. **a** The therapist presses down on his flexed spine and eases it into extension passively. **b** The patient lifts his hands from the stool and extends his back actively. The therapist indicates the activity with a squeezing movement of her thumb and fingers over his spine (right hemiplegia)

Trunk Extension with the Hips Flexed

The patient often needs help to flex his hips sufficiently and to bring his trunk forwards with his spine extended. The therapist achieves the extension for him passively at first, by pressing gently down on his spine with the weight of his arms supported. She can place one of her feet on a stool in front of him and rest his arms across her knee, or the patient can place his clasped hands on the stool (**Fig. 6.22 a**). When passive extension feels freer, she asks him to straighten his back actively and lift his arms into the air (**Fig. 6.22 b**).

The patient must also be taught to bring his extended trunk forwards with his arms at his side and his scapulae adducted. If he does not learn to keep his shoulders back and his upper trunk extended, his paralysed arm will medially rotate and hang constantly in front of his body when he stands or walks.

To facilitate the movement, the therapist sits beside the patient and first helps him to extend his thoracic spine. With one hand over each of his shoulders, she draws his scapulae back towards each other and asks him to keep them there (**Fig. 6.23 a**). Placing one of her hands in front of his chest and the other over his thoracic spine to stabilise his thorax, she assists the forward movement of his trunk (**Fig. 6.23 b**). The patient maintains the adduction of his scapulae actively and keeps his arms at his sides.

After moving back into an upright position, the patient brings his trunk forwards again, but this time he lifts his seat off the plinth until his weight is over both legs, with the hips and knees remaining flexed. He stays in the half-standing posture while still maintaining extension of his trunk and keeping his shoulders back in position (**Fig. 6.23 c**).

Patients whose tone is on the low side will often use the total extension synergy in the leg when they stand from sitting. As a result, the affected leg adducts and rotates inwardly, and the heel may be pushed off the floor by the overactive plantar flexors. To facilitate the correct movement, the therapist kneels in front of the patient, crosses her hands over and places one on each of his thighs just above his femoral condyles. As he comes up to standing, she draws his knees forwards over his feet and away from each other (**Fig. 6.24**). She slowly withdraws her assistance, making the patient aware that he must not push against her hands, and gives less and less manual assistance.

Once in standing, the patient maintains his hips in extension with abduction and external rotation and bends his knees as far as he can without his heels coming off the floor (**Fig. 6.25**). With more advanced patients it is possible to go right down to the squatting position, or for them to sit down on a low step and rise to a standing position again with their knees apart.

Activities in Standing with Weight on the Hemiplegic Leg

For the patient to walk safely and in a more normal way, he must be able to support his weight on his hemiplegic leg with selective extension of his hip and knee. Careful preparation is necessary for dynamic weightbearing in the stance phase of gait, either before walking is commenced or to improve the gait pattern of a patient who is already walking.

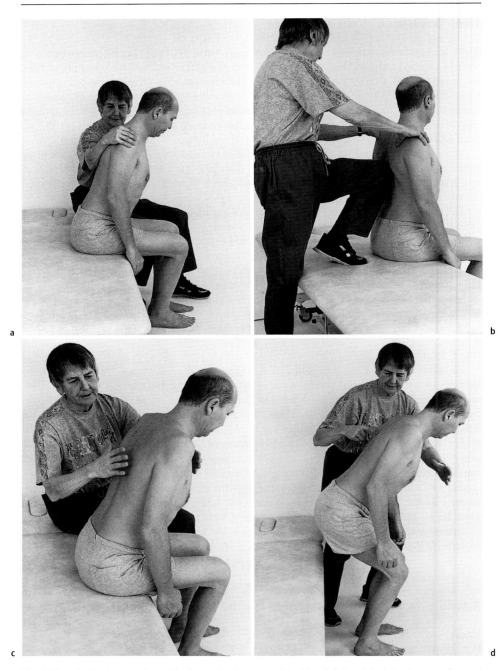

Fig. 6.23 a–d. Trunk extension with the patient's arms at his sides (left hemiplegia). **a** Leaning forward with his shoulders back. **b** The therapist uses her knee to help thoracic extension while mobilising scapula adduction. **c** Keeping his scapulae actively in position when the trunk is brought forwards. **d** Shoulders and arms remain in position when the patient lifts his seat with his trunk extended

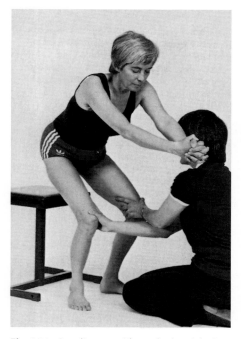

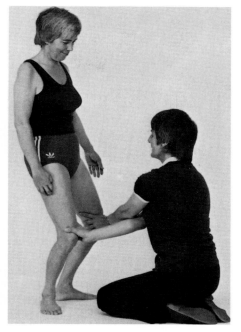

Fig. 6.24. Standing up without the hemiplegic leg adducting. The therapist facilitates the correct movement and the patient tries to keep her knees apart (right hemiplegia)

Fig. 6.25. Standing with the hips in extension, abduction and external rotation. The patient flexes her knees and practises tilting her pelvis selectively (right hemiplegia)

Pelvic Tilting with Selective Flexion/Extension of the Lumbar Spine

The patient stands with his feet apart and both knees flexed. He tilts his pelvis rhythmically anteriorly and posteriorly, keeping his upper trunk, shoulders and head still. The patient's knees should remain at an angle of about 40° throughout the activity, because it is almost impossible for him to tilt his pelvis back and forth if they are fully extended. The pelvic movement continues while his weight is gradually shifted over towards his hemiplegic side, far enough for him to be able to lift his sound foot off the floor.

To teach the patient to tilt his pelvis selectively, the therapist will need to progress gradually from a mass movement to a localised one. The therapist sits in front of the patient and places her knees one on either side of his hemiplegic leg. Adducting her knees against his femoral condyles, she maintains the degree of flexion by drawing his knee forwards with her knees. She instructs the patient to bring his seat forward towards her and uses her hands to help him do so. She places one hand over his lower abdominal muscles just below his umbilicus and the other round behind both his buttocks (**Fig. 6.26a**). The untrained patient will at first be able to perform the movement only by leaning his whole trunk backwards.

When trying to tilt his pelvis up at the back, instead of extending his lumbar spine the patient brings his whole trunk forwards by flexing his hips (**Fig. 6.26b**). The thera-

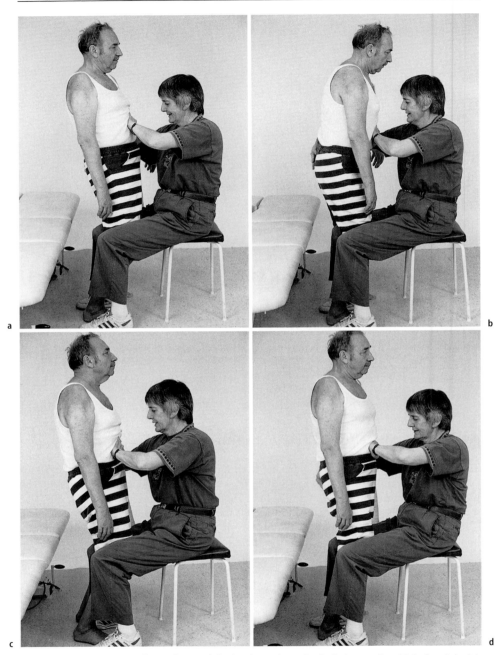

a

b

c

d

Fig. 6.26 a–d. Learning to flex and extend the lumbar spine selectively in standing (right hemiplegia). **a** At first the patient leans his whole trunk backwards when trying to flex his lower back. **b** Pushing his hips back instead of extending the lumbar spine. **c** Stabilising the thorax with the therapist facilitating selective flexion of the lumbar spine. **d** The patient keeps his knees slightly flexed while extending his lumbar spine selectively

pist accepts the compensatory movement at first because the patient clearly understands what is expected of him but cannot yet isolate the movement. He is then told to try and keep his chest quite still and move only the part below his navel. The therapist facilitates the movement with her hands and uses different verbal phrases to help him until he finally succeeds. When he is flexing his lumbar spine she uses the hand behind his buttocks to tense the gluteal group as if he were tucking in his tail. Her other hand assists the contraction of his lower abdominal muscles (**Fig. 6.26 c**). When he is extending his lumbar spine in isolation she gives him the feeling of lengthening the lower abdominals and lifting his buttocks up at the back (**Fig. 6.26 d**).

When the patient is tilting his pelvis rhythmically back and forth selectively, the therapist uses her legs to move him gradually over towards his hemiplegic side. Once all his weight is on the affected leg, he lifts the sound foot off the floor without interrupting the pelvic movement (**Fig. 6.27 a**). His sound leg should not swing back and forth to compensate for insufficient control of flexion and extension of the hemiplegic hip, as it will tend to do. Instead, the therapist asks the patient to hold his leg motionless in front of him with the hip and knee flexed (**Fig. 6.27 b**).

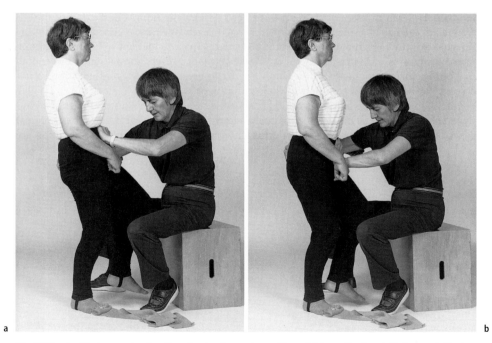

a   b

Fig. 6.27 a, b. Flexing and extending the lumbar spine with weight on the hemiplegic leg. **a** Flexing with the sound foot lifted from the floor. **b** Selective extension with the thorax stabilised (From Davies 1990)

Standing with a Rolled Bandage Underneath the Toes

Without the necessary training, almost all patients have difficulty in extending their hemiplegic leg selectively when standing upright. Not only does the knee hyperextend in the mass pattern of extension, but the foot plantar flexes and the toes flex strongly, a problem particularly obvious during the stance phase of walking, when all the weight is on the hemiplegic leg. If the problem is not prevented by specific treatment from the beginning, or overcome should it already exist, not only do the muscles become increasingly hypertonic, but an actual loss of range of motion is likely to develop. Until the patient has regained sufficient selective extension it is most helpful and effective to place a bandage rolled to an appropriate size under his toes during activities to train weight-bearing on the hemiplegic leg **(Fig. 6.28)**. With the toes held in dorsal extension by the bandage, plantar flexion of the ankle and flexion of the toes are inhibited and the full extensibility of the relevant muscle groups, including the intrinsic muscles of the foot, can be maintained.

If the Achilles tendon is allowed to shorten or become very hypertonic, the foot will supinate or invert strongly in the swing phase and the patient will have to wear a brace when walking, either to maintain dorsiflexion or to prevent his ankle from being injured. Without intensive prophylactic treatment the problem may very easily develop; Garland (1995) goes so far as to say that, "Equinus is the most common deformity of the hemiplegic lower extremity."

Hypertonicity or shortening of the toe flexors causes clawing of the toes, and the resultant deformity can be most painful, as well as impeding walking. Corns develop on the pads beneath the toes as they press so hard against the floor. The flexion of the interphalangeal joints can lead to reddened areas or even open sores forming on the dorsal aspect of the toes due to the constant pressure against the patient's shoe. In addition, any contractures of his calf muscles or toe flexors will prevent the patient from feeling his foot in normal contact with the floor, a sensation which provides information so necessary for balance and confidence when standing or walking.

Merely by using the simple procedure of having the patient stand on the rolled bandage and helping him to move proximally against the distal hypertonus, the therapist can prevent the development of hypertonicity and avoid loss of range of motion. In

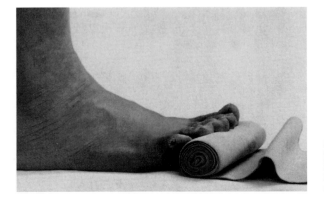

Fig. 6.28. Bandage placed under the patient's toes to inhibit flexion. The size of the rolled bandage is gradually increased as tension decreases (right hemiplegia)

fact, plantar flexion of the whole foot is so effectively inhibited by the activity that it will often be possible for her to stimulate active dorsal flexion of the patient's ankle and toes immediately afterwards. The patient can also be shown how to perform the movement on his own at home after cessation of physiotherapy (see Figs. 16.8 and 16.9).

Without fully understanding the biomechanics of the foot, some therapists are unwilling to place the rolled bandage beneath the patient's toes because they are afraid of damaging his metatarsophalangeal (MP) joints or even causing them to sublux. Their fear is unfounded, however, because of the joint construction itself and the protection provided by the plantar fascia and the arrangement of powerful ligaments. With regard to the MP joints themselves, "In marked contrast to the condition in the hand, the range of extension is greater than the range of flexion, and this is associated with the requirements of walking. This is especially the case in the metatarsophalangeal joint of the great toe, where flexion is limited to a few degrees of flexion but extension may be possible up to 90° (Johnston and Willis 1954). During walking, when the heel rises off the floor in terminal stance, the MP joints dorsiflex (extend) 21°, and with the toes remaining in contact with the supporting surface, the metatarsal shafts angle upwards as the hind foot is lifted (Bojsen-Moller and Lamoreux 1979). In her comprehensive gait analysis, Perry (1992) describes how, "This motion continually increases throughout preswing to a final position of 55° extension" and states that, "Freedom for the foot to roll across the rounded metatarsal surfaces depends on there being adequate passive mobility of the MP joint and yielding control by the flexor muscles". She goes on to explain how the plantar fascia, extending from the calcaneus to the fascia about the base of the toes, provides passive stability in terminal stance and pre-swing, illustrating clearly how, "This fascial band is tightened by metatarsophalangeal (MP) dorsiflexion."

Clearly, then, the MP joints will not be damaged by stationary weight-bearing activities with the patient's toes in some degree of dorsiflexion maintained by a rolled bandage placed beneath them. The size of the roll can be carefully adjusted if the therapist observes any deviation in the position of the foot or if the patient expresses any discomfort. Based on her observations, the height of the rolled bandage is gradually increased as tension and stiffness release and range of movement increases.

Certainly, the prophylactic activity is infinitely preferable to having to resort to surgical intervention to overcome the problems later. Any such interventions, even those described so positively by Garland (1995), are complicated, expensive and painful, prolong the period of rehabilitation and in some cases may even have detrimental consequences.

Flexing and Extending the Weight-bearing Leg

With the patient in sitting, the therapist places the rolled bandage beneath his toes and mobilises his foot passively to inhibit any hypertonus, thus enabling the sole to be in a normal position in contact with the floor (**Fig. 6.29 a**). She places one hand over the dorsum of his foot and moulds it down medially to overcome any supination tendency. With her other hand on his knee, she moves his leg from side to side while still holding his foot firmly in the corrected position on the floor (**Fig. 6.29 b**). When all tension has been released and the foot stays relaxed in position, the therapist helps the patient to stand up, facilitating the forward movement of his knee over his foot. Once in standing, the patient should first try to remain in a symmetrical, upright posture, without tension

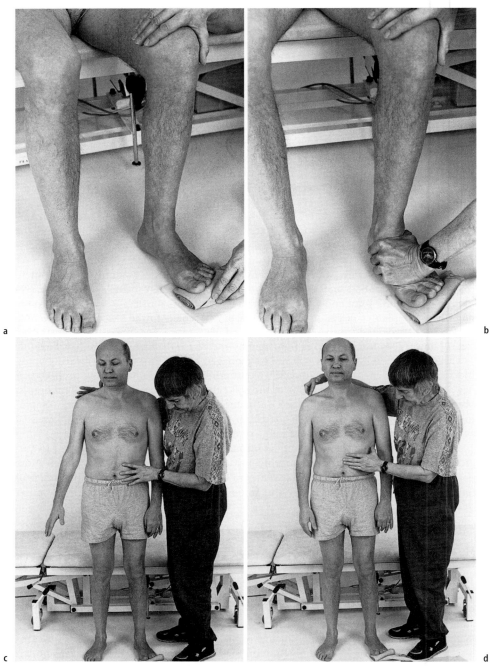

Fig. 6.29 a–d. Standing with a rolled bandage under the toes (left hemiplegia). **a** Placing the bandage rolled to the appropriate size. **b** Mobilising the foot by moving the knee. **c** Excessive activity in the sound arm and foot. **d** Able to relax and stand confidently with the rolled bandage in place

in unnecessary muscle groups and without compensatory movements of his arms or sound foot (**Fig. 6.29 c, d**). He transfers his weight over his hemiplegic leg before lifting his sound foot off the floor. The therapist helps him to maintain his balance while he slowly flexes and extends the supporting leg, taking care that his knee does not snap back into hyperextension.

■ **Facilitation for the Patient with Disturbed Sensation.** Patients with disturbed sensation in the hemiplegic leg need to feel correct weightbearing so that they can learn to reproduce it themselves. At first the therapist may have to facilitate the movement with total support. She stands on the patient's hemiplegic side and supports his knee on that side between both her knees or thighs. With her arms round him, she draws him towards her and asks him to lift his sound leg in the air (**Fig. 6.30**). She then moves his supported knee into flexion and extension by alternately adducting and abducting her legs. When she feels him helping actively, she moves her knees slightly away from his knee and gives him the verbal feedback that he is performing the correct movement. With his knee in the slightly flexed position, she removes her knees form his altogether and, helping him only to maintain balance, asks him to continue on his own.

■ **Facilitation for the Patient Who Is Afraid.** If a patient is afraid to stand on his hemiplegic leg, or feels he can do so only with the knee hyperextended, the therapist can help him to gain confidence by sitting right in front of him and supporting his leg and trunk. She sits on a stool and holds the patient's affected knee between her knees in such a way that, when she adducts her legs, her femoral condyles prevent his leg from pushing back into hyperextension. In this position the therapist has both her hands free to facilitate

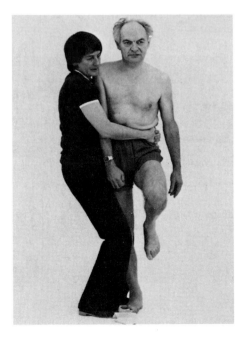

Fig. 6.30. Weightbearing on the hemiplegic leg with full support. The therapist uses her legs to facilitate flexion and extension of the knee, and the patient starts to join in actively. His weight must be transferred right over the hemiplegic leg (right hemiplegia)

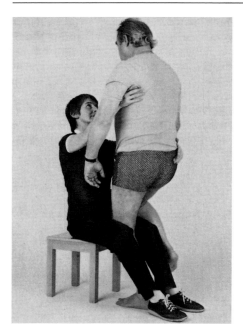

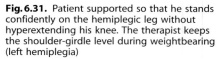

Fig. 6.31. Patient supported so that he stands confidently on the hemiplegic leg without hyperextending his knee. The therapist keeps the shoulder-girdle level during weightbearing (left hemiplegia)

hip extension and to adjust the position of the pelvis and the posture of the patient's trunk (**Fig. 6.31**). Using her knees, she moves the patient gently over one side and then the other and asks him not to press against her leg with his good leg. He does so in order to use adduction to reinforce extension in the total synergy. When he feels more confident, the patient lifts his sound foot from the floor or can take steps sideways or backwards with his sound leg. The therapist slowly reduces the amount of support by releasing the pressure of her knees.

Coming off a High Plinth onto the Hemiplegic Leg

The patient moves to the edge of the plinth and places his hemiplegic foot flat on the floor, with the leg outwardly rotated. The therapist guides his foot to the floor, holding the foot and toes in dorsiflexion. Pausing in this position, he extends and flexes his knee selectively, moving it as far as he can into extension without it snapping back, and without his toes clawing. The therapist facilitates the knee movement with her other hand and ensures that the patient remains vertically upright and does not lean over the plinth towards his sound side, or support himself with his hand. The therapist stands up beside the patient so that she can facilitate the correct movement as he lifts his sound buttock off the plinth and comes to stand with his feet together, still with his affected knee in some degree of flexion. She uses the hand furthest from him to help him extend his hip and bring his weight forwards over his foot when his seat leaves the plinth. Her other hand on the opposite side of his pelvis rotates the sound side forwards. The patient tries to remain standing with his weight only on his hemiplegic leg and the other

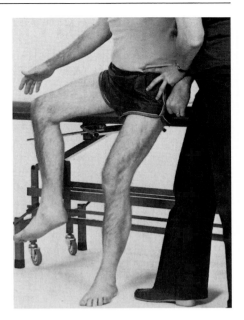

Fig. 6.32. Weightbearing on the hemiplegic leg alone while standing up from a high plinth or sitting back on it again. The knee remains slightly flexed throughout the activity (left hemiplegia)

foot still in the air, while bringing the sound side of his pelvis forwards until it is on line with the other. The activity required to adjust the pelvis will then take place in the muscles of the hemiplegic hip and the trunk on that side. In order to return to a sitting position, the patient lifts his sound leg into the air and rotates his pelvis back to place his sound buttock on the plinth again (**Fig. 6.32**). The activity, either to stand up from the plinth or sit back on it again, is valuable because it requires extension of the affected hip independent of the rotation component.

Stepping Up onto a Step with Weight on the Hemiplegic Leg

Patients often find it difficult to take weight on their hemiplegic leg without fixing the knee in a certain position, either in hyperextension or in too much flexion. To give the patient the feeling of mobility during weightbearing, his affected foot is placed on a step in front of him and he then steps up and places his other foot on the next step. He steps down again, moving his sound leg well back and putting his foot down on the floor as slowly as possible. To facilitate the activity, the therapist first helps the patient to place his hemiplegic foot correctly on the step. Using her hand over his thigh with the thumb on the outer side of his leg, she draws his knee forwards over his foot as he moves up on to the step. Standing close to the patient, she presses the near side of her pelvis firmly against his hip from behind to supplement the extensor activity during the upward movement of his body. Her arm and shoulder passing round behind him with the hand resting on his sound side prevent his leaning backwards and thus help him to bring his whole trunk vertically forwards over the foot in front (**Fig. 6.33**).

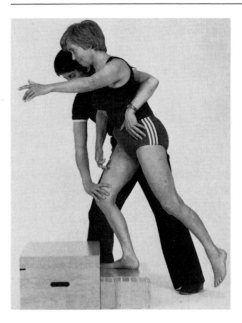

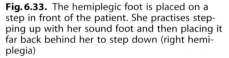

Fig. 6.33. The hemiplegic foot is placed on a step in front of the patient. She practises stepping up with her sound foot and then placing it far back behind her to step down (right hemiplegia)

When the patient's ability has improved sufficiently and he requires less support, the height of the step can be increased (**Fig. 6.34 a**). The higher step demands more activity from the hip and knee extensors. The therapist facilitates the upward movement in the same way as she did before and asks the patient to keep his sound foot in the air for a while instead of placing it immediately on the step with the other one (**Fig. 6.34 b**).

Activities in Standing with Weight on the Sound Leg

Patients have difficulty in taking a step with their hemiplegic leg and often bring it forwards without flexing the hip and knee sufficiently, if at all, because of extensor hypertonus. They therefore hitch the pelvis up on the affected side, as if they were wearing a full leg brace, and use the activity of the contralateral hip to swing it forwards in one piece. Other patients lift the leg actively forwards in the total flexor pattern, with the foot supinated. Many patients are unable to transfer weight correctly, diagonally forwards, over the sound side, and attempt to move the hemiplegic leg while it is still bearing some of their weight. In preparation for the swing phase of walking, the therapist includes activities aimed at enabling the patient to stand on his sound leg and teaching him to move his hemiplegic leg selectively when the foot leaves the floor.

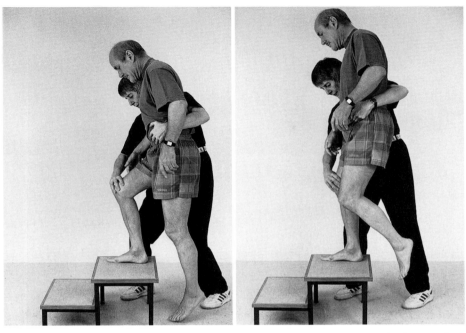

a   b

Fig. 6.34 a, b. Stepping up onto a higher step with weight on the hemiplegic leg. **a** The therapist facilitates the forward movement of the knee. **b** Delaying placing the sound foot on the step demands increased extensor activity (right hemiplegia)

Releasing the Hip and Knee

The patient stands with his feet together and lets the hip and knee of his hemiplegic leg relax and fall forwards. The pelvis relaxes downwards and forwards at the same time. The therapist, kneeling in front of the patient, facilitates the movement, with one hand guiding the pelvis forwards and downwards while her other hand draws the knee forwards from the front (**Fig. 6.35 a**). If her hand pushes behind his knee it might stimulate his pushing back against her hand. The patient carries out the same activity with his hemiplegic foot placed behind him, as it would be at the initiation of the swing phase in walking. The movement is more difficult in this position, as with the hip in extension, extensor hypertonus in the whole leg is increased. When the knee and hip fall forwards now, the heel must leave the floor, and the therapist helps to prevent the foot pushing into inversion as it does so, asking the patient to let his heel fall inwards (**Fig. 6.35 b**). As the knee flexes, the leg tends to abduct in the total flexor pattern, and the patient should try to let the knee relax medially towards his other knee. Because the coordination between the two sides is often difficult, most patients bend both knees in order to allow flexion of their hemiplegic knee. If the patient is unable to prevent the simultaneous flexion of his sound leg, the therapist can sit on a stool and block his unaffected knee with her knee, while facilitating the flexion movement of the affected leg with her hand (**Fig. 6.36**). When she feels that his sound leg is remaining in extension, she gradually withdraws her supporting knee.

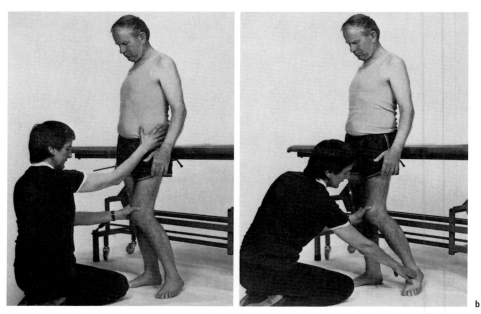

a   b

Fig. 6.35 a, b. Standing with the weight on the sound side and relaxing the extensors of the hemiplegic leg (left hemiplegia). **a** With the feet parallel the activity is easier, as there is less extensor hypertonus. **b** With the hemiplegic foot behind, as in walking, extensor hypertonicity increases in the whole limb. The therapist prevents the foot from pushing into plantar inversion

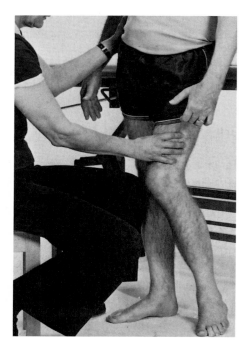

Fig. 6.36. Preventing the sound leg from flexing simultaneously as the hemiplegic leg relaxes (left hemiplegia)

Taking Steps Backwards with the Hemiplegic Leg

The ability to walk backwards is necessary for many functions, for example moving to sit down in a chair, or moving out of the way when a door opens or when other people approach at speed. Being able to take quick steps backwards is also most important for maintaining or regaining balance and preventing falling in normal life. Practising the movement teaches the patient to move his hemiplegic leg selectively and to transfer his weight fully over the sound leg, both of which will also improve the way in which he walks forwards. The patient stands with his weight on the unaffected side and takes a succession of small steps backwards with the hemiplegic leg. The therapist kneels at his hemiplegic side and, with one hand on his iliac crest, prevents him from hitching his pelvis up as he would otherwise do, using the total extension pattern to move his leg back instead of flexing his knee. With her other hand the therapist holds his toes and foot in dorsiflexion and facilitates the normal action of taking a step backwards, i.e. with the knee flexing actively while the hip extends (**Fig. 6.37**). If the therapist is unable to guide the leg in a normal pattern of movement because there is too much resistance, the patient supports himself lightly with his sound hand on a plinth and she asks him to do nothing at all except allow her to move his leg. She then moves the leg in the correct movement pattern, taking very small steps backwards one after the other with his foot touching the floor lightly each time, so that he can feel what should hap-

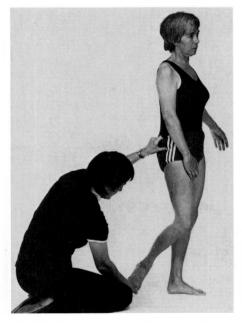

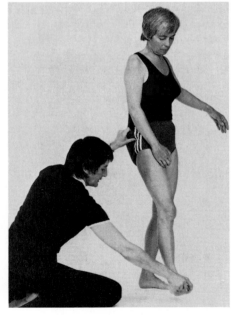

Fig. 6.37. Small steps back with the hemiplegic foot. The patient does not hitch the side of her pelvis up or move it backwards (right hemiplegia)

Fig. 6.38. Swinging the hemiplegic foot forwards like a pendulum, without lifting the leg actively (right hemiplegia)

pen. When she feels there is no longer any resistance, she gives him the feedback that the movement is now correct and asks him to move his leg actively with her. When the foot is behind him, the patient is asked to leave it there, without pushing against the floor. The therapist then guides the foot forwards like a pendulum, as in normal walking **(Fig. 6.38)**. She does not ask the patient to take small steps when he brings the leg forwards, as this would encourage active hip and knee flexion, which is not a part of the normal pattern. Once he has learnt to carry out the whole activity he must also try to do so without supporting himself with his hand. When the patient can take steps backwards in this way, the therapist stands up and facilitates automatic steps backwards with her hands on either side of his pelvis (see Chap. 9).

Placing the Hemiplegic Leg

In order to take a free normal step forwards with his affected leg, the patient needs to be able to stand on his sound leg without the hemiplegic leg participating in maintaining balance. The patient stands with his back to a high plinth and maintains his balance while allowing the therapist to move his hemiplegic leg freely in the air. He then actively controls the leg using eccentric activity of his hip flexors as she guides his foot gradually downwards, until it can rest on the floor without taking any weight **(Fig. 6.39)**. Placing the patient's leg while he is standing erect is much more difficult for him than when he is lying down because he has to hold himself upright against gravity, and extensor tone in the leg is therefore increased. He also has to stabilise his trunk, whereas in lying his spine is totally supported by the plinth.

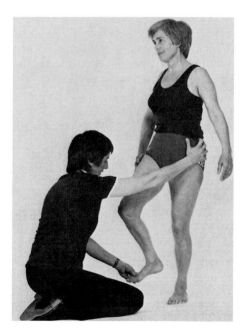

Fig. 6.39. Standing on the sound leg, the patient holds her hemiplegic leg actively throughout range until it rests on the floor (right hemiplegia)

Extensor spasticity in the entire leg increases still more when the leg is behind the patient with the hip extended. To inhibit the hypertonicity and also to give the patient the ability to stand easily on the sound leg, the therapist stands behind him with one arm supporting his body and flexes his knee by lifting his foot up. She holds his lower leg between her knees, using her hands to help him to keep his pelvis level and to let his thigh drop down towards the other knee (Fig. 6.40 a). When she feels that the affected leg is no longer pulling up with flexion of the hip or pushing down into extension, she lowers the foot slowly to the floor. The patient concentrates on not pushing his foot downwards and tries instead to let his toes just rest lightly on the floor behind him (Fig. 6.40 b).

Allowing the Leg to Be Drawn Forwards Passively

The patient's hemiplegic foot is placed on a broad bandage and, while he tries to inhibit activity in his whole leg, the therapist draws his foot forwards with the bandage. The movement is that of the swing phase of walking; it improves the release of the hip and knee behind and facilitates the knee extension in front. Because the patient is trying to remain inactive, the foot is not pulled into supination by the overactivity of the anterior

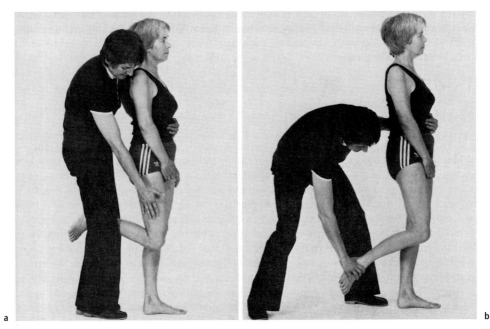

a   b

Fig. 6.40 a, b. Inhibition of extensor hypertonicity with the patient standing on the sound leg (right hemiplegia). **a** Standing behind the patient, the therapist clasps the patient's hemiplegic leg between her knees so that the knee is kept flexed despite hip extension. **b** When the hemiplegic leg is relaxed the therapist lowers the foot slowly to the ground. The patient concentrates on not letting the leg push into extension

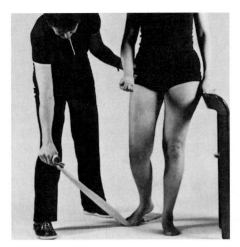

Fig. 6.41. Relaxing the hemiplegic leg and allowing the foot to be drawn forwards on a bandage without resisting the movement (right hemiplegia)

tibial muscle as the leg comes forwards. Such relaxation of the leg muscles is necessary for the swing, and the patient may need to hold lightly on to the back of a chair for support at first in order to allow his leg to relax sufficiently **(Fig. 6.41).** Later, he must also learn to relax his leg without holding on to anything, as he will need to in order to walk freely without a cane.

Considerations

When the patient has reached the stage of moving about independently, he will become increasingly spastic if he does not move selectively and without effort. His learning to move without using the primitive mass synergies requires an enormous amount of concentration and exactness from both therapist and patient. The therapist must know the exact pattern of each normal movement sequence before she can help the patient to avoid using only the stereotyped abnormal synergies when he moves. It is not practising walking per se that will improve walking, but rather the regaining of the missing components. The selective movements required for the stance and swing phases, which include the dynamic stabilisation of the trunk, need to be worked on intensively during therapy. The same principles apply to regaining or improving functional use of the patient's upper limb "The ability to control the body's position in space is essential to being able to move one part of the body, in this case the arms, without destabilizing the rest of the body" (Shumway-Cook and Woollacott 1995). In addition, regaining selective movements of the arm is equally important because, "Functional performance in the arm is most closely associated with the ability to move in space. Arm movements in space are complex movements that rely on well coordinated and calibrated movements of the shoulder, elbow, forearm and wrist to position the hand efficiently for function" (Ryerson and Levit 1997). These authors also emphasise important role of the trunk in the reeducation of arm movements. "Since changes in trunk alignment and loss of trunk movement control interfere with arm function in the upright positions, they have to be addressed as part of the rehabilitation of the hemiplegic arm."

The success of the activities described in this chapter is entirely dependent upon the exactness with which each is performed and upon the patient not using excessive effort. The more a patient struggles desperately to perform an activity which is beyond his capability and with too little assistance being given, the greater is the risk that he will use compensatory mechanisms to carry out the therapist's instructions, with tone increasing as a result. "Pathological influences will generate unwanted programs, leading to abnormal postures and limited movement capability. Just as repetition of good programs leads to good results, repetition of poor programs leads to bad results and the need to 'unlearn' them" (Brooks 1986). The therapist must therefore observe carefully, modify her voice and the words she uses when giving instructions or feedback, and always provide adequate support with her hands and other parts of her body to enable the patient to succeed without the need for such compensatory or alternative movements.

7 Retraining Balance Reactions in Sitting and Standing

A very important aim of treatment is that the patient may eventually walk in the street again, unafraid and unnoticed by other people. To achieve this aim the patient must be trained to react against gravity in all positions, quickly and automatically. He will also need to regain some form of protective or saving reaction so that he can save himself from falling, should he lose his balance.

Adequate balance is necessary, not only for walking but also for every activity the patient carries out during his waking hours. The ability to maintain equilibrium in a great variety of positions provides the basis for all the skilled movements that are required for self-care, work and enjoyment. The longer the period of immobilisation in bed after onset of stroke, during which the patient is totally supported and does not have to react to gravity at all, the more will be his fear when he is brought to the upright position later. Therefore, from the earliest opportunity, preferably within the first week, the patient should be helped out of bed and become used to being moved away from the midline, in all directions. He must also be taught how to return to the vertical position again. Maximum care must be taken that he does not fall over when he is still incapable of saving himself, because such a frightening experience will certainly increase his anxiety. In addition, fractures of the upper or lower limbs sustained during falls not only lengthen the duration of rehabilitation considerably but may compromise the outcome significantly. The patient must therefore never be left alone when he is sitting unsupported, even for a short time, while the nurse or therapist goes to fetch something, answer the telephone or speak to another patient or colleague. The need for extreme care is certainly emphasised by the disturbing numbers of falls experienced by stroke patients. In a study investigating the incidence, characteristics and consequences of falls in an inpatient stroke rehabilitation setting revealed that most occurred when the patient was sitting or during transfers. Of the 161 patients studied, 62 suffered falls. "The total number of falls was 153, which corresponds to an incidence of 159 falls per 10,000 patient-days" (Nyburg and Gustafson 1995).

Right from the start the therapist includes specific activities in the treatment aimed at regaining lost balance reactions. Not only will the activities enable the patient to maintain his balance safely in every situation, but, if performed accurately, they also provide an excellent way of retraining selective activity in his trunk and limbs.

Activities in Sitting

The following activities can be carried out with the patient sitting on the edge of his bed or on a plinth in the physiotherapy department and later in a chair. If balance reactions are retaught in sitting, with the feet unsupported at first, more activity in the head and trunk is stimulated. With the feet on the floor, the sound leg overreacts and prevents or alters normal reactions in other parts of the body. It is important, however, to train the reactions with the feet supported on the floor as well, because that is the position in which we normally need to maintain our balance in daily life.

Activities aimed at transferring the weight sideways should be practised towards both sides. Most patients, if untrained, are not able to transfer weight correctly over to their sound side either, and can do so only by supporting themselves with their unaffected hand. The same activities are also useful for patients in later stages of their rehabilitation when the reactions are still inadequate or too slow. The amount of support given is reduced and the speed increased as the patient's ability improves.

Moving to Elbow Support Sideways

The patient leans over until his elbow is in contact with the plinth, then brings himself up to sitting again. The therapist facilitates the movement by standing in front of the patient and supporting his uppermost shoulder with her forearm. Her other hand guides the patient's hand or arm in such a way that his elbow reaches the plinth first (**Fig. 7.1 a**). By pressing down on his shoulder with her forearm she facilitates the head-righting reaction. When the patient comes up from the sound side, the therapist holds his unaffected hand lightly from above so that he does not push off with it, and his hemiplegic side has to work actively instead (**Fig. 7.1 b**).

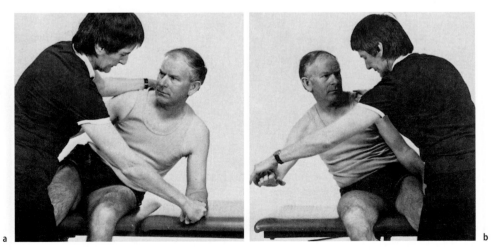

a   b

Fig. 7.1 a, b. Sitting, moving to elbow support sideways (left hemiplegia). **a** To the hemiplegic side; **b** to the sound side. The patient does not use his hand to return to the upright position

Transferring the Weight Sideways

The therapist's facilitation of the correct activity differs considerably according to which side the patient is moving. However, whether weight is being transferred to the left or right, his trunk should remain upright and his shoulders be on the same level and in line with one another. Furthermore, as is the case in the normal balance reaction, the pelvis and the shoulder girdle should remain parallel to one another, neither side rotating backwards or forwards (see Chap. 2).

■ **Towards the Hemiplegic Side.** The therapist sits on the patient's affected side and brings his weight over towards her. That side of his trunk should not shorten as it often tends to do, so her hand in his axilla prevents a downward movement of his shoulder girdle. There are three possible reasons why the trunk shortens on the hemiplegic side, and the therapist should analyse which one is causing the problem for the individual patient. Most commonly, the shoulder girdle on the sound side is elevated hyperactively by the patient in his attempt to maintain an upright position, and the impaired shoulder therefore moves downwards. It may be that the elevators of the shoulder girdle are hypotonic and inactive on the affected side and the shoulder sinks down as a result. Another possibility is that the patient leans over to the side instead of actually transferring his weight, which he may not feel secure enough to do. To facilitate the correct movement of the sound side, the therapist places her other hand over the side flexors to stimulate their contraction as she draws the patient towards her (**Fig. 7.2 a**). Before the patient is able to move freely and safely to the impaired side, the therapist should never pull on his hemiplegic arm, as the shoulder is easily traumatised, particularly in abduction.

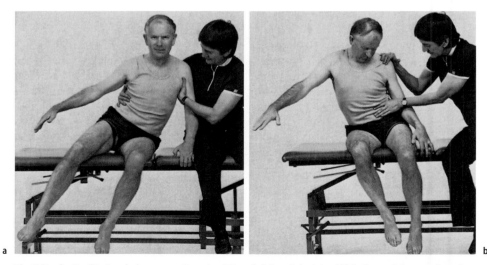

a   b

Fig. 7.2 a, b. Facilitating balance reactions in sitting (left hemiplegia). **a** With the weight transferred to the hemiplegic side; the therapist prevents the hemiplegic side from shortening. **b** With the weight transferred to the sound side; the therapist stimulates the activity of the trunk side-flexors

The movement is repeated, and the patient starts participating more and more actively. The therapist can ask him to hold the position and stay there while she reduces her support, or to move into the correct position without her assistance.

■ **Towards the Sound Side.** When the patient transfers his weight over the sound side, an active shortening of the hemiplegic side with the head righting to vertical is required to hold the body against gravity. Using the web of her hand, the therapist applies firm pressure to the trunk side flexors to stimulate their activity. With her other hand she presses down on his shoulder to facilitate the righting reaction of the head and to prevent the shoulder girdle from being pulled upwards as the patient moves his weight sideways (**Fig. 7.2 b**). The therapist asks him not to support himself with his sound hand, but to reach out with his hand in line with his body instead. As the patient's ability improves, the therapist once again reduces the amount of support she is giving and the patient participates more actively.

Progressing with the Activity to Include All Components of the Balance Reaction

Once the correct activity in the trunk is occurring spontaneously and the patient can transfer his weight freely and confidently to both sides, the range of movement is increased. The patient moves further and further sideways and the therapist facilitates the normal reactions of the head, trunk and limbs.

■ **Moving Far Over the Hemiplegic Side.** The therapist stands up and cradles the patient's arm against her body, holding it in place with her arm. Her hand supports the humerus from below to ensure the correct alignment of the glenohumeral joint and prevent any trauma to his shoulder. The patient then transfers his weight well over to the hemiplegic side. When he is sufficiently far over the supporting hip his other leg should lift reactively off the plinth, his hip flexors and abductors and his knee extensors holding the leg in the air. At first the therapist will need to ask the patient to lift his leg up or guide it into position with her free hand (**Fig. 7.3 a**). Unless he receives careful training, the patient invariably uses typical compensatory movements when his weight shifts over the affected hip, the most common being those which can be seen in **Fig. 7.3 a**:

- The patient's thorax is translated laterally to the supporting side, without an isometric contraction of the abdominal muscles on that side to hold the ribs down in place. Their activity is also required to provide a stable anchorage for the muscles of the opposite side, which have to hold the body against the pull of gravity (Davies 1990).
- His hemiplegic knee flexes involuntarily so that the foot is drawn back underneath the plinth.
- The weight-bearing hip remains in some degree of medial rotation, which prevents the weight from being transferred fully over that side.
- The sound leg does not lift spontaneously into the air; instead, the patient uses it to hold on to the plinth by flexing his knee.
- The shoulder girdle on the sound side elevates, so preventing the side of the trunk from shortening.

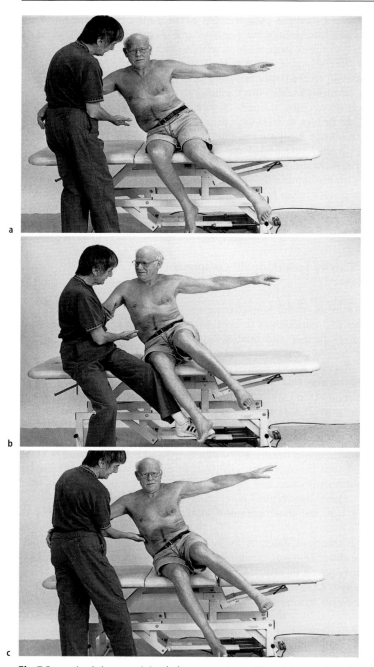

Fig. 7.3 a–c. In sitting, retraining balance reactions with weight transferred far over the hemiplegic side (right hemiplegia). **a** Difficulties most frequently encountered in treatment. **b** With her toes beneath the patient's heel, the therapist facilitates knee extension and lateral rotation of the hip. **c** The therapist corrects any remaining difficulties, e.g. inadequate contraction of the abdominal muscles

The therapist needs to observe and analyse the reactions of the patient's whole body carefully and then strive to eliminate any such compensatory movements by facilitating the normal components of the reaction appropriately. Following is a way in which balance reactions have been retrained successfully with many patients: Supporting herself against the plinth behind her, the therapist places the foot nearest to the patient underneath his heel. As he transfers his weight towards her, she guides his hip out of the medial rotation by moving his foot medially with hers. At the same time she prevents his knee from being pulled into flexion, and with a slight pressure upwards under his heel she assists the necessary extension for the supporting side (**Fig. 7.3 b**). With the fingers of her free hand she indicates to the patient that he should tense the muscles in the region of his waist and move his lower ribs away from her. The movement sideways is repeated several times, and when the therapist feels with her foot that the patient's leg is no longer resisting the corrected components of movement, she gradually takes her foot away from his heel. She then stands up again and asks the patient to repeat the activity, using her hands to assist whichever part he still has difficulty in controlling adequately on his own, for example, the tensing of the abdominal muscles on the hemiplegic side (**Fig. 7.3 c**).

■ **Moving Far Over the Sound Side.** The typical difficulties encountered by the patient when he transfers his weight right over the sound side must also be analysed and overcome (**Fig. 7.4 a**):

- The trunk side flexors on the hemiplegic side do not shorten to hold the body up against gravity, and the shoulder girdle elevates.
- The hemiplegic leg does not lift off the bed reactively.
- The arm does not abduct in extension.

To facilitate the normal balance reactions, the therapist sits on the plinth beside the patient, on his impaired side. She places one hand on top of his shoulder and the other over the patient's lower ribs and trunk side flexors, in such a way that the web between her thumb and index finger is against his side. She asks him to move away from her and presses down on his shoulder to prevent the shoulder girdle from elevating. At the same time she applies pressure with the web of her lower hand to assist the side flexion of his trunk and stimulate activity in the abdominal muscles on that side (**Fig. 7.4 b**).The therapist should not instruct the patient to lift his hemiplegic leg into the air at this stage, because before he has regained sufficient control of hip and trunk, he will be obliged to use compensatory movements. Typically, with enormous effort, the patient flexes his whole trunk and lifts the lower limb in the total flexion pattern. The pelvis retracts and tone increases as a result. Instead, the movement to the sound side should be practised meticulously until the patient can activate the side-flexors of his trunk adequately. Only when he can transfer his weight far enough over the sound side with ease does the therapist help him to lift the leg off the plinth or give him a verbal command to do so himself. She uses words which inhibit hyperactivity, for example, asking him to "just let it float into the air" and "just let it stay up there". Even when the patient's leg is lifting reactively without her assistance, the therapist may still need to facilitate the action of the trunk and position of the shoulder girdle (**Fig. 7.4 c**). She must be sure that her position allows the patient to move far enough over to the side before his leg lifts. As was the case when the patient moved towards his hemiplegic side, the therapist once again gradually reduces the amount of help she is giving and increases the speed of the move-

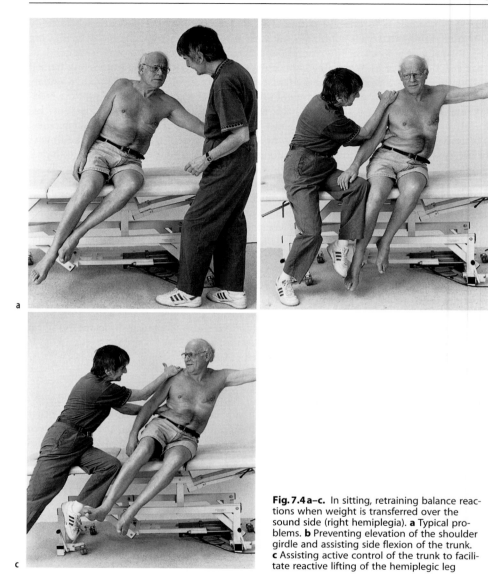

a

b

c

Fig. 7.4 a–c. In sitting, retraining balance reactions when weight is transferred over the sound side (right hemiplegia). **a** Typical problems. **b** Preventing elevation of the shoulder girdle and assisting side flexion of the trunk. **c** Assisting active control of the trunk to facilitate reactive lifting of the hemiplegic leg

ment. She also makes unexpected changes in direction, not always moving him several times in exactly the same way to one side before practising towards the other as if it were a separate exercise. The balance reactions need to become quick and automatic if they are to prevent his falling.

Sitting with Legs Crossed – Weight Transference Towards the Side of the Underneath Leg

The patient requires stable balance when sitting with one leg crossed over the other, as he will need to use the position when putting on his trousers, socks and shoes. The activity is important for retraining the selective lateral flexion of the lumbar spine with

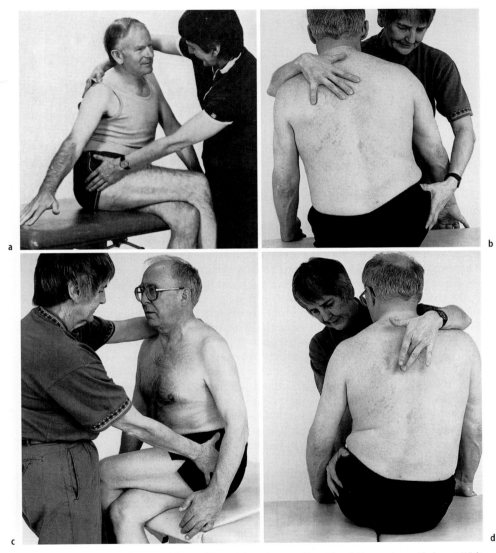

Fig. 7.5 a–e. Sitting with crossed legs with weight taken on the side of the underneath leg. **a** With weight on the hemiplegic side the righting reaction of the head is facilitated. **b** Helping the patient to lift his sound buttock off the plinth. **c** Keeping the hemiplegic leg in place. **d** Stabilising the thoracic spine and lifting the affected buttock (left hemiplegia)

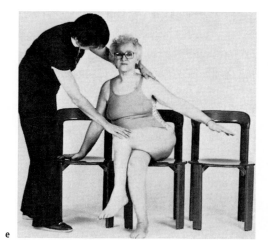

Fig. 7.5 e. With the hemiplegic foot on the floor lifting up the sound buttock (right hemiplegia)

the thorax stabilised, so necessary for walking. It also facilitates selective extension with outward rotation of the leg over which the weight is being transferred The patient transfers his weight towards the side of the underneath leg and lifts the contralateral buttock off the supporting surface, with lateral flexion of the lumbar spine. His shoulders remain on the same level with his thoracic spine extended and vertical to the ground. There should be no necessity for overt balance reactions of the head or arms, and the movement should be performed rhythmically and fluently, without undue effort.

To facilitate the correct movement with weight taken on the hemiplegic side, the therapist first helps the patient to bring his impaired foot into the midline, an adjustment which is normally made automatically before one leg is crossed over the other. She holds it in place while he lifts his other leg to place the sound knee over the other one. Standing in front of the patient, the therapist places her arm over the top of his shoulder, in such a way that the crook of her elbow can facilitate the head-righting position (**Fig. 7.5 a**). Her hand rests on his thoracic spine so that her fingers can stimulate its extension. Her other hand under the trochanter on the opposite side assists with weight transference and helps the patient to lift his buttock off the plinth (**Fig. 7.5 b**). She asks the patient to repeat the movement and to try not to press his head against her arm. She later withdraws her support gradually until he can reproduce the movement correctly on his own.

To facilitate the correct movements when the patient is transferring his weight to the unaffected side the therapist helps the patient to lift his hemiplegic leg and cross it over the sound one. The leg will often keep sliding off the sound knee due to the retraction of the pelvis and the hypertonicity in certain muscle groups. The therapist will then need to hold it in place with her thigh at first (**Fig. 7.5 c**). With the fingers of one hand the therapist stimulates extension of the thoracic spine while her other hand helps the patient to lift his buttock off the plinth (**Fig. 7.5 d**). As the patient moves over the side and back again, she will feel the resistance in his leg gradually decreasing until it can remain in place when she withdraws her supporting thigh.

Once the activity is possible with the patient's feet in the air, it should also be practised towards both sides with the foot of the underneath leg placed flat on the floor. If the height of the bed or the plinth is not adjustable, the patient sits on a chair with an additional chair on either side of him (Fig. 7.5 e). The chair at the side gives the patient a feeling of security and can also be used for activities to practise weightbearing through the hemiplegic arm.

Reaching Forwards to Touch the Floor

Many patients are afraid to lean forwards if there is nothing in front of them even when sitting with both feet on the floor. Before the patient can attempt to transfer his weight forwards actively he must be helped to overcome his anxiety and be able to lean down easily and confidently in different positions. The movement is necessary for many functional tasks, and certainly it is a prerequisite for his learning to stand up from sitting in a normal way again. To facilitate the movement the therapist kneels down right in front of the patient, whose feet are supported on the floor. She guides his hands forwards to touch his toes, making him aware that his hemiplegic hand must arrive first (Fig. 7.6 a). Both the patient's feet should stay flat on the floor without pushing, an activity which often requires careful progression. At first he should move only so far forwards that he is able to return to sitting upright without his heels coming off the floor. The activity is practised until the patient's hands can be placed flat on the floor. He should learn to relax his neck, trunk and arms completely even when the therapist is helping him to sway gently from side to side (Fig. 7.6 b).

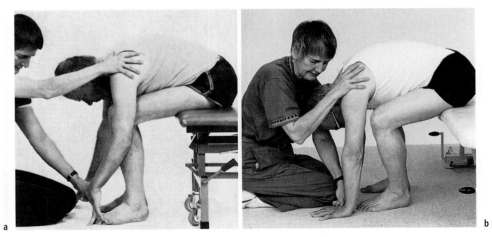

a   b

Fig. 7.6 a, b. Sitting, bending forwards (left hemiplegia). **a** The patient touches his toes without his heels lifting off the floor. **b** Placing both hands flat on the floor

Reaching Forwards with Clasped Hands and Trunk Extended

The patient stretches his clasped hands forwards and in all directions, while his feet remain flat on the floor, at first with the therapist supporting the hemiplegic knee. Interest and automatic reactions can be stimulated by letting him push a ball away in various directions or by hitting a balloon to another person.

Activities in Standing with the Weight on Both Legs

Shifting Weight from Side to Side with Both Knees Flexed

Standing upright but with his hips and knees slightly flexed, the patient transfers his weight from one side to the other, rotating his body as if he were skiing. His arms swing relaxed at his side. The therapist facilitates the movement with her hands on either side of his pelvis, keeping the supporting hip forward each time and assisting the rotation of his body (Fig. 7.7 a).

Pushing a Ball Away with Clasped Hands

Patients are often afraid of bringing their weight forwards, but when concentrating on an activity such as pushing a ball away, they do so spontaneously. The therapist facili-

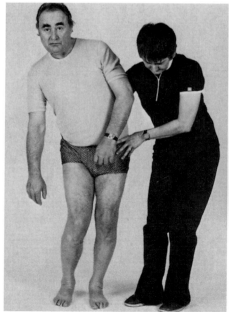

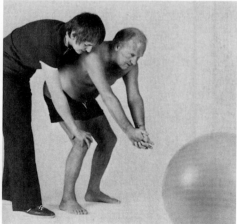

a

b

Fig. 7.7 a, b. Shifting weight in standing. **a** From side to side with both knees flexed (left hemiplegia). **b** Leaning forwards to push a ball away

tates the movement with her hands on either side of the pelvis, steadying the patient while keeping his weight over both legs (**Fig. 7.7 b**). The activity can also be practised while he is standing with one foot in front of the other, to encourage balancing with a narrower base of support and the weight moving forwards over one leg.

Playing with a Balloon

The patient plays with a balloon, hitting it away or tapping it repeatedly into the air with his clasped hands or with his hemiplegic hand on its own. As balance and the ability to take steps improve, he can be encouraged to step forwards while he keeps the balloon up in the air (**see Fig. 8.11 d**).

Being Tipped Backwards

The patient must relearn the normal balance reactions that should take place when weight is displaced behind the line of gravity. At first the therapist gives him total support, as she draws his body backwards and guides the forward movement of his trunk and arms. Without careful training, the patient's hips continue to extend when he is off balance, and with no hip flexion to bring his trunk forwards as a counterweight he will be in constant danger of falling over backwards. The correct movement is facilitated, slowly at first, with the patient voluntarily correcting the position of his head, trunk and arms. The speed is later increased until the reaction occurs automatically, even when the therapist suddenly shifts the patient backwards from the pelvis without giving him any warning (**Fig. 7.8**). Because dorsal extension of the feet is a normal component of the balance reaction, the movement is also useful for stimulating the activity in the hemiplegic foot.

Activities in Standing with the Weight on the Hemiplegic Leg

If the patient is to walk confidently without support, he needs to be able to bear weight on the hemiplegic leg without fear of losing his balance. Taking weight through the leg makes him aware of it, improves sensation and normalises tone. The hip should remain extended, and at no time should the affected knee hyperextend.

Hyperextension of the knee may be caused by the retraction of the pelvis on the hemiplegic side, insufficient active hip extension or exaggerated plantar flexion of the ankle, pushing the tibia backwards. The leg becomes a rigid pillar as a result, all the muscle activity being in the total pattern of extension. Because the support is then static, it makes normal dynamic balance reactions impossible, and to take a quick step with that leg to regain balance is difficult if not impossible.

During weight-bearing activities with all the weight taken on the hemiplegic leg, the therapist helps the patient to prevent his knee from hyperextending by assisting hip extension with outward rotation and by moving his pelvis forwards over his foot. One way in which she can achieve the correct alignment of the supporting limb is by placing her

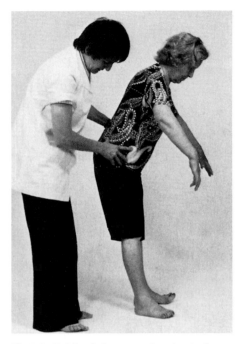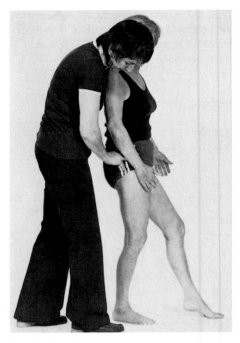

Fig. 7.8. Training balance reactions by tipping the patient backwards while she is standing (right hemiplegia)

Fig. 7.9. Standing on the hemiplegic leg, taking steps forwards and backwards with the other foot. The therapist facilitates hip extension (right hemiplegia)

thumb on the head of the femur from behind and easing it forwards and outwards over the long axis of the patient's foot.

1. Standing with his weight on the hemiplegic leg, the patient takes small steps forwards and backwards with his other foot, and also to the side. He does not transfer his weight immediately onto the sound leg, but remains steadily on the hemiplegic leg (**Fig. 7.9**). To add interest to the activity, the patient can be asked to write numbers or different letters on the floor with his sound foot.

2. The patient places his sound foot on a small step in front of him. He puts it slowly and carefully on the step, without rushing or banging it down (**Fig. 7.10 a**). While balancing on the hemiplegic leg he can tap the sound foot lightly and rhythmically on the step, later tapping his foot first to one side and then to the other as his control improves.

   By raising the height of the step far greater activity in the hip extensors is demanded, particularly if the whole foot is placed flat on the step and not just the forefoot (**Fig. 7.10 b**). The therapist will often need to help the patient to stabilise his thorax to facilitate the abdominal muscle activity which is now required. She places one of her hands over the lower end of his sternum and her other over his thoracic spine at about the level of the 10th thoracic vertebra. She then asks the patient to lift his sound foot and hold it in position directly above the step for a moment before re-

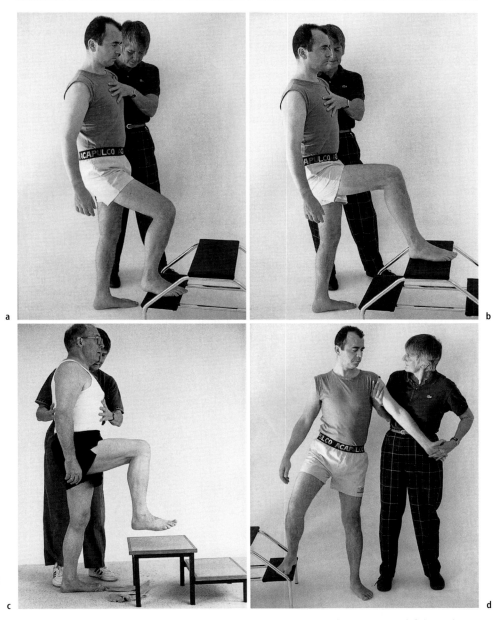

Fig. 7.10 a–d. Standing on the hemiplegic leg and placing the sound foot on a step (left hemiplegia). **a** With the step in front, the therapist stabilises the patient's thorax. **b** The height of the step increased. **c** Holding the foot directly above the step. **d** With the step at the side

placing it again, which requires still more activity from both the abdominals and the hip extensors (**Fig. 7.10 c**). He repeats the lifting and replacing movement several times before putting his foot down on the floor (**Fig. 7.10 c**).

3. By placing the small step to the sound side of the patient, activity in the abductors can be stimulated with improved control of extension of the hemiplegic hip. He places his foot on the step without transferring his weight away from the affected leg (**Fig. 7.10 d**). Still more activity is demanded from the working muscles if the patient places his whole foot flat on the step and parallel to its edge instead of just touching it with his toes.

4. The patient places his sound foot on a scale, which can be placed in different positions in front or to the side of him. He tries to reduce the registered weight until he can achieve zero from the moment his foot touches the scale (**Fig. 7.11**).

5. Standing with his weight over the hemiplegic leg, the patient moves or kicks a football with his other foot. He kicks the ball against a wall or to another person, but only so vigorously that he is still able to control the hemiplegic leg and prevent it from pushing into the total extension pattern. Kicking the ball with the medial border of his foot will improve selective extension with outward rotation of the weight-bearing hip (**Fig. 7.12 a**). If the patient kicks the ball to someone standing on his sound side, he will be extending the supporting hip more selectively because his legs are in abduction (**Fig. 7.12 b**). Kicking the ball to a person standing to his affected side will demand more activity in the abductors of his hip as well as in the invertors of his foot (**Fig. 7.12 c**). In fact, in both cases small equilibrium reactions in the foot may be elicited with intrinsic muscle activity stimulated.

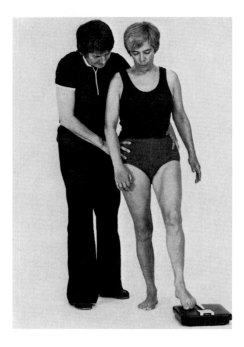

Fig. 7.11. Standing and placing the sound foot gently on a scale (right hemiplegia)

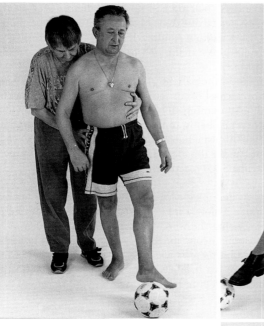

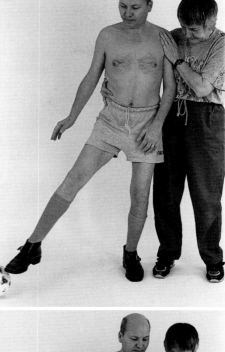

a

b

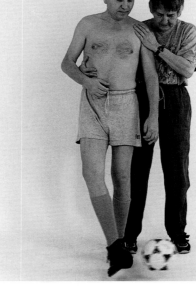

Fig.7.12a–c. Kicking a football with the sound foot (**a**) with the medial border of the foot to improve selective extension of the hemiplegic hip (right hemiplegia); **b** to the sound side, which includes abduction of the supporting hip (left hemiplegia). **c** Kicking to the affected side encourages turning the head to that side and intrinsic muscle activity is stimulated in the weightbearing foot (left hemiplegia)

c

The activities with both the scale and the ball are additionally valuable because they not only retrain weightbearing with selective extension but also encourage the patient to balance on his hemiplegic leg without holding his head in a fixed position to stabilise himself. He automatically looks at the ball to kick it, or at the scale to read the figures.

6. Standing with his back to a high plinth, the patient places his unaffected foot gently on the knee of the therapist, who is kneeling in front of him (**Fig. 7.13 a**). He then puts his foot behind him while still maintaining all his weight forward over the hemiplegic leg. The advantage of the therapist being in this position is that she can assist his hip and knee to encourage dynamic weightbearing as he extends and flexes his knee. She can also place her fingers under the toes of the hemiplegic foot, to prevent them from clawing and to facilitate balance reactions in the foot.

As the patient's ability to balance on his hemiplegic leg improves, the therapist can hold his sound foot with one hand and move it slowly into different positions while the patient adapts accordingly (**Fig. 7.13 b**). During the whole activity the patient's hands are left free and not clasped together, as spontaneous movements may occur while he balances on one leg. It is most important that there is always a table or plinth behind the patient because, should he suddenly lose his balance, from her kneeling position the therapist might otherwise not be able to save him from falling.

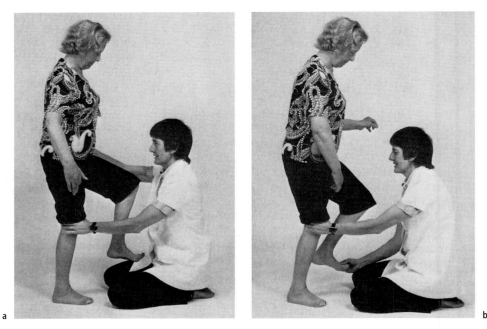

a   b

Fig. 7.13 a, b. Balancing on the hemiplegic leg (right hemiplegia). **a** Placing the sound foot lightly on the therapist's knee. The patient's knee does not hyperextend. **b** The therapist moves the patient's sound foot slowly in different directions

Activities During Which the Weight Is on Alternate Legs

Going Up and Down Stairs

Climbing stairs brings an automatic transference of weight, first over one leg and then over the other. It is a familiar activity for adults and often produces a very normal pattern of movement for the patients. The activity can be used with patients who may still not be able to walk unaided, and their walking improves as a result. The ability to negotiate stairs easily is also an important part of full rehabilitation, as we come across stairs frequently in our daily life. Right from the beginning the patient is helped to go up and down stairs in a normal way, which means that he moves forwards, placing only one foot on each step, and never with both feet coming onto the same step.

The procedure for going up stairs is as follows:

1. The patient holds on to the handrail with his sound hand if he or the therapist feels uncertain in any way. He should be encouraged to hold as lightly as possible and not support his whole forearm on the handrail. The patient transfers his weight over his hemiplegic leg and places his other foot on the first step. To facilitate the normal movement sequence the therapist has the hand furthest from the patient just above his knee, with her thumb and fingers on opposite femoral condyles. Exerting some slight pressure downwards, she draws his knee forwards over his foot as he steps up with his sound leg (**Fig. 7.14 a**).
2. As he transfers his weight well forwards over the sound foot in front, the therapist slides her hand down over his hemiplegic knee as far as the shin, and with a circular motion places that foot up onto the second step (**Fig. 7.14 b**). Most patients require such help at first because, with the hip in extension, extensor tonus throughout the leg is increased and sufficient active flexion of the hip and knee is not possible. The therapist places her arm round behind the patient so that her hand rests on the opposite side of his pelvis. She uses her arm to steady the patient's trunk when his weight is transferred over to the sound leg and his hemiplegic leg is lifted.
3. Immediately when the affected foot is in place, the therapist replaces her hand above the patient's knee, so that she can again help him to move it forwards over the foot as he steps up with the sound leg. At no time does either knee fully extend; instead, a rhythmical cycling-type movement takes place, as in the normal pattern.

As the patient's ability and confidence improve, the activity is carried out with his hands clasped together in front of him (**Fig. 7.14 c**) or, better still, with his arms free at his sides (**Fig. 7.14 d**). When the therapist feels that the patient is actively controlling the movement of his legs, she moves her hands and gives support only on either side of the pelvis. The amount of support is gradually reduced, until finally he is able to manage alone.

For most patients, going down stairs is more difficult than climbing up stairs, particularly when stepping down with the hemiplegic leg. As the leg is brought forwards, it tends to pull strongly into adduction crossing over in front of the other leg, with the foot inverting in the total pattern of extension. The patient is unable to place the foot flat on the next step, or has difficulty in doing so. He may also feel apprehensive, looking down the flight of stairs. The procedure is as follows:

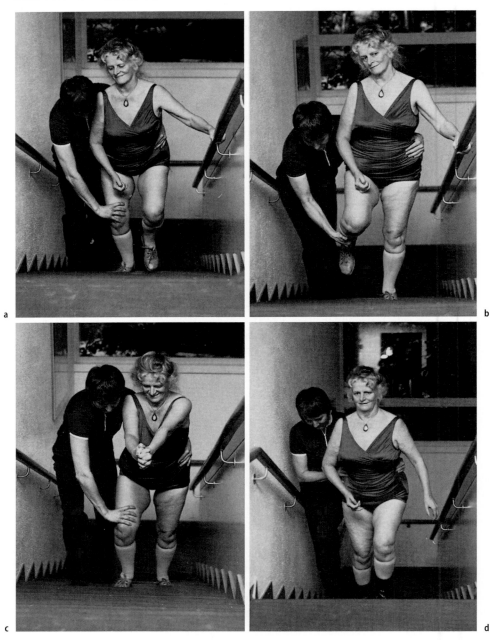

Fig. 7.14 a–d. Going upstairs (right hemiplegia). **a** With the weight on the hemiplegic leg, the patient brings her sound foot to the step above. **b** The therapist slides her hand down over the shin and with a circular motion helps to place the hemiplegic foot on the next step. **c** The therapist draws the patient's knee forwards as she steps up with her sound foot. Feeling more confident, the patient clasps her hands. **d** The patient no longer needs to hold on to the bannister, and the therapist has reduced her support

1. The patient holds the handrail lightly and the therapist, standing at his hemiplegic side, asks him to step down first with his sound leg. To facilitate the normal movement sequence she places the hand furthest from him just above his affected knee and draws the knee forwards into sufficient flexion, with the heel lifting, to enable his other foot to reach the step below (**Fig. 7.15 a**). Her other hand rests on the far side of his pelvis, and her arm around his sacrum helps to bring his hips forwards over the foot in front.
2. The hand on the hemiplegic leg remains in the same position, as the patient brings it forwards. In order for the leg to move, the patient's weight must be transferred over to the sound side, and the therapist uses her shoulder against his thorax to facilitate the necessary weight shift. Her other arm on the far side of his trunk provides stability and enables him to move sufficiently over the sound side. If the hemiplegic leg starts to adduct as it moves downwards, the therapist guides it outwards, and once again uses her other arm from behind to bring his pelvis forwards (**Fig. 7.15 b**).
3. When the patient's foot is correctly placed on the step below, the therapist at once draws his knee forwards to prevent the leg from pushing into total extension as he starts to bear weight on it (**Fig. 7.15 c**). The patient then steps forwards with the sound leg.

The patient must be carefully instructed and encouraged to place only one foot on each step right from the first attempt. Should the inversion of the foot be too difficult to control at first, the foot can be bandaged firmly for protection during early training to give patient and therapist confidence (**Fig. 7.15 d**).

When the patient has learnt the correct movement sequence he no longer needs to hold on to the handrail. As an intermediate stage he can steady himself by placing his sound hand on the wall at his side (**Fig. 7.15 e**). When he feels sufficiently secure he stops using the hand for support, and the therapist facilitates balance and movement from the pelvis. Once again, she gradually withdraws her support until he can go confidently up or down stairs without requiring help at all, which will be important for his life outside the protected environment of the hospital or rehabilitation centre (**see Fig. 9.26**).

Transferring Weight Sideways on a Tilt-Board

The tilt-board can be useful when retraining balance reactions in standing and for teaching the patient to shift his weight from one side to the other confidently. Even patients who are not yet able to walk without assistance learn to transfer their weight correctly as they feel and see the movement of the board, and the controls are very clear. The board tilts sideways until it meets the absolute resistance of the floor. To avoid any anxiety for the patient, the therapist can give him complete support at first by placing both her arms around him, if necessary, and drawing him towards her until he feels more confident. She then gradually withdraws the assistance.

The patient learns to tilt the board from one side to the other while standing with his feet apart and placed parallel to the edges of the board. He steps onto the board with his hemiplegic foot first and the therapist helps him to place it in the correct position. Standing close to him on the affected side, she supports his hip with her hip and stabi-

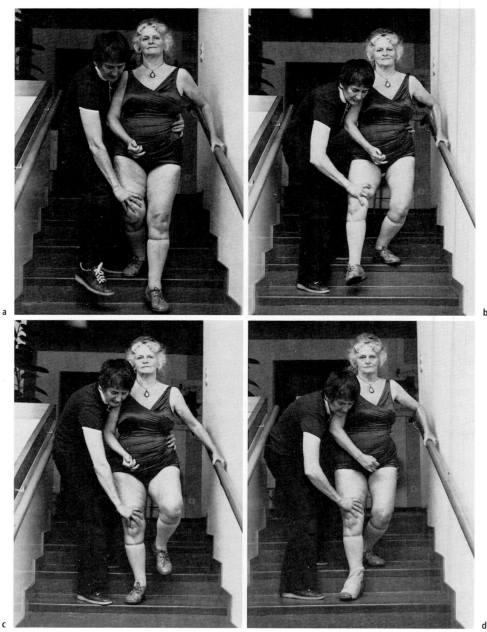

Fig. 7.15a–e. Going downstairs (right hemiplegia). **a** The patient steps down first with her sound foot. The therapist draws the hemiplegic knee forwards. **b** As the patient steps down with her hemiplegic foot the therapist prevents adduction. **c** When the hemiplegic foot is in place the therapist helps the patient to bring her weight forwards without hyperextending the knee. **d** A bandage prevents supination of the foot during early training

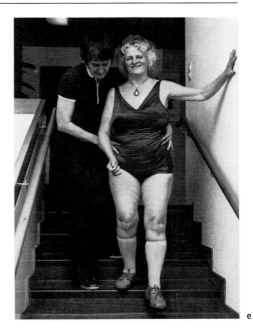

Fig. 7.15 e. The patient steadies herself with the sound hand on the wall as she no longer needs to hold the handrail

e

lises his knee with one hand as he brings his other foot into place (**Fig. 7.16 a**). Once the patient is safely standing on the board, the therapist helps him to stand upright with his weight evenly distributed over both legs and the board level. Still standing at his side, the therapist asks the patient to bring his weight towards her, with his hip moving first, and facilitates the correct movement for him.

With one hand in his axilla she lengthens the hemiplegic side, while with her other hand she shortens the unaffected side (**Fig. 7.16 b**). The patient's arms remain freely at his sides. When he can repeat the movement correctly towards the hemiplegic side, the therapist moves round to his other side and the same sequence is practised in the opposite direction (**Fig. 7.16 c**). Many patients will have just as much difficulty in coming correctly over the unaffected side and will need the ability in order to take an easy step with the hemiplegic leg during the swing phase of walking. When the movement to both sides becomes easier, the therapist can stand behind the patient, making small adjustments to his posture and facilitating the transference of weight from his pelvis (**Fig. 7.16 d**).

Transferring Weight Forwards and Backwards in Step-Standing

Many patients will soon learn to balance when standing with their feet wide apart but will find it difficult to stand with one foot in front of the other in a position similar to that of the mid-stance of walking. The base is much narrower, and far more muscle activity of the trunk and the hip abductors is therefore required. Learning to balance in step-standing will help to retrain activity in these muscles and also enable the patient

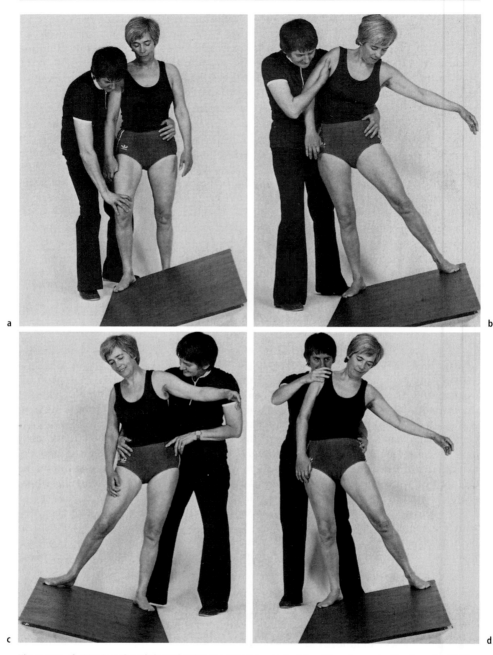

Fig. 7.16 a–d. Moving the tilt-board sideways (right hemiplegia). **a** Stepping onto the board with the hemiplegic foot first. The therapist guides the knee forwards. **b** Transferring weight to the hemiplegic side. The therapist lengthens the side of the trunk, and her hip maintains extension of the patient's hip. **c** Transferring the weight to the sound leg. The therapist has changed her position so that the patient moves towards her. **d** The therapist reduces the amount of support

to walk with a more normal stride width instead of with his feet too far apart as he will otherwise tend to do. In addition, he can practise transferring his weight forwards over the foot in front without using typical compensatory movements or adopting abnormal postures of his trunk.

The patient stands with a wall at his sound side and rests his unimpaired hand on its surface just above shoulder level. The therapist kneels slightly behind him on the hemiplegic side, and he takes a step forwards with his sound foot, placing only his heel on the floor with the ankle held in dorsiflexion (**Fig. 7.17 a**). The therapist encourages him to extend the hip of the weight-bearing leg as he tries to maintain his balance even when lifting his hand slightly away from the wall. His shoulder girdle and pelvis remain parallel to one another with no rotation backwards on either side. Maintaining the position of his trunk, the patient transfers his weight fully over the sound leg in front, trying to use plantar flexion of the hemiplegic foot to push him forwards. Most patients will bend the sound knee so that they can pull themselves forwards with their hamstrings on that side. The therapist therefore instructs the patient to keep his sound leg quite straight during the forward movement while she assists the push-off with the impaired foot (**Fig. 7.17 b**). She supports his heel to prevent the foot from inverting and thus ensures that it remains on line with his other foot. The patient's knee should remain extended, because he has not yet brought all his weight forwards over the leg in front. Only when the therapist has helped him to move his pelvis and everything that is above it over the supporting leg should the knee behind start to flex as it would normally do for the initiation of the swing phase of gait (**Fig 7.17c**). The patient transfers his weight back over the hemiplegic leg again, letting his heel sink down onto the floor with the therapist once more facilitating the movement of the heel as well as the activity of the hip and knee extensors. When the patient has his weight on the hemiplegic leg the foot in front should dorsiflex and only the heel should be on the floor. The movement is repeated back and forth and the patient tries to use his sound arm less and less, until he can take his hand off the wall altogether. Once the patient's foot is no longer pushing strongly into plantar inversion during the push-off phase, the therapist stands up to facilitate the movement forwards, using her foot beneath his to assist the necessary plantar flexion activity. She places her forefoot under his heel, and as he transfers his weight over the foot in front she helps him to lift his heel. With one of her hands on each of his shoulders she stabilises his thorax in extension, adducts his scapulae and can facilitate the forward movement of his whole body over his pelvis (**Fig. 7.17 d, e**).

The activity is also practised with the hemiplegic foot in front and the sound foot remaining behind, parallel to it, without turning outwards. The therapist again kneels beside the patient to assist with the correct positioning of his legs and feet as he transfers his weight forwards. When he brings his weight over the hemiplegic leg, he may have difficulty in controlling the selective extension of his knee. The therapist stimulates the co-contraction of the muscles acting to support his weight by applying pressure, tapping firmly with her hands simultaneously, one hand in front and the other behind his knee. For the best effect she cups her hands and brings them down briskly on to the muscles anterior and posterior to his knee with a firm downward pressure when he has all his weight on that leg (**Fig. 7.18 a, b**).

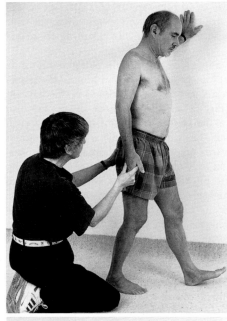
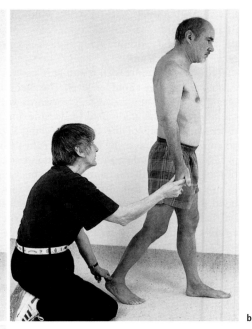

a

b

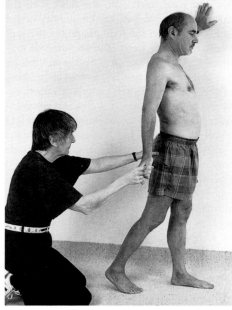

c

Fig. 7.17 a–e. Step-standing with weight transference forwards and backwards (right hemiplegia). **a** Weight back on the hemiplegic leg,
with only the heel of the sound foot on the
floor. **b** Pushing off with the hemiplegic foot.
c Weight right forward over the sound leg.
d, e The therapist's foot under the patient's heel
facilitates push-off to transfer his weight forwards

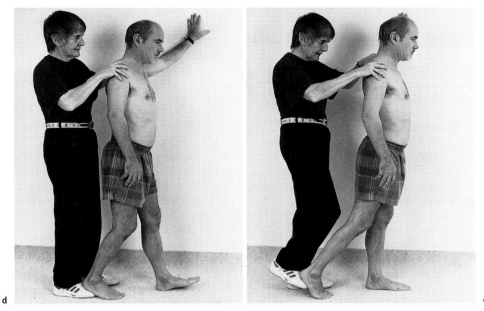

Fig. 7.17 d, e. (Legend see page 190)

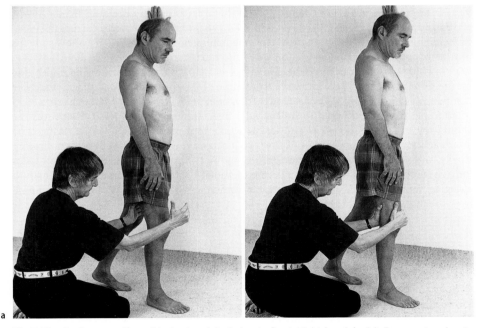

Fig. 7.18 a, b. Step-standing with the hemiplegic leg in front (right hemiplegia). Pressure tapping to stimulate activity in the muscles which stabilise the knee. **a** The patient brings his weight forwards and the therapist holds her hands a slight distance away from his knee, one in front and one behind. **b** She taps her cupped hands firmly down onto the anterior and posterior muscles of the knee

Stepping Sideways with One Leg Crossing Over in Front of the Other

The ability to take protective steps sideways is normally an essential part of our balance and saving mechanism. Practising the activity will also teach the patient how to transfer his weight freely to either side. It is first carried out slowly and correctly with facilitation, and then practised until the patient is able to take rapid automatic steps when he is displaced sideways in either direction.

■ **Moving Towards the Hemiplegic Side.** The patient brings his weight over the affected leg, and steps across in front with the other leg, taking care that his knee does not snap back into hyperextension as he does so. The movement requires considerable adduction of the supporting hip, with the trochanter moving far over the foot and the hemiplegic side elongating. With one hand in the patient's axilla the therapist prevents the side from shortening as he brings his weight well over the affected leg. Her other arm behind him presses down over the pelvis on the opposite side to assist the lateral movement of the trochanter towards the hemiplegic side (**Fig. 7.19 a**).

■ **Moving Towards the Sound Side.** The normal movement sequence is the same but, because of the typical difficulties which most patients experience, the facilitation required is different. When the patient takes a step across sideways with the impaired leg the pelvis retracts, the hip abducts with outward rotation, and the foot supinates as a result of the mass flexion pattern initiated by hip flexion to move the leg at all. The patient needs help to adduct it and to release the whole side in order to place the foot flat on the floor despite the tendency for it to supinate. The therapist assists by pressing firmly downwards and forwards on the iliac crest and then, when the foot is in the correct position, by helping him to transfer his weight over the hemiplegic leg (**Fig. 7.19 b**). She also helps him to maintain hip extension as he takes the next step sideways with the sound leg. Walking sideways with both of the patient's feet being placed accurately behind a line on the floor in front of him increases the degree of control and difficulty. He otherwise compensates by walking sideways along a diagonal path. An unrolled bandage or a strip of adhesive tape can be used to indicate the line. As the patient's ability improves, he should try to take bigger steps and let his whole foot meet the floor at the same time after each step sideways, instead of first the toes and then the rest of the foot following slowly, and put his feet down parallel to one another (**Fig. 7.19 c**). When the patient takes long rhythmic steps to the sound side the therapist's arm against his trunk can help to elongate the side as well as giving him the confidence to transfer his weight far enough over the supporting leg (**Fig. 7.19 d**).

Activities in Standing with the Weight on the Sound Leg

The patient must be able to stand effortlessly on the sound foot with the hemiplegic leg relaxed as a prerequisite for the normal swing phase of walking. To practise the ability the therapist kneels in front of the patient and lifts his affected foot into the air, with increasing rapidity and with less and less warning or preparation. He tries to offer no resistance to the movement of his leg and then to control its descent actively throughout

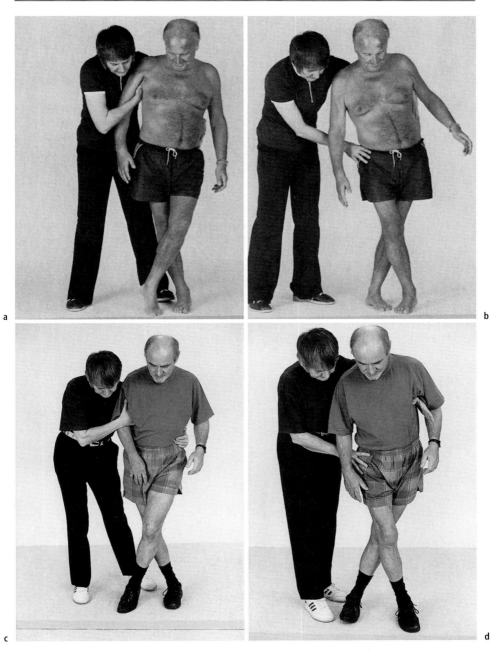

Fig. 7.19 a–d. Walking sideways with one leg crossing in front of the other (right hemiplegia). **a** To the hemiplegic side. The patient steps across with the sound foot without hyperextending his hemiplegic knee. The therapist facilitates the elongation of the side. **b** To the sound side. The therapist assists the forward and downward movement of the pelvis. **c** Moving sideways with the feet always behind a line. **d** Longer steps with the whole foot placed simultaneously on the floor

the range as it is placed down on the floor again. At first there should be a high plinth or table immediately behind the patient for safety reasons, and also so that the activity can be practised while his seat is resting against it until his balance and control of the leg have improved. Finally, the patient should be able to stand erect without the support of the plinth and allow his foot to be lowered right to the floor without its pushing down at all (**Fig. 7.20**).

For the many patients who have difficulty transferring their weight adequately over the sound side in order to leave the hemiplegic leg free to swing forwards, activities in which the hemiplegic foot moves an actual object will often enable him to transfer his weight spontaneously.

Kicking a Football

The ball is placed in front of the patient in such a position that he can step forwards first with his sound leg and then swing his hemiplegic leg forwards to kick the ball. Alternatively, the therapist can help him to place his foot behind him prior to the kick. He should not attempt to kick when his feet are next to each other, as he will then flex his leg actively to do so, instead of swinging it forwards as in walking. Kicking a ball is a very familiar movement, learnt in childhood, and it is amazing how it enables a patient to produce a normal movement, even though he may be unable to move his leg on command (see **Fig. 14.19a, b**). Patients of all ages enjoy the activity enormously.

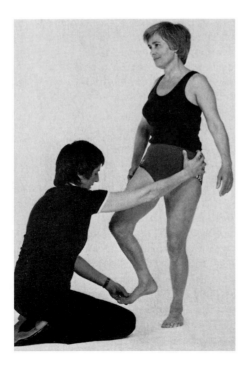

Fig. 7.20. Standing on the sound leg, the patient controls the hemiplegic leg through range without it pushing into extension (right hemiplegia)

Sliding a Towel or Piece of Paper Forward

With his foot placed on a towel the patient slides it forward and is helped to bring it back again. If the movement is difficult for him at first because he pushes against the floor with his foot in the total extension pattern, or because he lifts his foot too high off the towel with total flexion, the therapist teaches him the correct movement by asking him to allow her to carry out the activity for him. The patient rests his foot on the towel, trying to offer no resistance while the therapist pulls the towel gently forwards, his foot remaining in contact with it (**Fig. 7.21**). By feeling the correct movement he learns how to carry it out himself and slowly takes over actively. The same activity can be practised with a piece of firm paper under his foot, which will slide easily on even a carpeted floor.

Considerations

Human beings have an innate fear of falling; this is more marked in some people than in others. That the fear is innate and not due to some psychological predisposition is illustrated by its presence even in the very young baby. During the first 3 months of life, a Moro reflex (McCarthy and Atkinson 1986) or "startle reaction" (Bobath 1974) can be

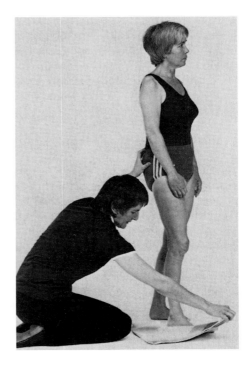

Fig. 7.21. The hemiplegic foot is drawn forwards on a towel while the patient concentrates on giving no resistance to the movement (right hemiplegia)

observed if the supporting surface suddenly moves or if the baby's head is allowed to drop about 10° into extension while it is being held in supine, supported behind the chest and head, using the so-called head-drop method. Through actual experience of falling and suffering pain as a result, some people will learn to fear even more. Many people with disabilities such as hemiplegia will experience such an increased fear, for which they are often mistakenly admonished or even sent to a psychiatrist, although their fear is quite natural and appropriate. In fact, fear of falling is a protective mechanism and will help to prevent the patient from falling and injuring himself.

It is often very difficult for the therapist to understand why a patient is so afraid even though during therapy sessions he appears to have sufficient motor control to maintain his balance. As one young patient exclaimed to her husband after he had chastised her for not walking across an open space similar to that which she had crossed only the day before, "But you don't know what I see and feel!" Most patients, like the one in this example, who experience inordinate and incomprehensible fear suffer from perceptual disturbances which cause the world around them to seem unfamiliar and unstable because the information they receive through the various sensory channels is confusing and contradictory. In addition to such a state of "neural mismatch" (Reason 1978), it is perhaps easier to understand the fear experienced by hemiplegic patients if we consider that usually all or most of the normal reactions for maintaining or regaining balance are reduced, if not absent altogether, unless they are carefully retrained.

To summarise:

1. The head is held in a fixed position by hypertonus, by over-activity on the unaffected side or by a posture which the patient adopts to stabilise himself, and so it cannot move freely to help him to balance.
2. The trunk fails to shorten and lengthen appropriately due to hypertonus or hypotonus and over-activity of the unaffected side.
3. The legs fail to abduct to serve as a counterweight, and the patient is unable to take quick steps to save himself. The hemiplegic leg reacts too slowly, if at all, due to spasticity and/or concomitant weakness, and he is often unable to take a quick step with the sound leg because it would entail bearing weight on the hemiplegic leg, which he is afraid to do.
4. The hemiplegic arm is not able to react either in extension and abduction or in protective extension. Hypertonus pulls it against the patient's side, or hypotonus renders it incapable of springing into action.

The untrained patient is therefore left with only his unaffected hand to help him to maintain his balance, either by holding on to something or by pushing against a supporting surface. When he is standing or walking this means leaning on a stick, and even then he is not protected against falling to the hemiplegic side or backwards. Only a small movement away from the midline would be sufficient to cause him to lose his balance, as the stick will leave the floor.

If the patient is to move freely without fear and walk without a walking stick, his balance reactions must be re-established and some form of protective mechanism made possible. For all the tasks in his daily life he needs to be able to use his unaffected hand functionally, and he cannot do so when he is totally dependent on it for maintaining his balance. It would seem a pity to relegate the patient's one skilled functioning hand solely for the primitive task of maintaining balance. The restoration of balance reactions therefore plays an important role in successful rehabilitation. Even patients who show little return of voluntary muscle activity in the arm and leg can relearn the balance reactions remarkably well and recover the ability to take quick steps to regain balance when standing or walking. Only when balance is adequate will fear disappear.

Another important reason for retraining balance reactions in sitting and standing is that all active movements of the limbs require postural adjustment and preprogrammed reactions to provide "postural stability for the limb directly involved in the primary movement and equilibrium for the head and trunk" (Latash and Anson 1996). As the authors explain,

> "Any voluntary movement is by itself a postural perturbation mostly because of the mechanical coupling of the joints. The transmission of forces and torques from the moving segments through the body's linked segments is the primary reason for postural perturbations. Corrections for postural perturbations induced by a voluntary movement are termed 'anticipatory' if they are released prior to the movement. These corrections represent feedforward postural control associated with the movement control that prevents or alleviates the postural and equilibrium disturbances. They are preprogrammed, triggered internally, and time-locked to the future movement's initiation. Their mechanical effect counteracts the postural disturbance expected from the planned movement."

The anticipatory nature of the corrections for postural perturbations caused by movements of the upper limb is borne out by the findings of Jull (1996), which demonstrated the transversus abdominis muscle acting to stabilise spinal segments even before the arm was actually lifted in abduction by the deltoideus. The restoration of balance reactions is a prerequisite for active motor function of the hemiplegic upper limb, and activities to restore the reactions should be included in the treatment in conjunction with those aimed at retraining selective control of the arm and hand which are described in the following chapter.

8 Encouraging the Return of Activity in the Arm and Hand and Minimising Associated Reactions

In most hospitals and rehabilitation centres emphasis is placed on teaching the patient to walk again and on his becoming independent in the activities of daily living. As a result, his arm and hand often tend to be neglected, without specific treatment aimed at regaining functional activity. The patient becomes more and more skilled in managing all activities with his sound hand, and the full potential in the affected hand may never be fully developed. Even if no activity has appeared in the arm and hand it is important to treat them, as each part of the body affects the other parts. If the arm shows a marked associated reaction, pulling strongly in the spastic pattern of flexion, it will influence how the patient walks, hamper balance reactions and interfere with his ability to perform everyday tasks. Cosmetically, he will be distressed by the constant flexed position of his arm in front of his body which immediately draws attention to his disability.

With regard to improving the different perceptual disturbances which are invariably present to some degree following a lesion of this nature, intensive treatment of the upper limb is crucial. The input to the arm and hand will not only improve the sensation of the part itself but also have a beneficial effect on the patient's perception of his whole body and its relation to the surroundings. Referring to the muscular articular sense, termed in physiology the proprioceptive system, and its important role in motor control, Bernstein (1996) explains that "proprioceptive sense means 'sensing itself', that is, having a sense of one's own body". As has been described in Chap. 1, assisted interaction with the environment can help to improve many other cognitive abilities as well. It should also be remembered that for functional use of the hand, "the capacity of dexterity appears to be not in the movements themselves, but rather in their interaction with the environment" (Bernstein 1996).

From the onset of the illness, the patient's arm must be kept fully mobile and the spastic flexion pattern inhibited. As many of the following activities as possible should be carried out carefully even when the arm is still hypotonic. The full inhibition of hypertonus in the arm and trunk and the facilitation of any active movement possible is an integral part of the treatment during all stages of the rehabilitation. The following sequences, with the patient lying, sitting and standing, show how hypertonicity in the arm can be reduced by proximal and distal inhibition, and how active movement can be stimulated. If any of the movements are limited by painful shortening of the various muscle groups or other soft tissue structures, the therapist must work carefully but determinedly to regain the lost extensibility. The same applies if there is limitation of movement in the joints themselves. Whatever the cause, pain or contracture can inhibit the return of active movement or prevent the patient from being able to use what voluntary activity he has. Maitland (1991) describes 'pain inhibition' as being a factor which "can be responsible for apparent (not actual) muscle weakness, instability, limitation of range of movement".

Activities in Supine Lying

1. Before moving the patient's arm, the therapist reduces any hypertonus or hyperactivity in the patient's trunk to allow the scapula to move freely. She rotates the trunk, elongates the side and brings the pelvis forwards, placing the leg in a flexed position with the knee leaning across the other leg (**Fig. 8.1 a**). The therapist works until the pelvis remains forward on the affected side and the leg lies without having to be held in the required position. If the tone is really reduced, the leg and pelvis will stay in place without the patient having to hold the position actively, or the therapist having to place a sandbag or pillow to stabilise the buttock or foot. Should the leg push into extension or the knee fall sideways during the arm activities, the therapist must then repeat the inhibition of the side and the whole limb before continuing. The passive maintenance of the position is her indication that the tone is not increasing. The leg must therefore not be held in place mechanically. It would be counterproductive to hold it in position by means of an external fixation of some sort, such as a sandbag or a nonslip material, because the valuable source of information with regard to increasing tone would be lost. The muscles could be hypertonic, but, with the leg held in place mechanically, any movement normally caused by their contraction would be prevented and the increase in tension pass unnoticed.
2. Cradling the hemiplegic arm against her side, she uses her other hand to move the patient's scapula into elevation with protraction. With the ball of her hand below the spine of the scapula she moves the shoulder girdle on that side forwards and upwards, asking the patient to try to allow the movement without resistance (**Fig. 8.1 b**). As she moves the scapula the hypertonus is reduced both proximally and distally, and the therapist brings the arm slowly into outward rotation.
3. Once the scapula is moving easily, the therapist brings the patient's arm forwards and upwards through flexion into elevation while maintaining protraction of the scapula and extension at the elbow. With her elbow against that of the patient, the therapist applies the appropriate amount of pressure to ensure that his arm does not pull into flexion. She then opens his hand by drawing the thumb out of the palm and dorsally extending the wrist and fingers fully (**Fig. 8.1 c**). The therapist's thumb against the dorsal aspect of the patient's wrist gives counterpressure, enabling her to overcome any resistance offered by the flexors of the wrist and fingers (**Fig. 8.1 d**).
4. When full elevation of the extended arm has been achieved, the therapist should also move the arm into horizontal abduction with supination of the forearm. With her elbow beneath the patient's elbow she holds it in extension, while at the same time preventing retraction of the scapula and maintaining the correct position of the head of the humerus in the glenoid fossa (**Fig. 8.1 e**). The passive movement ensures that the flexors and internal rotators of the shoulder retain their full extensibility.
5. When hypertonus in the arm has been inhibited and passive movement is possible without resistance, the patient can attempt to move his arm actively, but without effort. The therapist asks him to let his hand remain against her forehead (**Fig. 8.2 a**). He can then take his hand to his other shoulder, with the appropriate amount of assistance, and try to let it stay there without the arm pulling into the total pattern of flexion (**Fig. 8.2 b**). Similarly, he can move his hand to his own head and let it rest there (**Fig. 8.2 c**), and then move it again to the therapist's forehead.

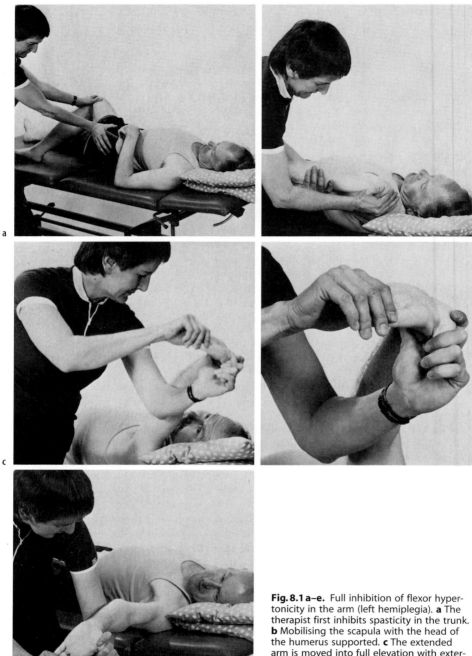

Fig. 8.1 a–e. Full inhibition of flexor hypertonicity in the arm (left hemiplegia). **a** The therapist first inhibits spasticity in the trunk. **b** Mobilising the scapula with the head of the humerus supported. **c** The extended arm is moved into full elevation with external rotation. **d** Inhibiting flexor spasticity in the hand. The therapist's thumb on the dorsum of the wrist gives counter-pressure. **e** The arm is taken into abduction at an angle of 90° to the body

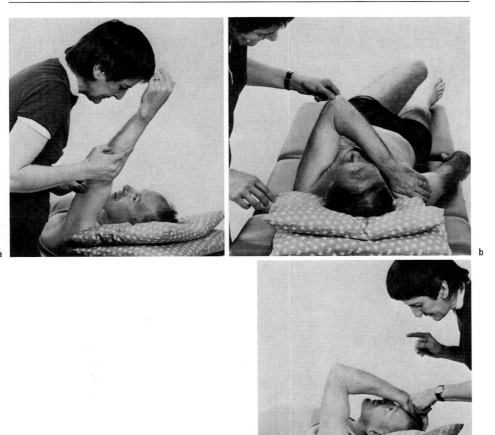

Fig. 8.2 a–c. The patient attempts easy active movements (left hemiplegia). He moves his hand (**a**) to the therapist's forehead (the fingers remain relaxed), (**b**) to his opposite shoulder and (**c**) to rest on his own head

6. More difficult for the patient is the attempt to let his hand remain inactive and relaxed when the arm is placed in different positions by the therapist (**Fig. 8.3 a**). He must learn to grade movement in this way if he is to use the arm and hand for different functions. The degree of difficulty is increased by placing the arm in more and more complex positions, those in which the spastic patterns or mass synergies exert a greater influence. For example, the patient slowly lowers the arm to his side without the elbow flexing or the hand clenching (**Fig. 8.3 b**).

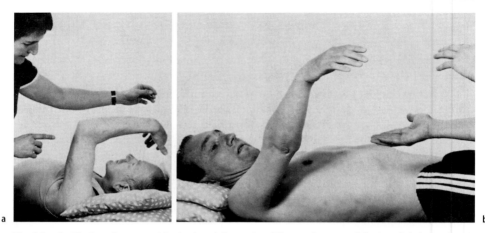

a   b

Fig. 8.3 a, b. Placing the arm with the hand free. **a** In different degrees of flexion (left hemiplegia);
b lowering it to his side with the elbow extended and the fingers relaxed (right hemiplegia)

Activities in Sitting

In our daily life we use our hands mainly when we are sitting or standing; we get dressed, eat, write, work and play in these positions. It is therefore preferable for the patient to be treated in sitting and standing positions rather than in lying when he is attempting to move his arm actively with facilitation. These positions also enable the therapist to use the valuable principle of inhibiting hypertonicity by moving proximal parts of the body against the distal spastic components.

1. The patient sits on the plinth with his arms extended behind him in outward rotation. He moves his weight from one side to the other while keeping both hands flat on the supporting surface. The therapist facilitates the necessary movement of the scapula with her hands, with the respective sides of the patient's trunk shortening and lengthening alternately. When the patient transfers his weight to the left, the left side elongates, allowing the left shoulder girdle and scapula to elevate. The right side shortens reciprocally and the shoulder girdle is depressed to allow the hand to remain flat on the supporting surface. When he moves his trunk to the right she assists the necessary depression of the left scapula. Throughout the activity, the therapist uses her elbows to keep those of the patient in extension until she is sure that he can maintain the position safely alone (**Fig. 8.4 a**).

2. The therapist places the patient's arm at his side, in outward rotation with the fingers extended. Using her forearm to support his elbow in extension and her hand to keep his shoulder forward, she helps him to bring his weight over that side (**Fig. 8.4 b**). Great care must be taken to avoid injuring the patient's wrist through excessive dorsiflexion. The therapist can avoid the danger by ensuring that the arm and hand are turned sufficiently outwards, so that when he moves from side to side, the weight is

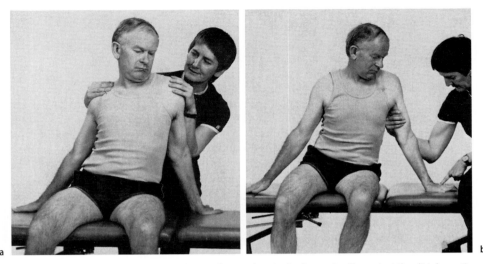

Fig. 8.4a, b. Inhibiting hypertonus in the arm by moving the body proximally against the distal spastic components (left hemiplegia). **a** With arms extended and his hands flat on the table behind him, the patient moves from side to side. **b** With the hemiplegic arm supported beside him in extension, the patient brings his weight towards the arm. The scapula elevates and the hand remains extended

taken through the medial and lateral aspects of his palm without the degree of dorsiflexion increasing at all. Once again, the scapula must move freely into elevaton and depression as he transfers his weight from one side to the other, moving proximally against the spastic arm. When the hypertonicity has been inhibited the therapist withdraws her support; she can then ask the patient to flex and extend his elbow selectively, i. e. without moving his trunk to produce flexion and extension at the elbow, and without using inward rotation of the shoulder to reinforce the extension attempt.

3. Because the scapula is very often the key to the spasticity in the whole upper extremity, the therapist must pay particular attention to the inhibition of hypertonicity in that area before active movements are attempted.

   a) Placing the patient's hands flat on the plinth behind him with his fingers pointing backwards, the therapist helps him to flex and extend his trunk. The proximal movement inhibits the hypertonicity, not only around the scapula but also throughout the arm and hand. As the trunk flexes, the scapulae are bought into full protraction. Standing behind the patient, the therapist presses downwards and backwards on his sternum to increase flexion of his thoracic spine, while with her other hand she moves both his scapulae as far forwards as possible. Both sides of the shoulder girdle must be brought forwards simultaneously because otherwise the scapula on the sound side will automatically be pulled backwards in a compensatory way. Once again, the therapist uses her elbow against that of the patient to maintain extension (**Fig. 8.5a**). When the patient extends his trunk, the therapist draws both his scapulae backwards in adduction and assists the extension of his thoracic spine (**Fig. 8.5b**)

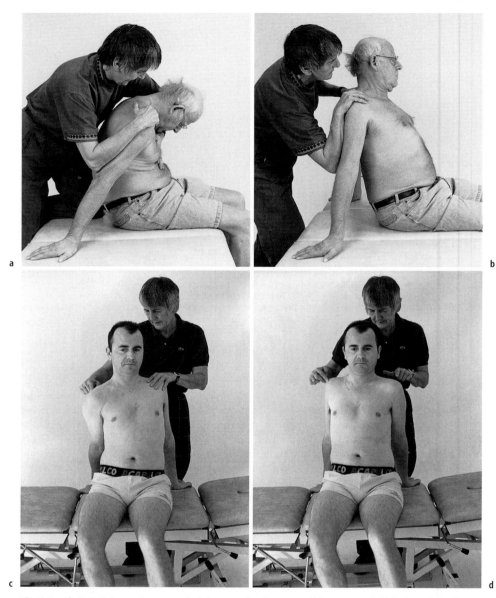

Fig. 8.5 a–d. Retraining active control of the scapula after normalising tone. **a** Full flexion of the thorax frees protraction of the scapulae. **b** Extension of the trunk with assisted adduction of the scapulae (right hemiplegia). **c** Moving the sound shoulder rhythmically back and forth while stabilising the other (left hemiplegia. **d** Learning to move the hemiplegic shoulder actively, with the therapist ready to help if necessary

b) Once the trunk and shoulder girdle are moving freely, the patient learns to move one shoulder back and forth while stabilising the other scapula. The therapist moves first the shoulder on the sound side back and forth rhythmically to a count of three, while keeping the contralateral scapula in position with her other hand (**Fig. 8.5 c**). She instructs the patient to let her move his shoulder easily and then asks him to move it with her without effort. The same movement is then performed with the hemiplegic shoulder. When she feels that the patient is moving actively, she gradually reduces the amount of help she is giving, but is ready to join in again at once should the movement become laboured or the rhythm be lost (**Fig. 8.5 d**).

4. Active control of the shoulder girdle can be encouraged further by teaching the patient to elevate and protract his scapula actively:

a) The therapist moves the point of the patient's shoulder in the direction of his nose, forwards and upwards, so working against the spastic pattern. She asks the patient to try not to resist the movement, and when she feels that there is no longer a resistance, he can assist actively. The therapist keeps the patient's hand in full dorsiflexion with finger extension, while he moves his scapula actively (**Fig. 8.6 a**). Most patients find it easier at first to maintain the passive elevation of the scapula with an isometric contraction and only later progress to moving it upwards from a neutral position into elevation isotonically.

b) With both arms flexed across his chest, the patient uses his sound hand to draw the affected scapula forward into protraction. The affected hand remains relaxed on the opposite shoulder as he rotates the trunk in a smooth continuous movement, back and forth (**Fig. 8.6 b**). Care must be taken that the patient's knees re-

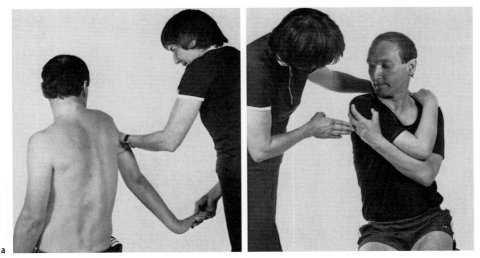

Fig. 8.6 a, b. Elevating and protracting the scapula (right hemiplegia). **a** With the arm in extension and external rotation the point of the shoulder is moved towards the nose. **b** With arms crossed the patient rotates his trunk to the sound side. His sound hand brings the hemiplegic shoulder forwards

main in the starting position, as the rotation will otherwise take place in the hips instead of the trunk. When the spasticity is inhibited sufficiently, the patient gradually gives less support to the hemiplegic arm, until it can finally remain in place without his holding it there. With the therapist's assistance, he brings the hemiplegic hand away from his shoulder and then back again actively.

5. The patient sits with his clasped hands supported on a table or plinth in front of him.
   a) Keeping his elbows extended, he moves his weight first over one side and then over the other, to inhibit the spasticity in the arm and hand. When he is leaning fully over one side, one hand lies on top of the other and he presses the underneath arm into lateral rotation of the shoulder with supination of the forearm (**Fig. 8.7 a**). Hypertonus in the pronators as well as in the finger flexors is reduced by the repeated movement of the trunk from side to side. When the thumb of his

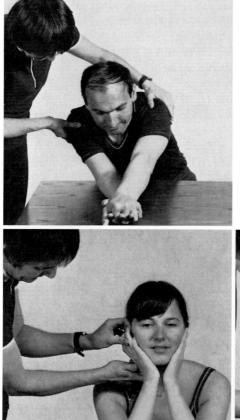

Fig. 8.7 a–c. Regaining active control of the arm (right hemiplegia). **a** Inhibition of pronation of the forearm. The patient moves his weight from one side to the other. **b** The patient rests her chin on her hands. The fingers remain relaxed. **c** The therapist moves the hemiplegic hand away and the patient brings it back to her face

a

b   c

lower hand is touching the table, the patient can hold it there until he feels there is less tension and then try to let the hand stay in position without his having to hold it there with his sound hand. He can also push both hands along the table far over to the sound side, which will bring the contralateral scapula into protraction. Pushing them towards the other side brings his weight over the hemiplegic side.

b) With the elbows remaining in place, the therapist helps the patient to place the balls of his hands under his chin, letting the fingers rest against the side of his face. As a precaution, she keeps slight contact with the tips of his fingers to prevent his face from being scratched should his hand flex unexpectedly (**Fig. 8.7 b**). When she feels that the fingers are relaxed, she brings his hemiplegic hand away from his face and then asks him to replace it gently (**Fig. 8.7 c**). The movement en-

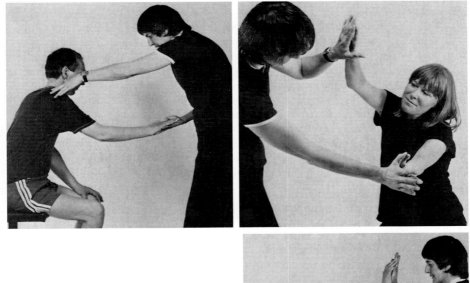

a   b

Fig. 8.8 a–c. Moving without effort (right hemiplegia). **a** With his hemiplegic hand resting on the therapist's hand the patient follows her movements. **b** With both of her hands against those of the therapist, the patient follows more complex movements. **c** The patient follows the therapist's hand forwards and upwards. The therapist gives quick repeated approximation through the ball of his hand

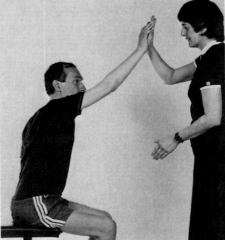

c

courages selective flexion of the elbow in supination without the fingers flexing. If the hand remains relaxed, the patient is asked to bring it further into extension before placing it under his chin again.

6. To help the patient to move smoothly and without overactivity, the therapist places his extended hand on her hand and asks him to follow her hand as she moves (**Fig. 8.8 a**). By increasing the speed of the movement and by changing the direction, the therapist can increase the degree of complexity according to the patient's ability. If he places both his hands on her hands and she asks him to follow the movement of both simultaneously, the activity becomes more difficult but has the advantage of preventing overactivity of the sound arm, as it must follow appropriately (**Fig. 8.8 b**).

7. The patient follows the therapist's hand as she moves it forwards and upwards, and she facilitates the movement with short, quick, approximating impulses through the ball of his hand (**Fig. 8.8 c**). Should the patient have insufficient activity in the muscles acting on his shoulder, the therapist can use her free hand to support his upper arm, assist elbow extension and prevent any injury to the shoulder through a sudden uncontrolled movement.

8. A ball will often facilitate activity for the patient because its movement is so familiar to him. The ball also adds interest to the treatment.

   a) The patient places his clasped hands on a gymnastic ball and pushes it as far forwards as he can (**Fig. 8.9 a**). He can also push it far over to the sound side, so bringing his shoulder forwards. The activity inhibits spasticity and also encourages the patient to bring his weight forwards. Not only is the arm being treated, but other movements are being retrained simultaneously. Bringing the ball towards his hemiplegic side will facilitate bearing weight spontaneously.

   b) When the hypertonus has been reduced, activity can be stimulated in the affected limb by helping the patient to move the ball with one hand. Selective movement is trained by his controlling the ball without the fingers flexing (**Fig. 8.9 b**). In the

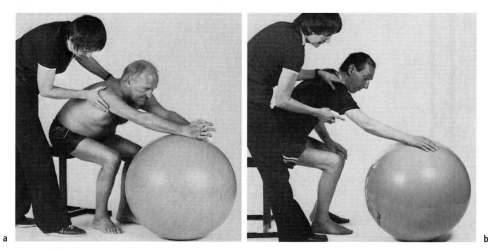

a   b

Fig. 8.9 a, b. Sitting, moving a ball to facilitate selective movement in the arm (right hemiplegia). **a** With both hands clasped; **b** with the hemiplegic hand

same starting position he can also move the ball from side to side, but this time stabilising his shoulder and moving only from the elbow. He can also roll the ball away with the dorsum of his hand and fingers.

Activities in Standing

With a Gymnastic Ball

1. Pushing the ball away with the back of his hand can also be practised with the patient standing. He is then able to swing his arm more freely, and will automatically bring his weight forwards without fear (**Fig. 8.10 a**). The therapist facilitates the movement and helps to prevent abnormal movements from occurring, e.g. adduction of the hip or retraction of the shoulder.
2. The patient can also drop and catch the ball using both hands, guided by the therapist, who holds his thumb and fingers in the required extension during the activity (**Fig. 8.10 b, c**).When necessary the therapist can at first guide the patient's sound hand as well, to prevent him from using the better arm overactively and to facilitate the correct movement.
3. The patient can learn to bounce the ball with the hemiplegic hand or with alternate hands, an activity which is more advanced than dropping and catching it. The therapist guides his affected hand to ensure a smooth, even rhythm (**Fig. 8.10 d**) and allows him to continue on his own if she feels that he is moving actively without undue effort (**Fig. 8.10 e**). Should the movement become strained or the rhythm be lost, the therapist should immediately take the patient's hand and allow the activity to proceed smoothly once again.

Both dropping and catching the ball and bouncing the ball are useful when combined with walking. The patient's walking becomes more automatic, and he looks at the ball instead of fixing his eyes constantly on the ground as he would otherwise do. Because he is reaching forwards to bounce or catch the ball in front of him, his weight will also be brought forwards and the steps he takes will then be reactive instead of active as they usually are.

With a Balloon

A balloon will often stimulate extensor activity in the patient's arm, wrist and fingers without exaggerated effort, and hand-eye co-ordination occurs spontaneously.
1. The patient with little to no voluntary activity in his upper limb can hit the balloon into the air with his hands clasped together and the therapist supporting his arm and shoulder.
2. To stimulate activity, the patient can be helped to hit the balloon with the hemiplegic hand alone. He should swing his arm forwards together with the whole side of his body and not attempt to lift it from the shoulder. With adequate facilitation, the movement is possible even if almost no activity appears to be present. The therapist stands behind the patient and rotates his trunk well back on the affected side

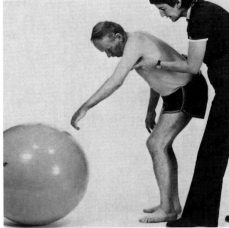

a

Fig. 8.10 a–e. Standing, using a ball to stimulate activity in the arm. **a** Pushing the ball away with the back of the hand (left hemiplegia). **b, c** Dropping and catching the ball. The therapist guides the patient's hemiplegic hand (left hemiplegia). **d, e** Bouncing a ball with alternate hands. The therapist first guides the hemiplegic hand until the patient can continue on her own

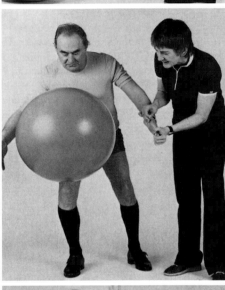

b

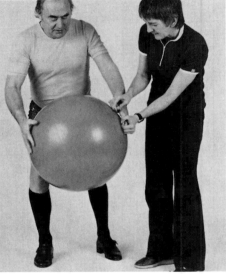

c

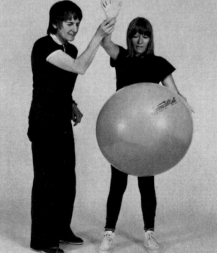

d

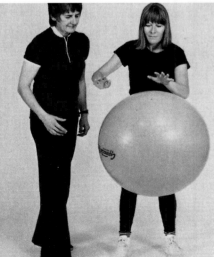

e

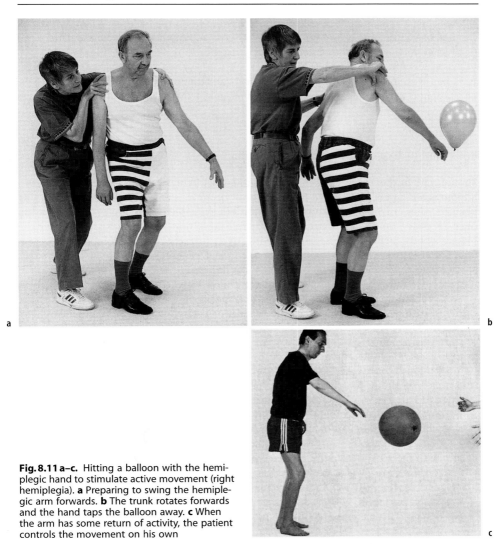

Fig. 8.11 a–c. Hitting a balloon with the hemiplegic hand to stimulate active movement (right hemiplegia). **a** Preparing to swing the hemiplegic arm forwards. **b** The trunk rotates forwards and the hand taps the balloon away. **c** When the arm has some return of activity, the patient controls the movement on his own

(**Fig. 8.11 a**). She instructs the patient to let his arm swing forward without effort as the helper throws the balloon towards him. With one hand on each of his shoulders, she facilitates the forward rotation of the patient's trunk by drawing the sound side back and thrusting the hemiplegic side forwards, so enabling him to hit the balloon back to the helper with a swing of his arm (**Fig. 8.11 b**). It is interesting to notice how often previously inactive muscles around the shoulder spring into action when the scapula is brought forwards during the swing to hit the balloon. When the correct movement has been learnt and sufficient muscle activity has returned, the patient can practise hitting the balloon without the assistance of the therapist (**Fig. 8.11 c**).

A patient with more controlled arm movement can attempt to keep the balloon in the air by tapping it up several times. Automatic steps are facilitated as he moves to follow the balloon.

Inhibition of Hypertonicity in Standing

Should tone in the arm increase during voluntary activity, spasticity will need to be inhibited again before the desired movement can occur in a more normal way. A standing position offers many opportunities for using the principle of moving proximally to reduce excessive tone in the extremities. For full inhibition the therapist must move the patient's body further than he can move it actively himself. After each inhibitory procedure some activity for the arm should be facilitated, making use of the improved tone.

1. The patient's hands are supported on a plinth or table in front of him, with the fingers extended. The therapist maintains the elbow in extension until the spasticity is reduced and the patient can keep the arm in position himself. In this position the patient can move his weight from side to side, or rotate his trunk while the shoulders remain fixed. He can also flex his thoracic spine fully, so bringing his scapula into protraction, and then extend the spine before repeating the flexion. He moves his thorax against the scapula to inhibit the hypertonicity.
   Stepping backwards and forwards with his sound leg while keeping the affected hip against the plinth, the patient brings his weight over the hemiplegic side, and active extension in the supporting arm is stimulated (**Fig. 8.12 a**). The arms can be placed in more and more external rotation with supination for the fullest inhibition. Selective elbow extension can be practised once inhibition has been achieved.

2. The patient stands with his back to the plinth and his hands are supported behind him with the arms outwardly rotated and extended. With the therapist's help, the patient brings his buttocks away from the plinth and extends his hips and spine as fully as possible (**Fig. 8.12 b**). The extension in the hips is increased if he is asked to straighten his knees. He can also move his weight from side to side in this position, or rotate his pelvis, emphasising bringing the affected side as far forwards as possible.

3. To elongate the side and free the scapula for movement, the therapist holds the patient's arm in full elevation with outward rotation. With one hand she maintains full inhibition of the patient's hand and with her other hand she keeps his shoulder forward and outwardly rotated. She will probably need to stand on a stool for the necessary height (**Fig. 8.13**). The patient then moves his weight over the hemiplegic leg and back again, to increase the elongation and inhibition. The spasticity in the whole arm is reduced by the proximal inhibition.

4. Patients have difficulty in maintaining extension at the elbow when abducting the arm. To inhibit fully the strong pull of the flexor muscles, the therapist stands behind the patient. With one hand she holds the wrist and fingers in full dorsal extension with the thumb abducted (**Fig. 8.14 a**), and with her other hand she prevents compensatory movement of the shoulder. While the arm is held in outward rotation and ex-

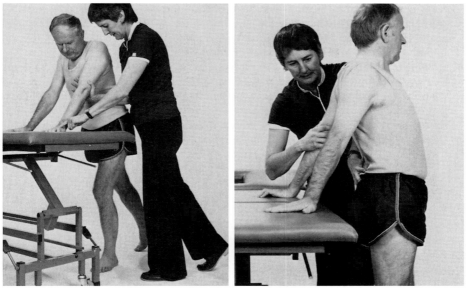

a　　　　　　　　　　　　　　　　　　　　　　　　　　b

Fig. 8.12 a, b. Inhibiting upper limb hypertonicity in standing (left hemiplegia). **a** With arms extended and the hands supported on a plinth in front of him, the patient takes a step backwards with his sound leg. The therapist helps to maintain elbow extension. **b** With the hands supported on a plinth behind him, the patient brings his hips as far forwards as possible and extends his whole spine

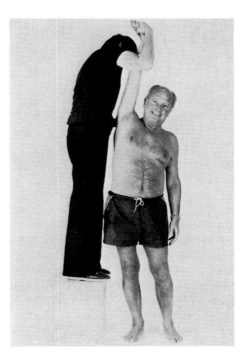

Fig. 8.13. Inhibiting hypertonicity around the scapula in standing. The therapist holds the extended arm in full elevation with external rotation, and the patient moves his weight over the hemiplegic side (right hemiplegia)

tension, the patient turns away with his other arm outstretched, as far as he possibly can (**Fig. 8.14 b**). He then brings the hand round forwards towards his affected hand again. He tries to go further back each time he repeats the movement as the tension in both the muscles and neural structures decreases.

5. Holding both the patient's hands in the same position, the therapist brings his arms sideways and upwards, and the patient tries to assist actively (**Fig. 8.14 c**). He also concentrates on not allowing the elbow to pull into flexion as the degree of abduction is gradually increased. As soon as the therapist feels that the elbows are about to flex, she lowers the hands again. If the therapist cannot reach both the patient's hands or if his shoulder is at all vulnerable, he can be asked to move his sound arm correctly

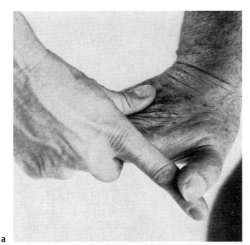

a

Fig. 8.14 a–c. Inhibition to allow elbow extension during active abduction of the arm (right hemiplegia). **a** Grip to inhibit flexor spasticity in the hand. **b** The therapist holds the extended arm in abduction while the patient turns away. **c** Abducting the arms without the elbow flexing

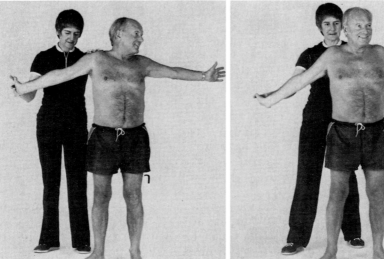

b   c

himself. The therapist can then assist or stimulate elbow extension with her free hand or maintain the correct alignment of the glenohumeral joint from below.

6. The patient first claps his hands together and then turns them over so that the palms face away from him. He places them against the therapist's chest while she helps him to protract the scapula and extend his elbows. With the hands in this position, they are brought above the patient's head until the shoulders are fully elevated. The patient pushes his hands upwards against one of the therapist's hands, while with her other hand she keeps his shoulder well forward. The patient then moves his weight sideways over the affected leg and elongates the hemiplegic side as much as possible **(Fig. 8.15)**. He repeats the movement sideways, and each time tries to elongate the side further. The flexor spasticity in the hand is dramatically reduced, and extension of the fingers can often be stimulated afterwards.

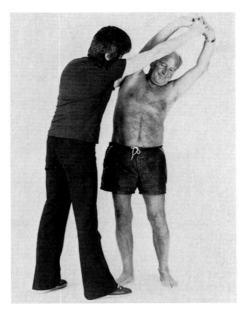

Fig. 8.15. Inhibiting flexor spasticity in the arm and hand (right hemiplegia). The patient's clasped hands are turned so that the palms face upwards. He leans them towards his sound side

Stimulation of Active and Functional Movements

By Applying an Excitatory Stimulus

To activate the finger extensors or increase existing activity the therapist can use three useful methods of stimulation.

1. Sweep tapping: Supporting the patient's arm with one hand, the therapist uses her other hand to sweep firmly and briskly over the extensor muscle group of the forearm, from its origin above the elbow to the fingertips (sweep tapping, Bobath 1978) (**Fig. 8.16 a, b**). As she passes the wrist, she gives pressure downwards on the dorsum of the hand, quickly sweeping upwards again over the fingers. The sweeping movement is performed with the therapist's fingers held firmly in extension, and the movement of her hand is so quick that it can be likened to that used to crack a whip. After a few sweeps, the patient may spontaneously extend the fingers, or otherwise can be asked to attempt the movement gently.

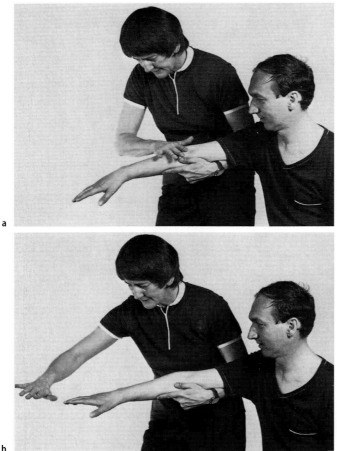

a

b

Fig. 8.16 a, b. Sweep-tapping to stimulate finger extension (right hemiplegia)

When re-educating finger extension, it is most important to avoid dorsal extension of the wrist until the patient can maintain active finger extension while extending his wrist. If he is encouraged to extend the wrist before he can extend his fingers, the tenodesis action reinforces their flexor spasticity and the hand cannot be opened or used functionally. During or after sweep tapping, the therapist should therefore ask the patient to try to lift just his fingertips, so that finger extension precedes wrist extension.

2. Immersion in ice: Placing the patient's hand in a mixture of crushed ice and water causes a reflex relaxation of the flexor spasticity of the fingers and wrist (**Fig. 8.17 a, b**). In many instances there is absolutely no resistance to passive dorsal extension immediately following the immersion in ice, and the patient may be able to extend his fingers afterwards. Although the effect will not last long on its own, the inhibition of the hypertonicity enables the therapist to use other inhibitory activities more easily and also to encourage active movement of the fingers and hand. Some patients without marked spasticity in the hand also seem to react well to the intense stimulation, and movement may be elicited as a result. The ice and water ratio must be correct for the best results, that is, only so much water as to allow the patient's affected hand to glide into the mixture without difficulty. The therapist holds the patient's hand in the ice mixture with her hand. She should not wear a rubber glove so that she can judge just how long the cold can be tolerated. It has been found that three immersions, each of about 3 s duration and following one after the other with only a few seconds' interval, are necessary before total inhibition of the spasticity is achieved.

3. A bottlebrush: The therapist draws a bottlebrush through the patient's hand while supporting his arm forward with the elbow extended. She tells the patient to hold the brush very gently and then, after pulling it out of his hand, she asks him to grasp

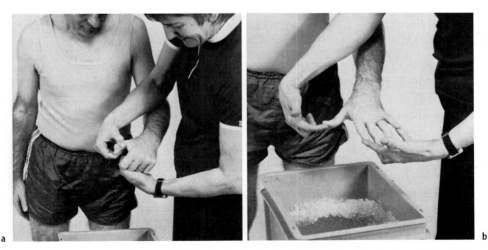

a   b

Fig. 8.17 a, b. Inhibiting flexor spasticity in the hand using ice (left hemiplegia). **a** The hand before inhibition; **b** the hand immediately following immersion in ice

it again. Often he is able to extend the fingers enough to do so **(Fig. 8.18)**. The extension of his fingers should occur in anticipation of the next grasp, and the patient should therefore not try to extend his fingers actively but rather think of taking the brush in his hand again.

When activity in the fingers has occurred with stimulation, the therapist chooses objects which help to produce the regained holding and releasing movements in ways which simulate those needed for performing actual tasks. For example:
1. The patient holds a wooden pole in front of him, either horizontally or vertically **(Fig. 8.19 a)**. With the therapist assisting where and when necessary, he releases the pole and moves his hemiplegic hand up and over the other hand to grasp the pole again. Then the sound hand makes a similar movement, while the hemiplegic hand

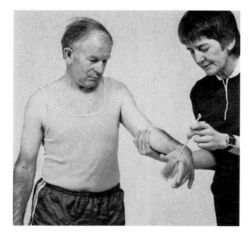

Fig. 8.18. Stimulating activity in the hand with a bottlebrush (left hemiplegia)
◁

Fig. 8.19 a, b. Grasping and releasing a wooden pole (right hemiplegia). **a** Moving the hands up the pole, one after the other. **b** Letting the pole drop down a fraction before catching it again
▽

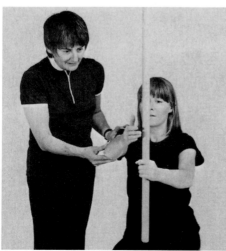

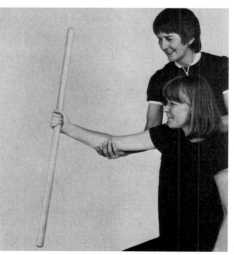

a   b

holds the pole in position. The therapist ensures that the affected arm does not pull into flexion, and the patient keeps his elbows extended.

As his skill increases, he can hold the pole vertically in front of him with his hemiplegic hand and, after releasing it slightly so that it falls, catch it again quickly (**Fig.8.19b**). The patient measures his improving ability by counting the number of times he can release and catch the pole before his hand reaches the top end.

2. A tambourine provides many opportunities for using the hand in different ways, with an acoustic feedback. The patient can beat it with his hand flat, stroke it with a circular movement and then beat it, or tap it with alternate fingers (**Fig.8.20**). By changing the position of the tambourine, supination and pronation of the forearm and lifting the extended arm are encouraged without the fingers flexing. Using a drumstick to play the tambourine requires still finer control of the wrist and fingers, such as finger flexion with different positions of the wrist and forearm.

By Using the Protective Extension Reaction

When overbalancing towards the hemiplegic side, most patients will be unable to save themselves with their affected arm. The so-called parachute reaction (Bobath 1990) fails because of insufficient extensor activity, particularly when flexor tonus increases due to fear of falling. With patients who have some active movement in the upper limb, protective extension can be facilitated. It is useful not only for protection, but also for stimulating extensor activity and speeding up existing motor function.

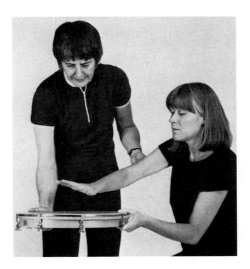

Fig.8.20. Playing the tambourine (right hemiplegia)

In Sitting

To prepare for the protective extension reaction in the arm, the patient is asked to lean towards his hemiplegic side and help to support himself with his arm. The therapist gives a gentle pull to bring him off balance and then, taking care not to increase extension of his wrist, pushes quickly up through the ball of his hand. In doing so she approximates the joints of the upper extremity, causing a stabilising contraction of the supporting muscles. At first she supports the elbow in extension with one hand (**Fig. 8.21 a**), and then as the activity increases she withdraws her support and reminds him verbally to keep his shoulder forward (**Fig. 8.21 b**).

Later, with the patient sitting on a plinth she draws him further and further to the side and then lets go of his hand, allowing it to rest quickly on the plinth. The activity can be carried out in various directions, and also in a standing position as the patient's ability increases.

In Standing and While Walking

The therapist holds the patient's sound arm and pushes him forwards or sideways in the direction of the plinth, a table or a wall. The patient saves himself with his extended hemiplegic arm, and the therapist controls the speed and prevents him from falling by guiding from his sound arm.

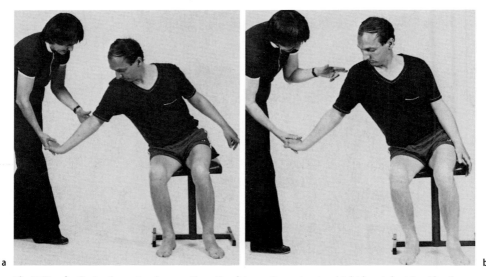

a   b

Fig. 8.21 a, b. Protective extension reaction stimulates active extension (right hemiplegia). **a** The therapist assists elbow extension. **b** The patient maintains elbow extension

In a Kneeling Position

Protective extension can also be practised on the mat. Kneeling has the advantage that it is very easy to bring the patient off balance to stimulate the activity. When the patient is kneeling the therapist can also control finger and wrist extension if she kneels in front of him and holds his hemiplegic hand open. He inhibits the reaction in his sound arm voluntarily, as it will otherwise dominate and reach the floor more quickly than the other.

Retraining Selective Flexion of the Arm and Hand

Most of the activities which have been described emphasise the regaining of extension of the arm, wrist and fingers. However, it should be remembered that, normally, for functional use of the hand in the activities of daily living, selective flexion of the arm and hand is in fact even more important. The ability to hold objects while flexing the arm is essential for many tasks such as washing, dressing, eating, drinking and personal grooming, to name but a few. Certainly, the ability is required for carrying the necessary items from one place to another, for example when laying the table or washing the dishes after a meal. When treating the patient it is therefore equally important to include activities to retrain selective flexion of the arm and hand. Describing the need to work for independent and controlled movements of the elbow, Bobath (1990) explains that "flexion of the elbow with supination brings his hand to his mouth and to the opposite shoulder or ear. In fact, he learns to control movements which he needs for the functional use of his hand later on," and also how "movements of the hand should become independent of the position of the arm at the shoulder and elbow". Equally important for hand function, but an activity frequently overlooked in the treatment, is the need to hold implements or items of clothing with finger flexion when the wrist is in varying degrees of flexion as well, for instance for picking up a knife or pen, or when pulling up trousers.

However, because hypertonicity or spasticity in the flexors of the elbow, wrist and fingers can create considerable problems for patients, many therapists are afraid of including any active flexion movements in the treatment. They fear that the flexor hypertonus may be further increased or a grasp reflex elicited or reinforced.

They therefore never allow the patient to hold objects in his hemiplegic hand, and in both physiotherapy and occupational therapy the upper limb activities are restricted mainly to those involving weightbearing through an extended arm. Most flexion movements which are practised are those requiring eccentric activity of the extensors of the elbow and not the flexors. During any activity where the patient is allowed to hold something in his hand, he may do so only with the wrist extended because the therapist is afraid of encouraging a primitive flexion grip.

The fear or misconception that flexor spasticity would be increased by retraining active flexion is, however, totally unfounded and in fact quite the opposite is the case. Voluntary movements performed in normal patterns, with facilitation if necessary, will actually inhibit hypertonicity. When the therapist "inhibits the unwanted parts of the abnormal total pattern" then "it is the restoration of this inhibitory control that makes permanent reduction of spasticity possible" (Bobath 1990) As the author so rightly explains, "Inhibition facilitates and facilitation inhibits."

In addition, the input to the hand achieved by handling real and familiar objects improves sensation, which in turn will help to overcome reflex grasping, because the reflex is present due to sensation in the hand being diminished or disturbed.

All voluntary movements must be selective, however, and not performed in primitive mass synergies which would serve to reinforce the abnormal patterns and indeed tend to increase tone in the muscles involved. It has even been suggested that, "what is usually called spasticity is, in most patients following stroke, unnecessary muscular activity which has become habitual" or that "practice of inappropriate muscle activity will result in the wrong movement being trained, and in a sense so-called spasticity is made up of habitual and unnecessary motor responses" (Carr and Shepherd 1982).

What is important for the patient is that adaptive motor behaviour should not be learned through unassisted repetition when a more effective and functional movement could otherwise become possible.

The therapist can help the patient to regain selective flexion of the upper limb both by including specific activities in her treatment programme and by helping and encouraging him to use his affected hand for simple tasks.

By Using Specific Therapeutic Activities

A short wooden pole, 2 cm in diameter, can be of invaluable help when facilitating and thus retraining selective movements of the upper limb. The diameter of the pole is significant, because with a thin gymnastic pole such as those generally available for purchase, the patient will have difficulty in forming his hand around it with an appropriate grip. It is therefore important that a pole of the correct size be obtained.

The patient holds the pole in his hand, with the therapist at first helping him to maintain the position of his fingers around it. He feels the weight of the pole and the contact with its firm rounded surface in his hand. When he is learning to move his arm in different ways, he should concentrate on moving the pole instead of trying hard to contract just the required muscles in an abstract way. If the pole remains correctly aligned it will indicate that unwanted components of the mass flexion synergy are not being activated. For example, when the patient is asked to bring the pole towards his head, which entails flexing his elbow, he tries to keep the pole level in a horizontal position and by so doing avoids pronating his forearm. By maintaining the pole on a line parallel to his chest, the components of medial rotation and abduction of the shoulder are eliminated, as is retraction of the scapula.

Some examples of activities with the pole are:

1. Holding the pole with the forearm supinated. The therapist stands beside the patient with her foot on a stool or the edge of the plinth and supports his elbow on her knee so that he does not have to stabilise his shoulder actively himself. The patient holds the pole and the therapist brings his forearm into full supination. Hypertonus in the pronators is inhibited if the patient flexes and extends his trunk slowly while the therapist maintains the fully supinated position of the arm. She reduces tone further by manipulating the soft tissues outwards to relieve the tension which is pulling the forearm towards pronation. When she feels that there is no longer any resistance,

she asks the patient to just let his hand stay in the position without her help. She takes her hand away from his and if necessary continues to assist him from a more proximal point near his elbow, her fingers guiding the movement gently (**Fig. 8.22 a**). As his control improves, the patient learns not only to hold the pole in position but also to move it slightly towards pronation and then back to supination again, gradually going a little further each time. The activity is intensified by increasing both the range of movement and the speed with which it is performed.

2. Moving the pole with selective elbow flexion. Once again, the therapist stands beside the patient and supports the weight of his arm on her thigh. She checks that he can hold the pole in position without pronation, and then asks him to draw it towards his head while keeping it level. During the movement he tries to let his elbow stay in place on her thigh, thus eliminating the tendency for the scapula to retract (**Fig. 8.22 b**). With her hand helping his hand to keep the correct position, the thera-

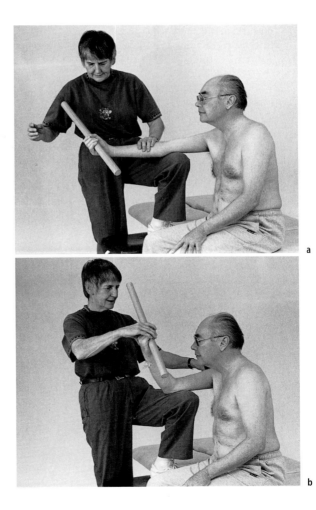

a

b

Fig. 8.22 a–d. Moving a pole to retrain selective arm movements (right hemiplegia). **a** Maintaining the pole in position with the forearm supinated. **b** Flexing the elbow without scapula retraction

pist moves the pole towards his head and then away again and asks the patient to move actively with her when she feels that there is no resistance (**Fig. 8.22 c**). It is easier for him at first to use a small range of movement so that he does not extend his elbow fully before flexing it again. Following each attempt the therapist can check that the movement is not being performed with undue effort or in a mass spastic pattern by asking the patient to let go of the pole (**Fig. 8.22 d**). If the patient is able to release his fingers easily, then the flexion was not a reflex grasping but an active holding. The activity can be increased by the patient gradually moving the pole further away from his head in a controlled, smooth manner before bringing it back towards his head again, and also by the therapist reducing the amount of assistance she is giving until he can eventually continue a few times unaided.

3. Holding the pole still in different positions. Often the patient can move the pole by flexing and extending his elbow but has difficulty in keeping it steady in one position, an ability which is also important for functional tasks. The therapist helps him to bend his arm without losing his grip and without pronation of the forearm and then asks him to stop in a certain position and to hold the pole in place when she takes her hand away. It is usually easier to begin with his elbow flexed to approximately a right angle (**Fig. 8.23**). Once he can keep the pole in place without its wob-

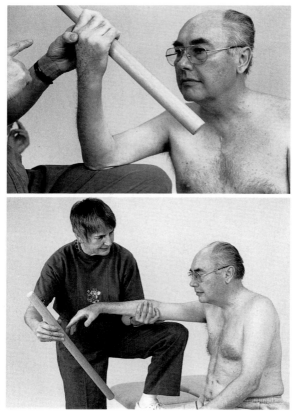

c

d

Fig. 8.22 c, d. c Selective elbow flexion keeping the pole parallel to the ground. **d** Always able to let go of the pole

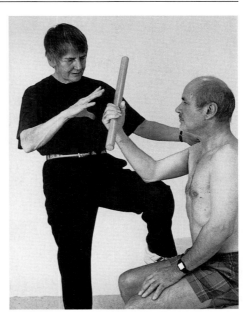

Fig. 8.23. Keeping the pole stationary with the elbow flexed to 90°

bling or turning towards the vertical, the same activity is practised with the therapist reducing the amount of proximal support. She moves her thigh away from below his elbow and asks the patient to maintain the position on his own. The activity becomes progressively more difficult with the elbow more and more extended.

4. Moving the pole with isolated flexion and extension of the wrist. The patient holds the pole lightly in his hand and the therapist asks him to let it move smoothly up and down without the arm moving at all. She stands in front of the patient and takes some of the weight off his arm by holding the pole with her hands on either side of his as the wrist flexes **(Fig. 8.24 a)**. He tries to keep his fingers in place despite the flexion movement of his wrist. He also concentrates on not pulling the pole away from the therapist, which would indicate flexion of the elbow and abduction of the shoulder in a total pattern of movement as he tries to flex his wrist by lifting up his arm. To allow the patient to experience the isolated activity of his wrist, the therapist facilitates the desired movement by using her index finger beneath his wrist and her thumb on the dorsal aspect of his hand. He then tries to let his wrist move downwards without pushing his arm down as well, while the therapist helps to make the activity smooth and effortless by pressing gently over the dorsum of his hand with her thumb and index finger **(Fig. 8.24 b)**. The therapist reduces the amount of assistance until he can continue a few times on his own. Once the patient is able to move his wrist selectively up and down, he should progress to being able to perform the same movement with his arm in different positions and without gravity assisting, as he will need to during functional use. The therapist supports his arm in front of his body with the elbow flexed and the forearm supinated. The patient tries to flex and extend his wrist without altering the position of the arm **(Fig. 8.24 c)**. The activity becomes increasingly more complex when the patient is required to stabilise his arm in the different positions himself while moving his wrist in isolation.

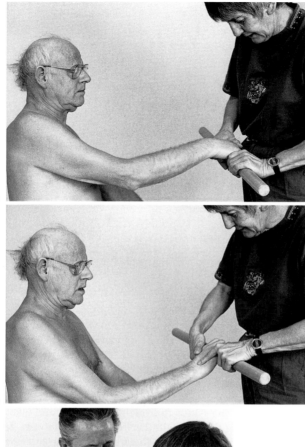

a

b

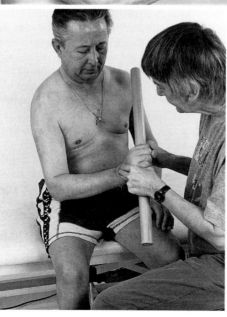

c

Fig. 8.24 a–c. Holding the pole while flexing and extending the wrist (right hemiplegia). **a** Flexing the wrist without releasing the grip. **b** Extending the wrist without pushing the arm downwards. **c** Moving the wrist with the elbow flexed and supinated

By Using the Hand for Simple Tasks

As described in Chap. 1, the patient can be helped to regain lost abilities by learning to move in appropriate familiar activities. The actual objects and events confronting him assist the retrieval of movement patterns from his storage systems or memory. During the performance of a real-life task with the actual objects to hand, verbal explanations become redundant, which is a great advantage. Movement is very difficult to explain and understand when put into words, and use of verbal commands can further add to the motor problems which the patient already has. In a study of three-dimensional arm trajectories involving normal adults performing movements following a verbal command, Morasso (1983), referring to the difficulty, makes the succinct comment, "simple experiments of this kind reveal the dramatic inadequacy of natural language to express movements and spatial relationships". Even more beneficial is the way in which using the hand can help to improve the control of the whole upper limb. The number of joints and the degree of freedom of movement to be controlled in order to yield the desired hand path and speed make it difficult to understand how the CNS plans and controls the trajectory of a movement and how one of a vast number of possible strategies is selected. In a study of human arm trajectory formation, it appeared that "these findings are consistent with the notion that trajectories are initially planned in terms of location of the hand and subsequently transformed into the required joint positions and torques" (Abend et al. 1982). As the authors mention, the same point of view had previously been advocated by Bernstein (1967). It would therefore seem reasonable to suppose that during treatment, bringing the hand in contact with stable surfaces or objects required for task performance would serve to provide points of reference and thus enhance active movements of the arm proximally.

When some active movement has returned in the hemiplegic arm or hand, the patient should be helped to use it as often as possible, not only during treatment but also in his daily life to perform actual tasks. The task performance is an important factor because "motor skill is not a movement formula and certainly not a formula of permanent muscle forces imprinted in some motor center. Motor skill is an ability to solve one or other type of motor problem" (Bernstein 1996), and even where active movement is still absent, the patient's hand should be guided during activities as a therapy. The sensation and awareness of the hemiplegic side can be improved in this way, and the return of potential active movement will be stimulated. Using the arm and hand even for very simple tasks is the best way to prevent associated reactions from occurring, as they do when the patient struggles to perform an activity with his sound hand alone.

The following are examples of activities during which the hemiplegic hand can be used, even at the stage when only slight return of voluntary movement is present.
1. Dressing provides several comparatively simple activities for the affected arm, i.e. activities where little stabilisation of the scapula and shoulder is required. (a) The patient picks his sock up with his hemiplegic hand (**Fig. 8.25 a**) before putting it on with his sound hand. (b) If at all feasible, the patient puts on his socks using both his hands, with the therapist giving minimal assistance (**Fig. 8.25 b**). (c) The patient uses both hands to put on his trousers (**Fig. 8.25 c**). (d) With very little activity in the fingers and thumb, the patient can tie his shoelaces, using the affected hand merely to hold one end of the lace (**Fig. 8.25 d**).
2. Other activities in his daily life provide opportunities for using the hemiplegic hand for easy tasks, such as: (a) eating toast or a bread roll (**Fig. 8.26 a**); (b) drinking

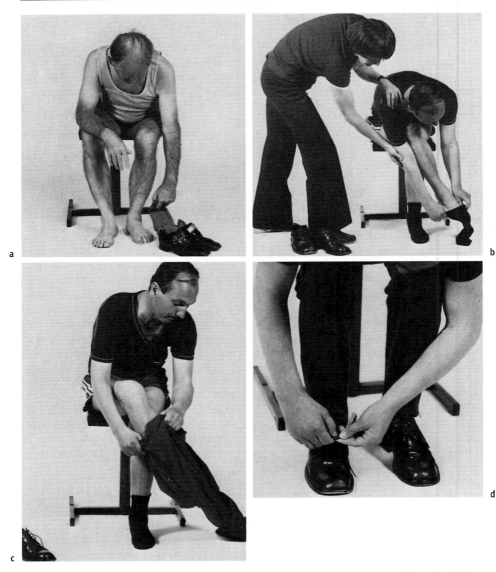

Fig. 8.25 a–d. Simple activities for the hemiplegic hand while the patient is getting dressed. **a** Picking up a sock (left hemiplegia); **b** putting on a sock with both hands (right hemiplegia); **c** pulling up a pair of trousers with both hands; **d** helping to tie shoelaces

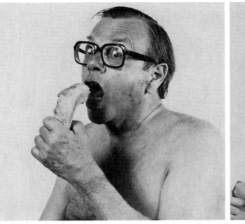

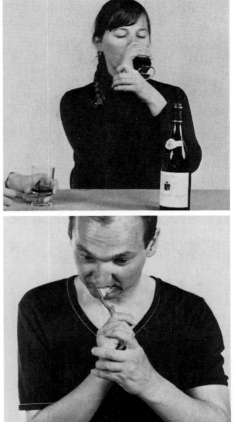

a

b

c

Fig. 8.26 a–c. Simple tasks for the hemiplegic hand in daily life. **a** Eating a bread roll (left hemiplegia); **b** drinking from a glass (right hemiplegia); **c** brushing teeth with the help of the sound hand (right hemiplegia)

from a glass (**Fig. 8.26 b**); (c) putting toothpaste on the toothbrush and brushing the teeth. The toothbrush is held in the affected hand while the toothpaste is being applied. The actual brushing action requires fine motor control, so that at first the patient will need to assist the hemiplegic hand with his sound hand (**Fig. 8.26 c**). When he feels he can manage some of the actions without assistance from the sound hand, he gradually withdraws its help at different stages of the procedure.

3. For more complex tasks which consist of several steps and require the use of both hands, the therapist guides the patient's hemiplegic hand to enable him to perform all the necessary movements in a normal manner. One example of such a task is cutting oranges in half (**Fig. 8.27 a**), pressing out the juice (**Fig. 8.27 b, c**), pouring the juice into a glass (**Fig. 8.27 d**) and then drinking it (**Fig. 8.27 e**). Clearing up after-

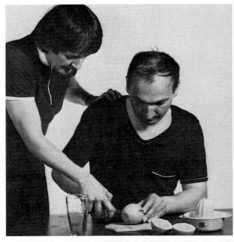

a

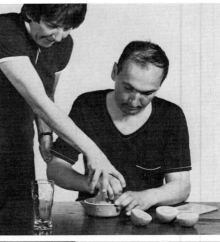

b

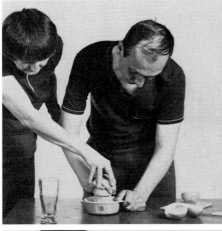

c

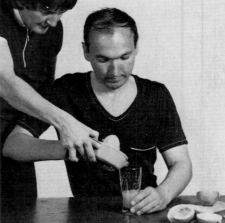

d

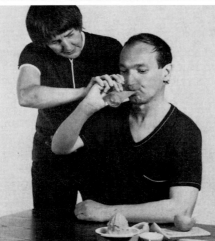

e

Fig. 8.27 a–e. Performing a complete task such as making orange juice, using both hands. The therapist guides the hemiplegic hand (right hemiplegia). **a** Cutting the oranges in half; **b** squeezing an orange; **c** standing to squeeze an orange (automatic standing improves balance); **d** pouring the juice into a glass; **e** having a drink of juice

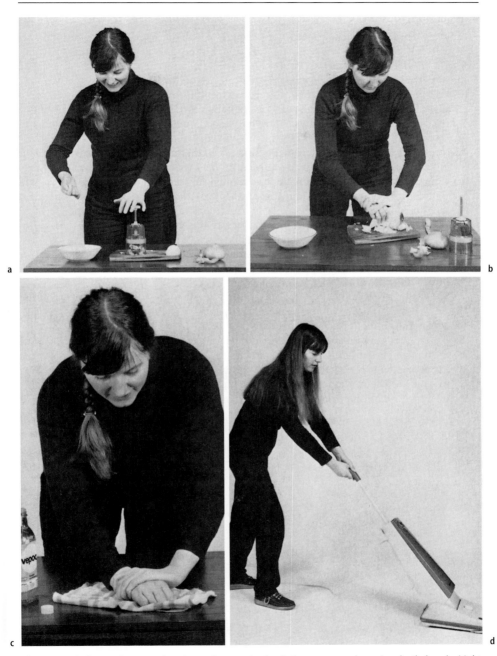

Fig. 8.28 a–d. Preventing associated reactions and stimulating recovery by using both hands (right hemiplegia). **a** Chopping up onions using only the sound hand causes the hemiplegic arm to pull into flexion. **b** Chopping onions using both hands; the arm takes part in the movement. **c** Polishing furniture. **d** Vacuum-cleaning

wards, cleaning the table and washing and drying the utensils are also part of the whole event. The patient should not struggle to use his hand in an abnormal way which may be the only way possible for him without the help of the therapist, because "if a student is only repeating his unskilled, clumsy movements, the exercise does not result in any improvement (Bernstein 1996). As the author so rightly points out, "The essence and objective of exercise is to improve the movements, that is, to change them. Therefore, correct exercise is in fact a repetition without repetition."

4. Using both hands to carry out an activity which could be done with only one hand prevents associated reactions in the hemiplegic arm and encourages the return of active control. The incorporation of the hemiplegic hand is therefore most important even before active movement has returned in the affected upper limb. For example:

a) Chopping up onions. If the patient uses only the sound hand, his hemiplegic arm pulls immediately into flexion (**Fig. 8.28 a**). If perhaps another type of implement is employed both hands are used, the sound hand holding the hemiplegic hand in place. The associated reaction is prevented; the whole body becomes more symmetrical and the movement more normal (**Fig. 8.28 b**).

b) Dusting or polishing furniture. The patient can use his clasped hands to dust or polish furniture or his motor car. If possible the hemiplegic hand lies flat on the duster and the other hand is placed over it (**Fig. 8.28 c**).

c) Shovelling snow, raking up leaves or vacuum cleaning. During these tasks, the hemiplegic hand also holds the handle even though it may need to be held in place by the sound hand during the activity (**Fig. 8.28 d**).

d) Ironing. Ironing takes a long time and, if done with the sound hand only, causes the affected arm to pull into flexion for a sustained period. Using both hands turns the activity into a beneficial therapy (**Fig. 8.29 a**) and the patient is sometimes able to continue the movement with his hemiplegic hand alone, as he smooths the garment in front of the iron with his other hand (**Fig. 8.29 b**). If necessary a protective

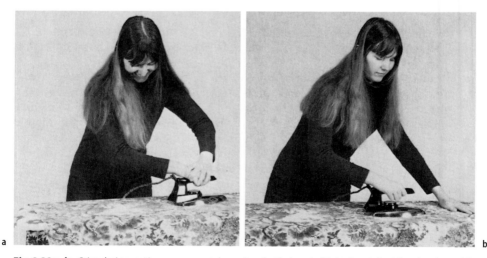

a   b

Fig. 8.29 a, b. Stimulating active movement by using both hands (right hemiplegia). **a** Ironing with both hands. **b** Continuing with the hemiplegic hand alone for a short time

strip of wood can be attached around the iron between the handle and the heated part, to avoid the danger of his fingers being burned.

5. Carrying something with the hemiplegic hand, e.g. a handbag or briefcase, even if only reflex activity is possible, helps to focus the patient's attention on the limb. Associated reactions are diminished and, in addition, the patient is free to use his other hand for more skilled activities (**Fig. 8.30**).

6. While walking, associated reactions can be inhibited by the patient holding his affected hand behind his back with outward rotation of the shoulder, using his sound hand to maintain the position (**see Fig. 9.10**). When walking out of doors with a close friend or relative, the patient holds hands with the other person, ensuring a natural appearance and a good arm swing without the arm pulling into flexion. The arms should swing forwards reciprocally with the contralateral leg and back again during the swing phase of the leg on the same side. It can easily happen that the helper and the patient both take their initial step with the same leg, for example both start walking with the right foot moving first. As a result the patient's arm swing will be out of phase – in the case of a right hemiplegia, his right arm swinging forwards with his right leg as his partner's left hand draws it forwards (**Fig. 8.31**). To ensure the recipro-

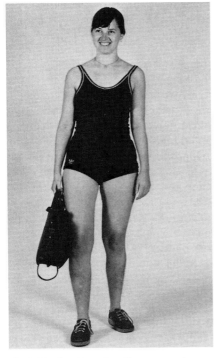

Fig. 8.30. Carrying a handbag, even when only reflex activity is possible, prevents flexion of the arm and side (right hemiplegia). Compare Fig. 3.14

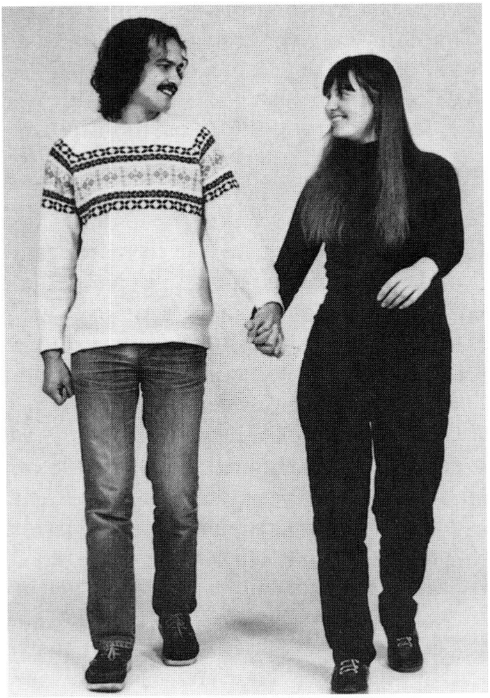

Fig. 8.31. Holding hands when walking prevents associated reactions in the arm

cal swing with the opposite arm and leg, the patient and his companion must commence walking with either the feet on the sides furthest from one another or those nearest to each other.

Considerations

If the arm and hand are not incorporated in movement and in the activities of daily life, they will have almost no experience or input at all. The sensation is not stimulated, and active movements may remain dormant. The hand becomes discarded as a useless tool, unlike the lower extremity, which has to be activated with every step the patient takes. It could be postulated that this is the reason why the sensation in the leg tends to improve, while that in the hand remains more impaired.

The patient should make it a personal rule always to use the hemiplegic hand for each and every function possible, even though it may be quicker and easier to use the sound hand on its own. "Of course some patients may not regain any function regardless of what is done, but it seems a shame to consign the arm to oblivion from the start before giving it a chance" (Semans 1965).

9 Re-educating Functional Walking

"The ability to walk upright on two legs has played a key role in human life-style for more than 3 million years" (Sagan 1979). The ability has broadened our lives and enabled us to acquire countless skills which would otherwise not have been possible." "Human gait is the most common of all human movements. It is one of the most complex totally integrated movements and yet is probably the most taken-for-granted. But walking does not come automatically like breathing. It must be learned" (Winter 1988). Because of our relatively small base in the upright posture, we require highly complex reactions to maintain our balance when walking. These balance reactions are dependent upon postural tone and the capacity to perform selective movements as described in Chaps. 2 and 3. Based on the results of animal experiments, it has been postulated that the basic movement synergies of locomotion are produced at spinal levels by so-called central pattern generators (CPGs) (Brooks 1986; Grillner 1981; Smith 1980) However, such spinal generating circuits, when stimulated by tonic activity, "produce, at best, a bad caricature of walking due to the lack of important modulating influences from the brain-stem and cerebellum" (Shumway-Cook and Woollacott 1995). In reality, as is the case with human movements in general, the movements required for functional walking arise from the interaction of multiple processes, including both perceptual and motor, as well as from the interaction between the individual, the task and the environment. "In respect to legged locomotion, the level of synergies can generate the intra- and inter-limb patterns but not actual, functional locomotion, which requires continuous and meaningful adjustments in anticipation of upcoming circumstances," and "the level of synergies' facility in guaranteeing the internal coherency of a movement contrasts with its inability to adjust the complex and harmonious movements which it produces to changes in the environment" (Turvey and Carello 1996). In real life, the movements involved in walking are dictated by plans, intentions, the wish to perform a task or solve a problem, and of course the necessity of adapting to the environment and the objects within it. Within each step cycle, the movements are finely tuned according to the needs of the task (Grillner and Zangger 1979). Because human locomotion is essentially so complex and dependent upon many higher centres, the re-education of walking entails far more than merely stimulating activity in the lower limbs or strengthening relevant muscles. It is easy to understand why some patients may require long and intensive treatment before learning to walk again and why many others who, although able to get on their feet again quite soon, will need skilled therapy to improve the way in which they walk Regardless of the problems, the time and the effort required to ensure the best possible result should not be restricted.

For every patient who has suffered a hemiplegia, the restoration of walking plays a prime role in his rehabilitation. To be able to walk again is his greatest hope and expectation, an aim which he can fully understand. Some studies have estimated that

60%–75% (Lehmann et al. 1975; Marquardsen 1969; Satterfield 1982) of the patients disabled with hemiplegia following nonfatal strokes were able to walk unaided after hospitalisation; others put the figure even higher, at 85% (Skilbeck et al. 1983; Moskowitz et al. 1972). These studies did not include the speed of the walking, the gait pattern, or whether the patients were dependent upon walking aids such as orthoses or canes. It was also not clear if the patients were able to walk on different surfaces both indoors and out, and to walk safely while performing tasks in their daily lives. Walking 20 metres in a test situation is very different from walking while concentrating on the task in hand and adapting to an environment which is constantly changing. Mulder et al. (1995) warn of the significant risk of the patient's ability being overestimated because, as they explain, "The gap between the laboratory and the everyday world would seem to be very large". Kesselring et al. (1992) also stress the inadequacy of studying walking in the artificial world of the laboratory where environmental influences are eliminated as far as possible and only the contraction of individual muscles or separate phases of gait are taken into account. The authors believe that it is of particular importance to study the movement sequence of walking in the "real world", because locomotion constitutes a special type of interaction between the organism and the environment, one which characterises its behaviour. Thus, in the opinion of Kesselring and co-workers, those studies which involve walking on moving treadmills or with suspension apparatus to relieve body weight cannot be considered valid, because the technical provisions per se will cause the movement sequences to be unnatural.

Considerations for Treatment

With improved training, not only should a higher success rate with regard to independent walking be possible, but also a more normal and economic walking pattern achieved.

In order to be truly functional, walking needs to be:

- Safe, so that the patient is not afraid and in constant danger of injuring himself through falling
- Relatively effortless, so that not all the patient's available energy is required for moving from place to place
- Fast enough to allow the patient to cross a room or circumnavigate a supermarket within a realistic time frame, and at a pace which enables him to keep up with the people accompanying him
- Cosmetically pleasing, so that the patient can walk amongst other people without being constantly stared at
- Possible without the use of a cane, so that the patient can use his sound hand to carry out tasks
- Carried out at an automatic level to enable the patient to concentrate on other activities

If these goals are to be realised, the therapist will need to understand the separate components of gait and retrain the relevant movements so that the patient can be helped to achieve the most normal walking pattern possible for him. None of the goals can be met if the patient is allowed or encouraged to walk in what has been termed the "typical hemiplegic pattern", dependent upon on a cane or quadripod for support. Many years ago, it was thought that walking in this very limited way was the only possibility for stroke patients – a belief unfortunately still held by some today. Experience has shown, however, that with informed therapy a more fluid, safer and less effortful gait can be achieved.

As Bobath (1978) so rightly recommended,

> *"In order to prepare for a reasonably normal gait, balance, stance and weight transfer should be practised. For the swing-phase the patient needs release of spasticity at hip, knee and ankle to lift his leg and make a step. He also needs control of the extending leg when putting his foot down to the ground. If all this is first practised while in the standing position, he will develop a better walking pattern than if he is made to walk immediately without the necessary control of his leg."*

When to Start Walking

It is most important that walking be included in the treatment programme as soon as possible. A patient who is kept sitting in a wheelchair too long will be afraid of the new height when he starts moving in the upright position again. Even patients without neurological impairment who have been immobilised in bed for long periods due to illness or orthopaedic conditions have expressed fear when they are allowed to stand up and walk again. In addition, prolonged sitting in a wheelchair increases flexion throughout the patient's body, making it progressively difficult for him to extend against gravity later.

Although many of the movements required for walking and maintaining balance can be prepared for in lying, the acquisition of such relatively simple control is in no way equal to the rapid selection and deselection of opposing muscle groups necessary for maintaining balance in a vertical posture. "Thus, although lying may seem to provide a precursor to vertical function in the motor-impaired individual, it seems more probable that the strategies needed to control a vertical column of segments are so specific that they can be acquired only through experiences in the vertical position" (Butler and Major 1992).

When to begin walking with the patient can be a difficult decision for all concerned, because it is always individual and will depend upon a variety of factors if unsuccessful attempts and detrimental effects are to be avoided. However, the following useful guidelines and criteria can help the therapist to decide if she can start to walk with the patient:

- During early walking attempts, an excessive amount of manual support should not be necessary, nor should the therapist require an assistant to help her to hold the patient upright or move his legs passively.
- The patient can take weight on his affected leg, and therefore does not have to lean on a cane, a quadripod or crutch in order to step forwards with his sound foot.
- Before walking is practised, the patient must be able to take weight on his hemiplegic leg without the knee being constantly hyperextended and the foot plantar flexed. The

abnormal movement pattern with its many disadvantages will otherwise be learned through repetition and be difficult to change later because, as Bach-y-Rita and Balliet (1987) warn, "If unchecked, improper motor control can become a highly reinforced program". For this reason, should a patient still have difficulty in maintaining the correct position of his limb, the therapist must first overcome the problem, either by changing the way in which she is supporting him, or by retraining selective extension of his leg.

- When supported by the therapist, the patient can transfer his weight over the sound side and take a step with his hemiplegic leg without gross contortions of his trunk taking place and without the therapist having to push or pull his foot forwards.
- With appropriate assistance the patient is able to walk in a relatively normal pattern and without a marked increase in hypertonicity in his limbs.
- If the patient is thrown into panic each time walking is attempted, despite the therapist's encouragement and support, he should not be forced to proceed and certainly not be chastised for his lack of courage, even though his motor power would seem to be adequate. Disturbed perception is invariably the underlying cause of the problem and can make walking a terrifying experience. Practising walking in isolation will only tend to reinforce the reaction, leading to despondency and a lack of willingness to try again. The same applies if the patient complains of feeling dizzy or nauseous when he is moving while upright; these symptoms are most probably caused by the discordant motion cues he receives, the "neural mismatch" described by Reason (1978). In both cases, the unpleasant symptoms are best overcome by including goal-orientated tasks when the patient is walking and by continuing to overcome his perceptual disorders through the treatment described in Chap. 1.

The Facilitation of Walking

According to the shorter *Oxford Dictionary*, to facilitate means "to render easier; to promote, help forward, to lessen the labour of, assist (a person)", facilitation being "the action, process or result of facilitating". Even the type of shoe can help to facilitate walking, and the patient should wear sturdy shoes with a leather sole and low rubber heels right from the beginning. They give better support and he can be asked to listen to the rhythm of his own walking, the sound of his shoes on the floor. Slippers encourage a shuffling gait and provide no support for the feet. We all tend to walk differently when wearing slippers!

There are many different ways in which the therapist can help the patient to walk in a more normal pattern, each based on overcoming his own particular difficulties. Her choice will depend on how well he reacts to her handling and whether his walking pattern improves as a result. To facilitate normal movement sequences and balance reactions, Bobath (1990) recommends the use of what she terms proximal and distal "key points of control", proximal key points referring to the trunk, i.e. the spine with its connections to the head, shoulder and pelvic girdles, and distal key points being a part of a limb such as the elbow, knee, hand and foot. Both types are used in combination because, according to the author, their effect on tonus and movement overlaps. "The use of proximal key points facilitates movements of the limbs while distal key points facilitate movements of the trunk." When the therapist is deciding where her hands would be most effective when helping a patient, Bobath offers the following advice:

"Key points are interchangeable and have to be adapted to the patient's reactions. The control of sequences of movements needs the changing of key points while the patient moves and according to which patterns the therapist wishes to inhibit or facilitate during the movement. Therefore, no one key point can be made responsible or used for obtaining whole sequences of movement."

Where and how the therapist's hands are assisting the patient when the best result is observed will also indicate to her where his greatest difficulty lies and thus form an integral part of her assessment.

Instructing Nursing Staff and Relatives

Once the therapist has ascertained which way of facilitating walking is most satisfactory for the individual patient she should teach the nursing staff and his relatives how they, too, can best walk with him. He will then be able to walk more frequently than if he practises only during therapy sessions and can thus become independent of a wheelchair far sooner. With careful instruction, which must include practical experience, the danger of the patient developing unwanted habits can be avoided; without such instruction, those helping him will automatically walk on his sound side, allowing him to hold on to them tightly with his sound hand and lean towards them. The best way of teaching the correct facilitation is to let the assistant feel the therapist's hands on his own body first, so that he understands which movements she is assisting and in which direction she is giving pressure. Then, while the assistant is walking with the patient, the therapist places her hands over his hands and asks him to let them remain relaxed so that he can feel exactly what her hands are doing before he continues on his own (**Fig. 9.1**). The patient does not need to use a cane for support when someone is assisting him, because the assistant can maintain balance for him and ensure the correct weight transference while he is walking.

Important Features of Walking and Associated Difficulties

Whichever way the therapist chooses to assist the patient, she should bear in mind certain features of normal walking and anticipate the difficulties which the patient is most likely to experience. Observing the ways in which the patient's walking differs from the norm will also guide the therapist as to where his key problems for treatment lie. The following characteristics of normal gait provide the therapist not only with goals for her facilitation but also with a basis for comparison when she is analysing the patient's walking difficulties. The importance of observation for evaluation and treatment is underlined by Montgomery (1987): "The single most useful tool in the clinical assessment of hemiplegic gait dysfunction is a skilled observer. Use of this tool presupposes a thorough knowledge of the postures, joint motions, muscle activity, temporal characteristics and nuances of gait."

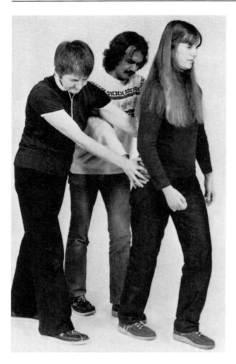

Fig. 9.1. A patient's husband learns to facilitate walking (right hemiplegia)

1. Standing Up From a Chair and Sitting Down Again

The ability to stand up and sit down easily and safely constitutes an integral part of normal functional walking. A correct upright posture has been described as the state of readiness to walk, and therefore as potential walking (Klein-Vogelbach 1976). When a person stands up from a chair, the extended trunk inclines symmetrically forward from the hips with the weight evenly distributed over both legs. The buttocks lift off the chair as the legs extend selectively, with the hips and ankles remaining flexed until weight has been brought over the feet. (see **Fig. 2.4**). Only then do the hips and knees extend to bring the trunk into the vertical posture. Sitting down entails similar movements of the trunk and limbs with regard to their joint angles and weight distribution, but the activity of the extensor muscles is eccentric as opposed to concentric when the seat is being lowered to the chair. Before a person starts to sit down, the feet move to align the body with the chair and the buttocks are placed on the supporting surface in a preselected position, which may vary according to the situation but which nevertheless affords balance and stability.

Common difficulties: If the patient does not bring his weight sufficiently far forward over his feet, standing up requires considerable effort, and hypertonicity in his arm and leg increase. Patients who stand up asymmetrically, leaning towards the sound side and with all their weight on the sound leg, have an incorrect posture on achieving

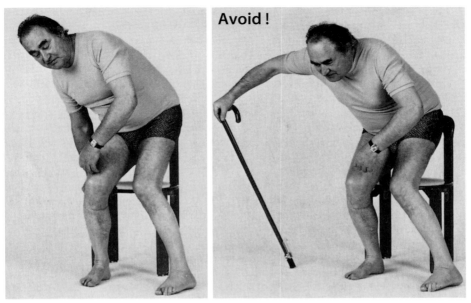

Fig. 9.2 a, b. Patient standing up asymmetrically (left hemiplegia). **a** Assisting with his sound hand; **b** using a stick

the upright position (**Fig. 9.2 a, b**). The walking pattern will be adversely affected from the very first step.

Sitting down on a chair again can be precarious because it entails several quite complex movement sequences to be really safe. Patients who fail to turn around completely to be in line with the chair, or who underestimate how far away the chair still is before sitting down, are in real danger of falling. Those who do not bring their weight sufficiently far forwards while lowering their buttocks onto the seat, but push back in extension and sit down too quickly, may cause the chair to move away or even tip over backwards. Due to disturbed perception, a patient will often sit down too far over to the hemiplegic side and may slip off the edge of the chair.

2. Forward Progression

The initiation of walking from a stance posture was shown by Carslöö (1966) to result from "the body losing its balance as a result of cessation of activity in postural muscles (including erector spinae and certain thigh and leg muscles)". The steps that follow are caused by a continuous shifting forward of the centre of gravity (Klein-Vogelbach 1976). "The various torques of the body weight displace the line of gravity, first laterally and dorsally, and then ventrally, to a position in which the propulsive muscles are able to contribute to and complete the first step" (Basmajian 1979). During the stance phase a propulsive force necessary to keep the body in motion is generated.

"The most common strategy used to generate propulsive forces for the progression in-
volves the concentric contraction of the plantar flexors (gastrocnemius and soleus) at
the end of the stance phase of gait. The ability of the body to move freely over the
foot, in conjunction with the concentric action of the gastrocnemius, means that the
center of motion of the body will be anterior to the supporting foot by the end of
stance, creating a forward fall critical to progression" (Shumway-Cook and Woollacott
1995).

The foot plantar flexes actively as the gastrocnemius shortens to provide the most important impulse of energy, with the soleus generating "an explosive push-off", according
to Winter (1988).

"The force that produces forward progression in gait is the potential energy obtained
as the body falls ahead of the supporting foot. Kinetic energy is gained in this fall
and then used to regain potential energy when the body is lifted up over the contralat-
eral foot in the next support phase" (Knuttson 1981).

Common difficulties: Most hemiplegic patients walk with their centre of gravity well behind the normal line, for several different reasons. The first step and those that follow
must therefore entail an active lifting of the leg and a placing of the foot, as the pendulum action is not produced spontaneously through the weight being transferred forward, or the body falling ahead of the supporting foot. Patients may have difficulty in
bringing their weight forwards over the standing leg due to the forces of the spastic extensor muscles and the loss of selective movement patterns. Many are quite simply
afraid of falling forwards, as the protective mechanisms are not adequate, and they
therefore feel safer when their weight is kept further back than in normal walking. Perhaps the most common contributory factor of all is the inability to plantar flex the
foot actively and selectively, a problem experienced by the great majority of patients.
Therapists tend to concentrate on regaining dorsal flexion of the foot, but without active
plantar flexion there is a loss or diminution of the propulsion forces required to bring
the body weight forwards. Many significant gait abnormalities were found to occur as
a direct result of gastrocnemius-soleus paralysis; "The abnormalities included changes
in step-length, walking speed, center of pressure advancement, timing of gait events,
ground reactive forces and joint moments", and knee stability was also affected (Lehmann et al. 1985). Without the push-off action of the plantar flexors the steps are far
shorter, because the knee does not extend at the end of the swing phase and the foot
thus makes contact with the floor far earlier. The speed of walking is therefore considerably reduced, and a reduction as great as 50% has been estimated (Waters et al. 1978).
To compensate for the loss of plantar flexion propulsion, the sound knee remains flexed
at initial contact and during loading, as the patient uses the leg muscles to pull his
weight forwards for the stance phase on that side.

3. Step Length

A normal step has been shown to be between 70 and 80 cm long, the individual length
being dependent upon several factors. Murray et al. 1964 found that subjects over
60 years of age took shorter steps than those in their twenties and that tall subjects ten-

ded to take the longest steps. However, as Klein-Vogelbach (1995) points out, "it would be an oversimplification to say that long legs take long steps and short legs short ones". The author explains that step length is dependent not only upon the length of the leg, but that the distance between the hip joints, the size of the feet and the amount of rotation and extension in the hips also play a role. She estimates that a hypothetical normal step length is between 2.5 and 4 times the length of the person's foot or, in other words, between about 60 and 96 cm when a person is walking at a normal speed.

Common difficulties: Patients take significantly shorter steps, both with the sound leg and the hemiplegic leg. Often the sound foot is placed adjacent to the hemiplegic foot or only a few centimetres in front of it. If the hemiplegic leg is brought forwards in a flexion synergy, the knee cannot be extended at the end of the swing phase and the step is thus far shorter. As a result, the walking is much slower and the energy expended to cover the distance far greater.

4. Speed and Rhythm

Normal gait is symmetrical with respect to both time and distance. The support times for right and left sides are equal, as are right and left step lengths. "The most comfortable walking speed lies close to 3.00 feet per second (0.91 m per second) to minimise 'energy consumption' and permit a reasonable propulsion speed" (Basmajian 1979).

An economically ideal walking speed is that which requires the minimum of effort for the relatively longest distance covered in a unit of time with energy consumption minimised, "when a subject is permitted to walk without the imposition of a pace frequency constraint, he selects a walking pace for the set speed in such a manner as to allow a minimum of muscular activity" (Basmajian 1979). The economic walking speed described by Klein-Vogelbach (1995) is approximately 108–120 steps a minute. In the large sample of subjects studied by Drillis (1958) the mean cadence was 112 steps per minute, while Murray et al. (1964) observed cadences of between 111 and 122 steps per minute. "An increase in velocity can be achieved by decreasing stride time (increasing cadence) or increasing stride length and is normally achieved by a combination of both" (Wall and Ashburn 1979). If the walking speed decreases to fewer than 70 steps per minute the rotation of the pelvis is almost entirely absent, and the arms will therefore no longer swing alternately (Klein-Vogelbach 1995).

Common difficulties: The hemiplegic patient walks asymmetrically with respect to both time and distance and the walking is arrhythmic. He takes a short quick step with the sound leg, possibly to avoid standing and balancing on the affected leg, but also to avoid the extension pattern of spasticity being provoked by the ensuing hip extension when the hemiplegic foot is behind. Walking slowly and carefully with a cadence way below the norm requires more balance and energy, and the patient tires quickly. Because of the reduced walking speed and the stiffness of the trunk, the rotation of the pelvis ceases and arm swing no longer occurs. Hypertonicity in the arm itself will also prevents the arm from swinging freely. Increasing the speed of walking by improving both step length and cadence is a most important aim of treatment and facilitation. The patient will otherwise have to walk alone, way behind the others with him, or they will have to adapt to his slow pace, which can be difficult and frustrating for all concerned. Although older people tend to walk more slowly in any event, research indicates that other changes in their gait may be the result of some underlying pathology rather than due to the ageing process alone. In one study, older adults without evidence of pathology in fact revealed no changes in the gait parameters tested (Gabell and Nayak 1984).

5. Stride Width

Stride width has been described as being a measure of the transverse distance between points on the central long axis of the feet during foot-to-floor contact. In a comprehensive study, the mean stride width was found to be 8 cm, with no systematic differences related to age and height of the subjects (Murray et al. 1964) The distance is considerably less than that between the hips joints, due to the inclination of the femur and to allow for economic walking, so that the feet are not directly beneath the hips during walking as could easily be imagined. Even for Murray and co-workers, their findings were unexpected: "Although the range of stride widths was large, we were surprised to see how narrow the stride widths were in many instances. Indeed, the mid-point of one foot of our normal subjects crossed over the other so that the stride width as measured was a negative value." In her inimitable style, Klein-Vogelbach (1995) avoids giving an absolute measurement but allows for individual differences in her definition: "Stride-width is the narrowest possible track which still allows the swinging foot to pass by the weightbearing leg without being impeded by it. As it does so, the medial side of the heel almost touches the medial malleolus of the standing leg."

The relatively narrow base is important, because if the limbs were parallel there would need to be considerable lateral displacement of the centre of gravity to transfer the weight over each supporting leg, which would decrease speed and increase energy expenditure (Saunders et al. 1953).

Common difficulties: Nearly all patients walk with their feet too far apart in comparison to their previous stride width, for several reasons. They may feel safer if their balance is inadequate; their weight is no longer right over the hemiplegic leg, or it may be easy for them to take a step with the affected foot if the legs are abducted. They may even be encouraged to walk more slowly and with a wider base by the therapist, who thinks it would be safer for them. However, far more selective muscle control is required to maintain balance during slow walking, and a recent study has revealed that for older patients, "Contrary to common expectation, a wider stride width does not necessarily increase stability but instead seems to predict an increased likelihood of experiencing falls" (Maki 1997). With the feet further apart than normal, weight has to be transferred not only forwards but also sideways from one foot to the other, which in turn shortens the step length. According to Klein-Vogelbach (1995), the gait resembles that of a sailor walking on board a swaying ship.

6. The Foot Angle

When the feet meet the ground, the angle which the long axis of each forms in relation to the midline or plane of progression is the same on both sides, but the angles show individual variability. The angle is dependent upon the trunk and the degree of inward or outward rotation of the hips. Houtz and Fischer (1961) showed that "a movement of the torso and hip region, that shifts their position over the feet, initiates the movement of each foot during walking. Movements initiated in the trunk lead automatically to changes in the position of the leg and foot." Although height did not influence the foot angles, subjects who were 60–65 years old showed a decidedly greater degree of "out-toeing" than did the younger subjects (Murray et al. 1964). The authors suggest that the increased foot angles of the older subjects could be their way of achieving additional lateral stability.

Common difficulties: Many patients are unable to stabilise their trunk adequately when walking, and lateral flexion or excessive rotation occurs. Others flex or extend their trunk in order to bring the hemiplegic leg forwards or use vigorous extension of the sound hip to do so. Distortion of the trunk- and hip-initiated movements causes the steps that follow to be abnormal too, so that even the sound foot does not adopt a normal position, but tends to be turned inwards toward the midline. The hemiplegic foot is frequently placed with the toes pointing laterally but the leg may be turned inwards with the opposite result.

7. The Forward Motion of the Hips

The movement direction of both hips, which can be observed at the level of the two femoral trochanters, is never backwards in normal walking, and there is no period when either hip is stationary. Throughout the gait cycle both hip joints move continually forwards through space along a wave-shaped path (Klein-Vogelbach 1976).

Common difficulties: The hips do not move forwards as in normal walking, but the direction of movement varies and often the hip joint actually moves backwards in the opposite direction to that in which the patient is walking. The backward movement occurs either during the stance phase, if the knee hyperextends, or during the swing phase, when the pelvis is hitched upwards in retraction to bring the hemiplegic leg forward actively in a flexion synergy.

8. The Swing Phase

"The swing phase of a normal gait is a low-energy phase. Once initiated the weight of the leg swings forward like a pendulum, but its course is regulated by several muscles of the thigh and leg" (Basmajian 1979). "The hip is laterally rotating during the entire swing phase due to pelvic rotation in conjunction with the leg's forward controlled momentum" (Basmajian 1979). Klein-Vogelbach (1984) agrees that the movement of the leg is always one of outward rotation at the hip throughout its swing phase and describes the forward movement of the limb as being reactive, brought about by the active stance phase on the contralateral side. Muscle activity in the swinging limb is therefore confined largely to the beginning and end of the swing phase, because the leg swings forward like a jointed pendulum under the influence of gravity. For the foot to swing through unhampered, the leg must shorten, and, according to Perry (1992), "In swing, knee flexibility is the primary factor in the limb's freedom to advance". At the end of the stance phase, the leg is rapidly unloaded and the knee flexes passively to an angle of approximately 30° to initiate the swing phase. The knee flexes further to about 60° by the time it passes the supporting limb at mid-swing. In addition, to allow the leg to shorten and swing freely forward its weight has to be suspended from above, which requires appropriate activity in the ventral muscles of the trunk to support the pelvis (Davies 1990).

In order for the toes to clear the ground easily during the swing phase, the foot needs to be actively dorsiflexed. It is important to note that dorsiflexion of the ankle is achieved by the tibialis anterior with the assistance of the extensor digitorum longus and extensor hallucis. The peronei are inactive during dorsiflexion. "At mid-swing the tibialis anterior becomes inactive for a period to allow the foot to evert and remain everted during mid-swing. This allows for adequate clearance, while the inactivity of the invertor fits the concept of reciprocal inhibition of antagonists" (Basmajian 1979).

The popular concept that supination of the foot is due to peroneal weakness should therefore be reconsidered. The peronei are active and most important during the stance phase to prevent excessive inversion of the foot, and thus maintain appropriate contact with the ground. The peroneus longus helps to stabilise the leg and foot during mid-stance, and Walmsley (1977) found the peroneus brevis to act synchronously with peroneus longus during ordinary walking.

Common difficulties: Patients with hemiplegia have difficulty in achieving a normal swing phase when walking. There is a great variety in the type and degree of difficulty, but for the majority of patients, inability to release the knee for the 30° of passive flexion at the initiation of swing and to increase the angle to 60° by mid-swing is the most significant cause of the abnormal forward movement of the hemiplegic leg. Three main factors contribute to the abnormal swing phase of the hemiplegic leg:

- Extensor hypertonus prevents the necessary shortening of the leg. After a step forwards is taken with the sound leg, the affected leg behind has a marked hypertonus in all the extensor muscle groups. The extension at the hip increases extensor hypertonicity throughout the leg in the total pattern of extension (**Fig. 9.3 a**). With flexion at hip, knee and ankle difficult if not impossible (**Fig. 9.3 b**), the patient hitches up the side of his pelvis and brings the extended leg forwards through circumduction in order to clear the floor (**Fig. 9.3 c**).
  Dimitrijevic et al. (1981) state that "the observed paralysis of the foot in hemiplegic patients seems to be, in the majority of cases, an 'active' paralysis due to the pull of the hypertonic triceps surae muscles". The foot is placed flat on the floor at the end of the swing phase, and often the ball of the foot makes contact with the ground first. The foot often remains outwardly rotated as the pelvis is retracted on that side. Some patients may succeed in bringing the whole side of the trunk forward, and the leg is then rotated towards the midline when it reaches the floor in front.
- Loss of selective movement with disturbed reciprocal inhibition. Where this problem predominates, the patient lifts his hemiplegic leg to take a step forwards, and in the mass pattern of flexion the side of the pelvis is lifted, the hip flexed in abduction and outward rotation, the knee flexed, and the ankle and foot dorsiflexed and supinated with the toes in flexion. The continuous activity of tibialis anterior without reciprocal inhibition causes the foot to remain supinated throughout the movement forward (**Fig. 9.4**). The leg is brought forward without the knee extending before the foot makes contact with the ground, and the step length is therefore greatly reduced.
- Inability to transfer weight adequately over the sound leg and free the affected leg for the swing. Most patients who have difficulty with the swing phase of gait will have difficulty in transferring their weight correctly over the sound leg while at the same time supporting the contralateral side of the pelvis from the trunk musculature above. When such activity is inadequate, too much weight remains on the hemiplegic

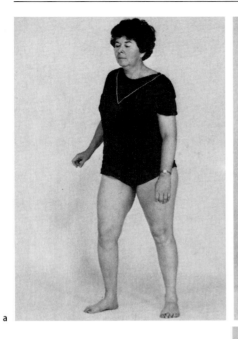

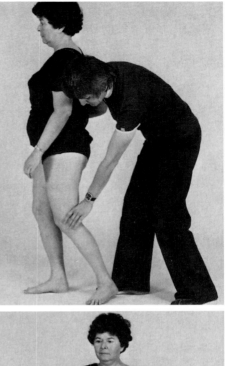

a

b

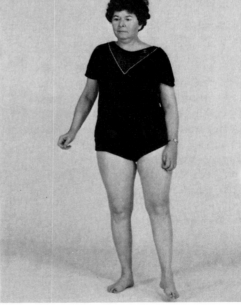

Fig. 9.3 a–c. Extensor hypertonicity in the hemiplegic leg prevents a normal swing phase (left hemiplegia). **a** Total pattern of extension after stepping forwards with the sound leg. **b** Marked resistance to hip and knee flexion. **c** The patient hitches her pelvis up and circumducts the extended leg to clear the floor

c

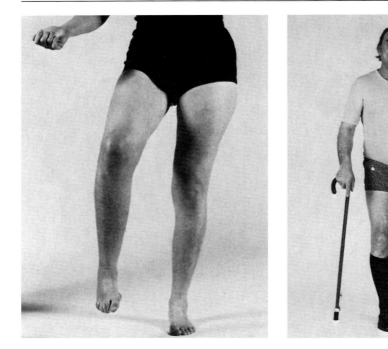

Fig. 9.4. Supination of the foot during the swing phase due to uninhibited activity in the tibialis anterior (right hemiplegia)

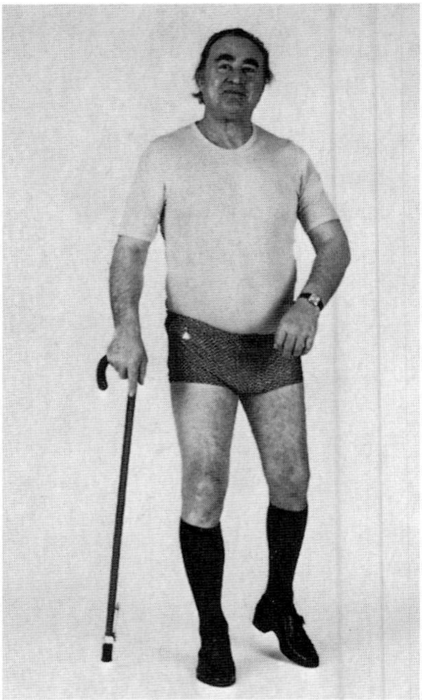

Fig. 9.5. The patient has difficulty in transferring weight over the sound side, despite using a cane (left hemiplegia)

leg because it has to support the side of the pelvis by propping it up from below (**Fig. 9.5**). The foot continues to push against the floor and cannot be relaxed in preparation for the swing phase. The patient has then to lift his leg actively with effort, releasing the weight either by leaning sideways toward the sound side or by hitching up the side of his pelvis before taking the step.

9. The Stance Phase

During the stance phase of gait, the supporting leg has to be stabilised to take the weight of the body; it has to provide the propulsive force necessary for progression, and it also needs to adapt to changes in speed, direction and the supporting surface itself.

The knee is never fully extended during normal walking. In certain phases where extension can be observed it is always between 5 and 10° short of the fullest possible range. The maintenance of this small amount of flexion serves as a shock absorber and also permits a smooth, easy transition from stance to swing phase. The greatest degree of extension occurs not during stance, but at the end of the swing phase to enable heel strike to be sufficiently far forward.

Common difficulties:

- A large percentage of patients, if not correctly trained from the beginning, will have a hyperextended knee during the stance phase of gait **(Fig. 9.6)**. Hyperextension of the knee has many disadvantages and should be avoided when the patient starts learning to walk again, or the problem should be overcome if he already locks his knee during weightbearing. Continued use of the total extension pattern can otherwise cause a progressive increase in extensor hypertonicity, shortening of the Achilles tendon and biomechanical changes at the ankle joint. Without the necessary amount of knee flexion during stance the leg will not move forward with momentum for the swing phase that follows, and many other functional activities which require flexion of the leg will be impaired as well, such as putting on shoes and socks, climbing stairs and getting into the bath. The hyperextended or "locked" knee usually occurs because:

- Active selective hip extension is not possible for the patient and he is therefore unable to bring his weight forwards over the hemiplegic foot. He steps forwards with the sound leg and the hemiplegic hip moves backwards, its continuous forward movement being interrupted. Because the femur is sloping backwards the knee hyperextends, and the weight hangs on the ligaments and soft tissue structures of the hip and knee.

- In the attempt to extend the hip and knee for weightbearing, the whole lower limb extends in a mass pattern, including plantar flexion of the ankle. The foot pushes down against the floor, and the resulting backward movement of the tibia produces hyperextension of the knee.

Knuttson (1981) has shown that during hemiplegic gait "the triceps surae activity may occur prematurely, starting immediately or shortly after foot-floor contact, since

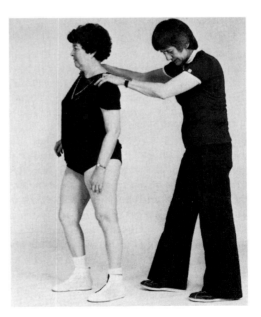

Fig. 9.6. Hyperextension of the hemiplegic knee during the stance phase. The hip has moved backwards (left hemiplegia)

the contact is often made with the foot flat on the floor, or with low toe elevation". The early activation of the triceps surae muscle usually leads to a tension increase sufficiently large to shorten the muscles before the body has passed ahead of the foot.

- Bobath (1978) describes how the heel of the hemiplegic leg is frequently placed down only after the toes have touched the ground. "The spastic resistance of the calf muscles makes full dorsiflexion in weight-bearing and weight transfer forward impossible. The patient therefore leans forward at the hip and bends it in order to transfer his weight over the standing leg. This results in hyperextension of the knee." Bobath also states that if the patient is made to extend his hip and bring it well forwards, his knee also extends but without hyperextending.
- With inadequate sensation in the leg, the patient locks his knee to be absolutely certain that it is extended and will support his weight. When the knee is slightly flexed, only very fine changes in soft tissue tension and joints provide information as to its exact position, but at the limit of its mechanical range of motion, the patient feels a total resistance which tells him that it is fully extended.

10. Balance

Walking can be thought of as a constant losing and regaining of balance, because weight is transferred forwards before the foot meets the ground at the end of each swing phase. "In walking, the center of gravity does not stay within the support base of the feet and thus the body is in a continuous state of imbalance. The only way to prevent falling is to place the swinging foot ahead and lateral to the center of gravity as it moves forward" (Shumway-Cook and Woollacott 1995). Repeated patterns of using, abandoning and regaining a balanced stance on the ground with alternate legs are therefore entailed (Brooks 1986). Balance strategies are adaptive, as they need to be for the performance of different tasks, or to avoid bumping into other people or objects, and for staying upright despite changes in the supporting surface. The ability to take quick automatic steps in whatever direction necessary appears to be the safest and most used strategy for maintaining or regaining balance while walking. Maki and McIlroy (1997) write that, "Contrary to traditional views, change-in-support reactions are not just strategies of last resort, but are often initiated well before the center of mass is near the limits of the base of support", and that subjects appear to select these reactions when given the option.

Common difficulties: Without specific training, the patient is usually unable to take quick reactive steps in all directions and as a result feels justifiably insecure. Increased tone and loss of selective activity prevent the reactive steps with the hemiplegic leg, and the inability to take weight on it impedes the steps with the sound foot. The patient may take a single step with his sound leg, but often one step is not sufficient to restore balance. This is particularly the case if he is falling towards his affected side, because once his sound leg has crossed over in front of the hemiplegic leg he is unable to flex the knee to free the foot in order to step quickly sideways with it. He therefore holds on tightly to stable objects in the vicinity with his sound hand or leans heavily on any form of fixed support.

11. Head Movements

In order to walk safely in and out of doors the head needs to be free to move independently without disturbing the walking pattern or its rhythm or speed. Balance is dependent upon information being provided by receptors in the cervical vertebrae and neck muscles, and such information is distorted or absent if the neck is held rigidly in one position (Wyke 1983). Being able to look to both sides is essential for avoiding collisions with objects, cars and other people, and normally when turning around, the head turns first as if leading the way. Free neck movements are necessary for performing tasks while moving in upright positions, and walking for pleasure entails turning the head to talk to companions, to window-shop or to enjoy nature in all its forms.

Common difficulties: The patient's neck is often held stiffly in one position, which contributes automatically to his poor balance, and if he cannot turn his head freely he will also be in danger of bumping into objects around him. The danger is accentuated if he has a hemianopia in addition because he will not be able to compensate for the visual field defect by turning his head. Many patients find it difficult to walk straight ahead if their head is turned to look at something, while others feel that they can walk only while staring fixedly at the ground or some point directly in front of them. When they are turning around, the head does not turn first but is kept in line with the rest of their vertebral column. Due to the influence of tonic neck reflexes, the position of the head will affect tone throughout the body, but particularly in the extremities.

Practical Ways to Facilitate Walking

When facilitating walking the therapist uses her hands in different ways, all aimed at preventing the common difficulties from occurring. Her hands can assist the selective movement patterns, inhibit or prevent unwanted activity and help the patient to transfer his weight appropriately. Facilitation would imply that the patient is enabled to bear weight on the hemiplegic leg without hyperextending his knee and to swing his leg forwards without hitching up his pelvis or circumducting his leg, and that the step lengths are more similar both in time and space. Facilitation should make walking less effortful, speedier and more rhythmic. Any form of facilitation that helps the individual patient to walk easily and rhythmically can be considered as being appropriate for treatment, but the following methods have proved to be the most useful.

For Standing Up

The preparation for standing up correctly from sitting has been described fully in Chap. 6. The activities should be practised carefully until the patient is able to bring his weight forwards over his feet without difficulty and come to a standing position without having to use his sound hand for support. When standing up in readiness for walking, the patient should be given the necessary amount of help to enable him to do so in a normal pattern. The therapist places her hands on either side of the patient's pelvis, and as he comes to the upright position, she helps him to extend his hip selectively,

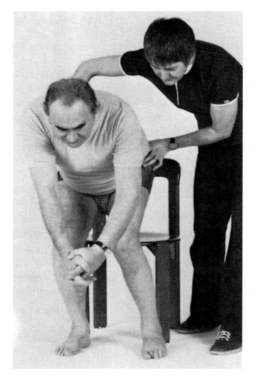

Fig. 9.7. Standing up from a sitting position without using the hand for support (left hemiplegia)

so that hyperextension of the knee is avoided (**Fig. 9.7**). If necessary, she uses her shoulder behind his thorax to prevent him from pushing back in the total pattern of extension as he stands up. She does not block the movement mechanically but instead asks the patient to try not to press against her shoulder.

Once he is standing upright, she encourages him to relax his arms at his sides, take weight equally through both legs and breathe out quietly before starting to walk.

For Sitting Down

The therapist reminds the patient not to sit down before he has moved into the appropriate position in relation to the chair and helps him to turn around first. As he starts to sit down she tells him to bend both knees and place his seat well back in the chair without a bump. With one hand on his hemiplegic knee, she draws it forwards over his foot and outwards to prevent the leg from adducting. Her other hand over the trochanter on the opposite side guides his buttocks slowly down to the middle of the chair. Her arm and shoulder behind his thorax regulate the speed of the movement by helping him to bring his trunk sufficiently far forwards over his feet.

For Walking

Preventing Hyperextension of the Knee by Assisting Hip Extension

For the patient who still requires assistance to extend his hip and so avoid hyperextending his knee, the therapist stands at his side and places one hand on each side of his pelvis. Her hand on his hemiplegic side is so placed that her thumb is directly behind the head of the femur, which is located approximately in the middle of the bulge formed by the gluteus muscle group (**Fig. 9.8 a**). The hip joint is more medial than is sometimes imagined, and careful palpation is needed to avoid the therapist mistakenly placing her thumb on the bony trochanter instead. Her fingers remain relaxed on the lateral aspect of the hip.

The therapist asks the patient to let both his knees flex slightly and then helps him to bring his weight over the hemiplegic side. As he steps forward with his sound leg, she guides his hip forwards into extension and lateral rotation, using her thumb behind the head of the femur to assist the correct movement. The pressure of her thumb is in a forward, downward and rotatory direction, which moves the patient's knee along the line of the long axis of the supporting foot. The reactive swing phase of the sound leg is facilitated by helping the patient to extend his hip and move his weight sufficiently far forwards over the supporting leg without his knee pushing back into hyperextension

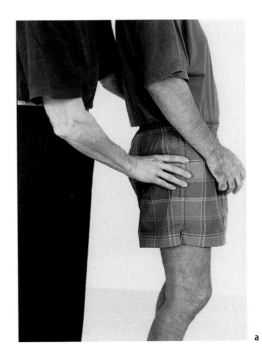

Fig. 9.8 a–e. Facilitating walking from the pelvic region (right hemiplegia). **a** The therapist's right thumb is directly behind the head of the femur

a

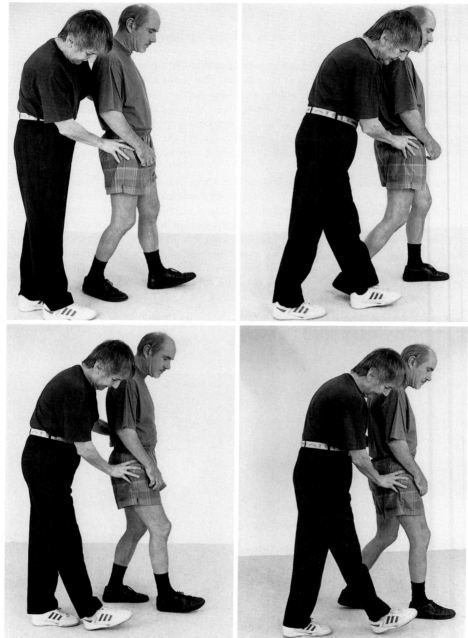

Fig. 9.8 b–e. b Pressing the hip forward and downward to prevent hyperextension of the knee in the stand phase. **c** Assisting flexion of the knee for the initiation of the swing phase with weight well over the sound leg. **d** Preventing the pelvis from being hitched up as the hemiplegic leg moves forward. **e** Pressing the head of the femur forward and downward with lateral rotation as soon as the foot meets the floor to ensure selective hip extension during weight acceptance

(**Fig. 9.8 b**). The patient is encouraged to take a step of as near normal length as possible and tries to put his heel down on the ground first with the foot dorsiflexed and turned slightly outwards.

The weight is then brought diagonally forwards over the extended sound limb, until the hemiplegic leg is free to flex for the initiation of the swing phase. The therapist's arm and hand supporting his sound side give the patient confidence to transfer his weight sufficiently (**Fig. 9.8 c**).

The patient releases his hip and knee and lets his heel fall inwards, i. e. in outward rotation of the hip, in preparation for the swing. The therapist presses downwards and forwards on the pelvis, along the line of the femur, as the hip and knee flex. She prevents the patient from hitching up the side of the pelvis and helps its forward rotation as the leg swings forward (**Fig. 9.8 d**).

At the very moment when the patient's hemiplegic foot reaches the ground in front again, the therapist quickly guides his hip forwards over that leg, to avoid the knee pushing back into hyperextension and its position having to be corrected (**Fig. 9.8 e**).

The sequence is then repeated, starting with the swing phase of the sound leg. The walking movements are carried out slowly and exactly at first, and the patient is given positive feedback to inform him when they are correctly performed. The therapist controls and organises the walking completely until the patient has learnt the sequence, timing and pattern of movement. She sets the rhythm with her hands and her voice and increases the tempo when she feels that the patient is ready to do so. As the patient's ability increases, she gradually reduces the amount of support, both manual and verbal, and once the speed has increased sufficiently, arm swing can be facilitated from the pelvis (**Fig. 9.9**).

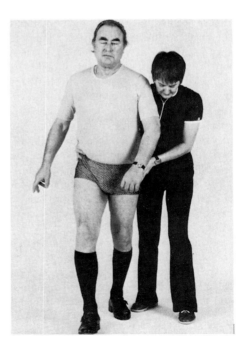

Fig. 9.9. Facilitating arm swing by assisting the correct rotation of the pelvis (left hemiplegia)

Helping the Patient to Stabilise his Thoracic Spine

If the patient cannot stabilise his thoracic spine adequately the movements of his legs will be abnormal. The therapist uses her hands to stabilise his thorax and move it forwards so that the steps follow reactively in a more selective pattern. Synergistic movements are eliminated when walking is facilitated in this way, even though the limbs themselves are not being manipulated directly. The patient who has difficulty in orientating his trunk correctly over his pelvis also benefits from feeling the therapist's hands in front of him and behind him as points of reference.

The therapist places one hand on the patient's thorax from behind at about the level of the thoracic vertebrae 8–10 and her other hand in front across the sternal angle and the lower ribs (**Fig. 9.10 a**). She presses her hands firmly against his chest, and with a slight lifting movement she moves his weight over the hemiplegic leg and then forwards to elicit the step with the sound foot (**Fig. 9.10 b**). Immediately the heel makes contact with the ground in front, the therapist transfers the patient's weight diagonally forwards over the sound leg for the new stance phase, and the hemiplegic knee flexes to initiate its swing phase (**Fig. 9.10 c**). The foot swings through as the therapist continues to move the trunk forwards and the knee extends with the momentum, heel-strike following after a normal step length (**Fig. 9.10 d**). Once the speed of walking is sufficient, the trunk rotates below the level of the therapist's stabilising hands and the arms start to swing reactively.

With One Arm Held Forward and Upward in External Rotation

A patient may be able to walk independently, but because of flexor hypertonus in the arm his gait is slow and effortful and his weight too far back To prevent the backward pull of the hemiplegic side and shoulder, the therapist can facilitate weight transference forwards by holding the patient's hemiplegic arm well out in front of him in an inhibitory pattern as he walks (**Fig. 9.11**). The patient must already be able to walk unaided and have enough active control of his hemiplegic leg to take weight on it during the stance phase, because with both the therapist's hands supporting his arm in the inhibited position, his shoulder could otherwise be damaged should he lose his balance or his leg give way.

The therapist first inhibits spasticity in the patient's arm by mobilising his scapula in elevation and protraction. With the hand nearest to the patient placed beneath his humerus just proximal to the elbow, she keeps his elbow extended and lifts the arm forwards and upwards in line with his trunk until the shoulder is flexed to an angle of 90°.

To stabilise the patient's trunk and to prevent the ribs being pulled upwards when she lifts the arm into position, the therapist presses her forearm firmly against his ribcage. Her other hand holds his wrist, hand and fingers in dorsal flexion using the inhibitory grip shown in **Fig. 8.14 a**.

Using a lumbrical grip, her hand supporting his arm from below guides the humeral condyles gently forwards as the patient takes a step with his sound foot and begins to walk. The web between her thumb and fingers supports the weight of the upper arm in slight outward rotation in order to maintain the correct alignment of the shoulder joint and prevent traumatising the soft tissue structures surrounding it.

With the patient's hemiplegic side no longer retracting and his weight brought forwards, the steps follow one another reactively in a flowing manner.

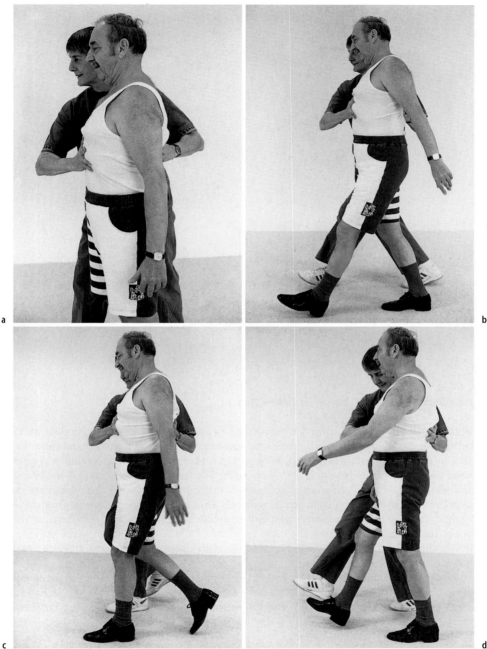

Fig. 9.10a–d. Stabilizing the thoracic spine to facilitate walking (right hemiplegia). **a** The therapist holds the patient's lower thorax firmly between her hands, with one hand against his sternum and the other against his thoracic spine. **b** Weight shifted over the hemiplegic side and forwards elicits a re-active step with the sound foot. **c** The whole body is moved diagonally forwards to the sound side for initiation of the swing phase. **d** A normal reactive step with the hemiplegic leg follows spontaneously

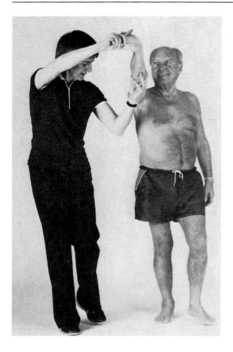

Fig. 9.11. Facilitating walking with the patient's arm held forward at an angle of 90° to his trunk (left hemiplegia)

With Both the Patient's Arms Held Behind Him

With the patient who can control hip and knee extension adequately, the therapist walks behind him, holding his arms in extension and outward rotation and his hands and fingers in dorsal extension (**Fig. 9.12 a**; see also **Fig. 8.14 a**). Her facilitation enables the patient to extend his hips and torso more easily by counteracting flexion of the trunk and shoulders. When the therapist holds the arms in one position as the patient walks, hypertonicity in the hemiplegic arm is reduced. The movement of the trunk proximally against the arm distally inhibits spasticity and counteracts associated reactions of the upper limb (**Fig. 9.12 b**). Using the same grip she can facilitate rotation while walking, by moving the appropriate shoulder forwards, with the arms remaining extended and outwardly rotated.

When facilitating walking in this way it is important that the patient's weight is not drawn backwards by the pull on his arms. With her fingers on the balls of his hands, the therapist therefore gives a slight but constant pressure upwards and forwards through his extended arms, which helps him to bring his whole body forwards over his feet throughout the gait cycle.

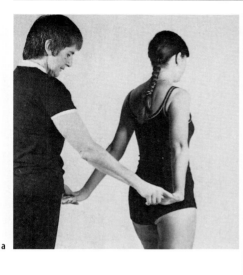

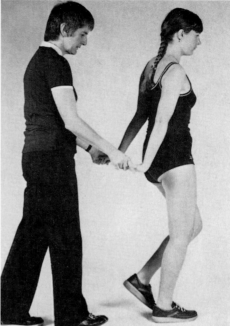

Fig. 9.12 a, b. Facilitating walking, with the patient's arms held behind her in external rotation (right hemiplegia)

Assisting Trunk Rotation from the Patient's Shoulders

When the therapist feels that the patient's arms have relaxed and he is walking at an appropriate pace, she can start to facilitate a reactive arm swing. She places her hands lightly on the patient's shoulders, with her fingers in front and her thumbs behind so that she can help the patient to adduct his scapula and extend his thoracic spine. With her thumbs the therapist moves the patient laterally and forwards over each successive weightbearing leg.

Helping the patient to stabilise his upper thorax, the therapist rotates alternate sides rhythmically forwards and then backwards in time with the swing phase of each leg, as they do in normal walking. The shoulders themselves should not move back and forth; instead, her hands ensure that the trunk rotation is taking place below the level of the 8th thoracic vertebra and the arms begin to swing as a result (**Fig. 9.13**). It should be remembered that the arms will swing only when the walking tempo is sufficient. If the patient is walking too slowly, he will move his arms actively in a stiff and artificial manner in his attempt to simulate an arm swing.

In certain cases, however, the therapist may need to ask the patient to allow his arms to swing actively in order to overcome the tendency either to fix his sound arm against his side or to hold it stiffly in one position for increased stability.

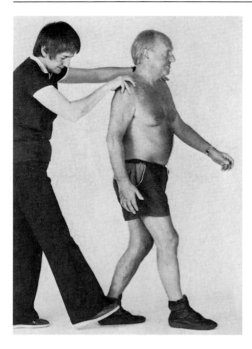

Fig. 9.13. Facilitating arm swing from the patient's shoulders (right hemiplegia)

With the Hemiplegic Arm Supported on the Therapist's Shoulder

Facilitating walking from in front of the patient with both his arms resting on the therapist's shoulders is not recommended, as the position increases flexion in the trunk and hips (**Fig. 9.14 a**). It is a normal compensatory reaction that when a person lifts his arms forward his hips flex to maintain equilibrium (Klein-Vogelbach 1976). The therapist therefore places only the patient's hemiplegic arm on her shoulder and splints his arm with her arm, her hand over his scapula to keep it forward. She can then use her other hand to help the patient to bring his hip forwards into extension over the supporting leg (**Fig. 9.14 b**). This method of facilitation can be useful for achieving rotation of the pelvis over the weightbearing leg, if the therapist asks the patient to rotate his pelvis back and forth rhythmically a few times before taking each step.

Facilitation of walking with the therapist in front of the patient has certain disadvantages. Free rhythmic walking is prevented, as the therapist is walking backwards. The patient tends to lean on the therapist, so gaining extension from his arms instead of from his hips. The position can also make him dependent on someone being in front of him, and in fact he has to learn to walk with space in front of him, as he must in his daily life.

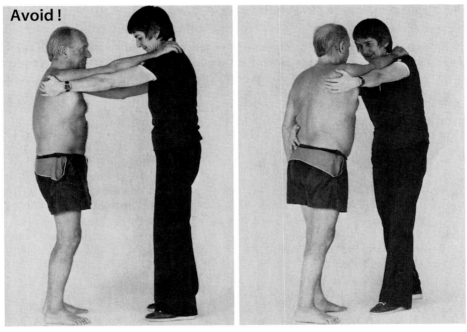

Fig. 9.14 a, b. Facilitating walking with the hemiplegic arm supported on the therapist's shoulders (right hemiplegia). **a** With both arms on the therapist's shoulders, increases flexion in the trunk and hips increases. The normal compensatory reaction is seen in the therapist's posture as well. **b** With only the hemiplegic arm supported, the therapist can use her other hand to assist hip extension

Avoiding Fixed Positions of the Arms

When learning to walk again many patients will hold their sound arm in a fixed position, either in an attempt to stabilise their trunk or because their balance is still inadequate. Associated reactions in the hemiplegic arm are common if hypertonicity is present, and the persistent flexed position is not only unsightly but will have a negative affect on the gait pattern as well. Introducing activities with objects which require that the patient use both his arms to perform them can help to overcome both problems. The activities can be enjoyable as well as making walking less frightening for the patient who is still rather afraid in upright positions.

The patient can bounce a ball in front of him as he walks, or throw it up in the air and catch it again (**Fig. 9.15**). The activity has the added effect of improving the rhythm of walking, if he bounces or throws the ball in time with each step he takes.

The patient can play a tambourine rhythmically as he walks. He taps out the rhythm of his own walking and tries to keep the beat regular. If he has active function in his hemiplegic hand he can hold the tambourine himself (**Fig. 9.16**), but otherwise the therapist holds it for him. By changing the position of the tambourine the therapist encourages the patient to move his head freely and not fix his eyes on the ground.

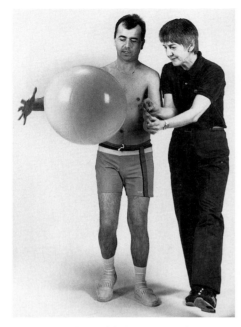 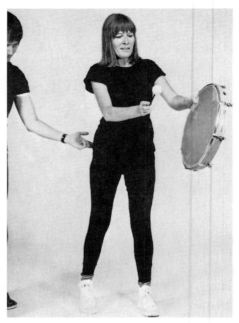

Fig. 9.15. Walking while bouncing and catching a ball inhibits associated reactions in the hemiplegic arm and improves rhythm as well. The therapist guides the patient's affected hand until he can manage on his own (left hemiplegia). (From *Right in the Middle*, Davies 1990)

Fig. 9.16. Walking rhythmically while keeping time with a tambourine, the patient does not look at the ground (right hemiplegia). Compare Fig. 3.16

Self-inhibition of Associated Reactions

If the patient's hemiplegic arm flexes strongly when he is walking, he or his therapist may inadvisably consider using the sound hand to prevent the spastic reaction, because it is unsightly and because they fear a further increase in tone.

The patient should not be asked to clasp his hands together in front of him when he walks, as the position will reinforce the flexion of the trunk and hips and prevent the arms from swinging. In addition, the force required to control the hypertonic limb will only accentuate the problem. Later, when balance and selective activity have been re-trained and the patient has learned to walk more confidently and without so much ef-fort, the arm will pull less strongly into flexion and remain at his side.

Some patients understandably choose to hold their hands behind their back when walking out of doors alone to prevent the abnormal posture of the hemiplegic arm, which draws attention to their disability. If a patient wishes to walk in this way when in public, he should be taught to hold the affected arm in outward rotation, so that his trunk is more upright and medial rotation of the shoulder is counteracted (**Fig. 9.17**). Al-though preferable to clasping the hands together in front, the fixed position of the arms has the same disadvantages.

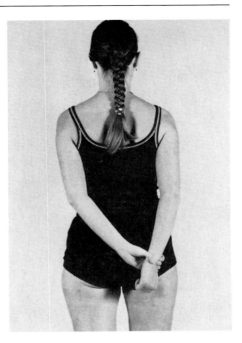

Fig.9.17. The patient inhibits flexor spasticity in her hemiplegic arm when walking on her own (right hemiplegia). Compare Fig.3.14

Protective Steps to Regain Balance

In order to walk safely and functionally, the patient needs to be able to take quick steps automatically in any direction necessary, and with either leg. Such steps often need to be practised slowly and carefully at first, and the speed gradually increased. The ability to take steps backwards and sideways is also essential for functional activities. To arrange his position to sit down at a table, on the toilet or when getting into a car, the patient must be able to manoeuvre his feet in any direction necessary.

Backwards

When the individual components of taking a step backwards described in Chap. 6 have been practised, the patient learns to walk backwards in a normal pattern. During quick protective steps backwards the body leans forwards from the hips. The therapist facilitates the movement by holding the patient's pelvis on each side and drawing it back towards her at increasing speed, and eventually without any warning or preparation (**Fig. 9.18**).

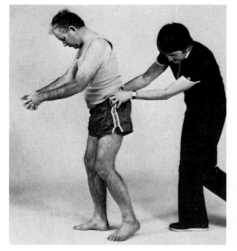

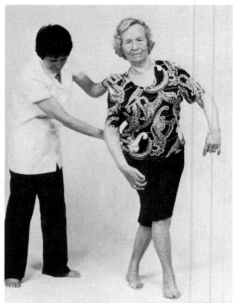

Fig. 9.18. Protective steps backwards
(left hemiplegia)

Fig. 9.19. Protective steps sideways (right   ▷
hemiplegia)

Sideways

Practising walking sideways will not only enable the patient to take protective steps but
will also improve the stance and swing phases of walking. The patient crosses one leg in
front of the other as he takes each step, and the speed is increased gradually **(Fig. 9.19)**.

Steps to Follow

To be fully confident and safe, the patient must be able to take quick automatic steps in
any direction. The therapist facilitates such "steps to follow" with her hands placed
lightly on the patient's shoulders. As he walks, she steers him unexpectedly in all directions and he follows without any resistance **(Fig. 9.20)**. The patient should also be able to
take the automatic steps when the therapist indicates the direction by moving his hemiplegic arm without giving a verbal command **(Fig. 9.21)**.

It is important to remember that normally, when we turn around, our head turns first
so that we can see where we are going. Many patients do not turn their head spontaneously in the direction of the movement, but hold it in one fixed position instead.
They face in the new direction only when the trunk has turned, bringing the head with
it. The correct rotation may have to be practised by turning the head consciously at
first. Practising rolling, which requires the same rotation, helps to retrain the movement. Activities such as bouncing a ball or beating a tambourine while turning round
will also help to overcome the difficulty.

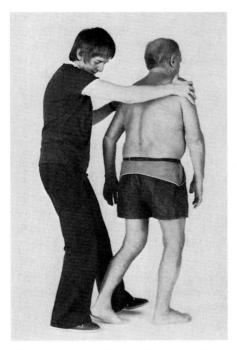 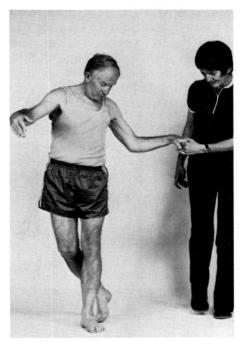

Fig. 9.20. Steps to follow in all directions (right hemiplegia)

Fig. 9.21. Quick automatic steps in an unexpected direction (left hemiplegia)

Supporting the Hemiplegic Foot

For a correct walking pattern the patient needs a certain amount of active dorsiflexion of the ankle and extension of the toes. He also needs to be able to inhibit the over-activity of the tibialis, which otherwise pulls the foot strongly into supination during dorsiflexion. For many patients the swing phase of gait, with its flexor components, is influenced by the total mass flexor synergy of the whole leg, which includes supination. Marked supination or plantar inversion at the end of the swing phase can easily lead to a sprained ankle or even a fracture if weight is prematurely taken through the hemiplegic leg, before the position of the foot has been adjusted.

With careful treatment, where the various components of walking are individually practised, the difficulties can usually be overcome. The decision to order a permanent calliper or some form of rigid foot brace should not be made too early, because most patients will learn to manage without one. The first consideration for the therapist is the patient's footwear, because shoes alone can make a big difference to both his safety and the pattern of his walking. Unfortunately, because present-day fashion favours sport shoes with popular brand names, many patients, regardless of their age, arrive for treatment wearing exactly these, obviously new and specially purchased for the occasion. But the rubber sole extending over the toes accentuates the problem of lifting the foot clear of the floor, and the cushioning effect for which the shoes are renowned detracts further from the amount of information that patients with poor sensation are able to perceive. Different types of shoes should therefore be tried out before any form of definitive support for the foot is deemed necessary. Although there may be surprising individual differences, most patients will be helped by shoes which ideally have the following features:

- A wide sole which extends further than the uppers on both sides
- Smooth leather soles which will not stick to the floor during the swing phase
- A heel about 2–3 cm high to assist forward propulsion in the absence of active plantar flexion
- A broad rubber heel for increased stability during weightbearing
- Uppers without rough stitching which might cause pressure sores
- Buckles or Velcro fasteners to avoid the frustration of grappling with shoe laces

A shoe with all these features was specially designed and made by Bally in Switzerland and has helped to improve the gait pattern of many hemiplegic patients and enabled others to walk without additional orthotic devices (**Fig. 9.22 a**). The shoe may be too expensive for some patients to afford, but it is possible to find similar shoes on the market which have many of the important characteristics (see **Fig. 10.21**). A half-boot type of shoe provides some lateral support in addition, which has helped other patients to walk more confidently (**Fig. 9.22 b**).

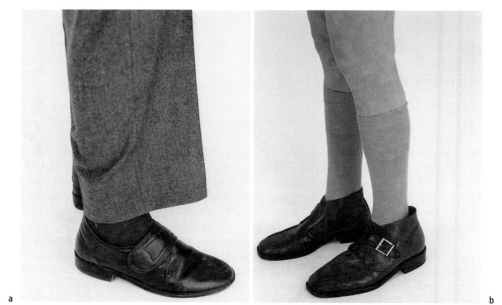

a   b

Fig. 9.22 a, b. Suitable shoes. **a** A shoe incorporating special features, made by Bally/Switzerland (right hemiplegia). **b** A half-boot provides some lateral support, which gives confidence (left hemiplegia)

Using a Bandage for Provisional Support

Before the patient has regained sufficient active control of his leg, the foot must be held in the correct position, both when gait is being facilitated by the therapist and when he is walking on his own. He will otherwise be afraid to walk freely and will, in fact, be in danger of injuring his ankle (**Fig. 9.23 a**). If active dorsal flexion is absent or insufficient, the patient will tend to flex his whole leg too strongly in order for his toes to clear the ground. The swing phase becomes distorted, and the natural cadence of walking is lost.

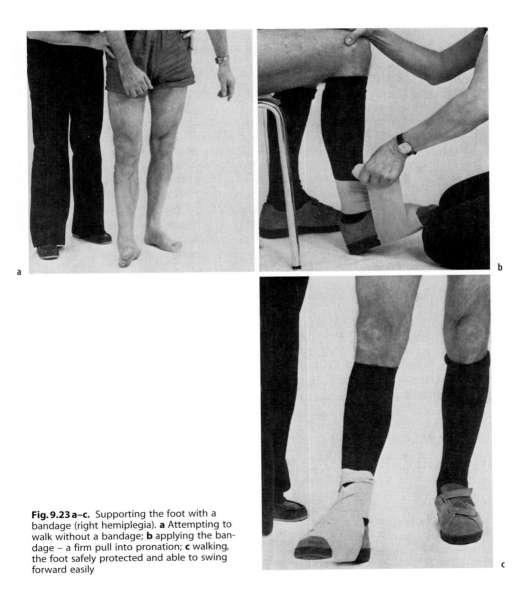

a

b

Fig. 9.23 a–c. Supporting the foot with a bandage (right hemiplegia). **a** Attempting to walk without a bandage; **b** applying the bandage – a firm pull into pronation; **c** walking, the foot safely protected and able to swing forward easily

c

Walking, however, need not be delayed until the patient can control his foot actively. A crepe bandage, bound firmly over the shoe, will hold his foot in dorsiflexion and prevent supination despite hypertonicity and/or loss of selective activity. With the bandage applied outside it, the shoe still fits comfortably and the patient experiences a normal contact between his foot and the sole. The bandage, which must be only slightly extensile, can also be bound tightly enough to maintain the correct position, because the firm sole of the shoe protects the circulation.

Applying the bandage

- The patient sits on a chair and the therapist kneels in front of him and inhibits hypertonicity in his foot.
- With the patient's knee flexed to a right angle, the therapist mobilises his foot until his heel stays firmly on the floor with his toes propped on her knee.
- She wraps the bandage twice around his forefoot to gain a good hold, the direction of the bandage being from medial to lateral underneath the foot.
- The therapist pulls the bandage up tightly at the lateral border of the shoe and then crosses it over in front of and around behind his ankle. While doing so, she presses down firmly on the patient's knee to prevent his heel from being lifted off the floor (Fig. 9.23 b). The bandage is not pulled tightly when it passes around the ankle, but only where it acts on the sole of the shoe.
- The bandaging continues, and extends along the sole of the shoe from the level of the fifth metatarsal head to where the heel of the shoe begins. The heel itself is left uncovered, so that the danger of slipping is eliminated. Particular attention is paid to supporting the area immediately below and anterior to the lateral malleolus, where the supination tendency can best be controlled.

With the bandage correctly applied in this way, the patient is enabled to bring his foot forwards easily in a plantigrade position during the swing phase of gait (Fig. 9.23 c). If the patient is in constant danger of hurting his ankle, the bandage should be applied first thing in the morning, as the ankle may otherwise be injured even during transfers during the day or due to the prolonged incorrect position of the foot while he is sitting in the wheelchair. Such patients often have a localised oedema of the foot and lateral side of the ankle, caused by repeated traumas. The oedema disappears rapidly after a few days if the ankle is protected at all times, but the bandage must be removed every few hours to relieve pressure and then put on again.

Indications for Using the Bandage

1. Dangerous supination or inversion of the foot in sitting, standing or walking
2. Inadequate active dorsiflexion of the foot during walking
3. For early attempts at learning to go up and down stairs correctly (Chap. 7)
4. For young patients, where the decision to order a permanent calliper or ankle brace is delayed in the hope that sufficient control may be achieved with intensive treatment

5. As a temporary aid for patients who have worn an ankle brace for some time and are trying to learn to walk without it (the bandage is made progressively less supportive)

Choosing an Orthosis

The word orthosis, although not appearing as such in the *Oxford* dictionary, seemingly derives from the Greek root *ortho*, meaning "straight, right, correct". It is a term which through common usage has come to mean any one of a great variety of foot splints and supports, ranging from different types of plastic ankle-foot orthoses (AFOs) to braces with metal uprights and straps to hold the foot in position. For purposes of clarity, in the text that follows, the term brace will be used to indicate some type of plastic AFO and the word calliper (Hornby 1975) when referring to a support which includes a metal upright(s).

The decision to order either a calliper or brace carries a great deal of responsibility, because most patients will find it difficult to manage without it at a later stage, once they have become used to the foot being supported. Some patients do, however, discard the support when they have become more confident through walking freely with it. It is particularly important for the patient to be able to walk short distances at home without his foot being supported mechanically, e. g. for walking to his bed after having a bath or walking to the toilet at night. A brace or calliper is seldom required if the patient has learnt to bear weight correctly on his hemiplegic leg without using the spastic mass pattern of extension with the knee hyperextended. Selective extensor activity of the hip and knee during the stance phase eliminates excessive plantar flexor activity and enables the patient to release the knee before bringing the foot forwards. With sufficient knee flexion during the swing phase, very little active dorsiflexion is required, and the activity is usually possible for the patient when it is part of the walking pattern.

If, however, despite intensive and informed training for all phases of walking, the supination persists and no active dorsiflexion returns, his foot will need to be supported in some way. It is certainly preferable for a patient to wear a brace or calliper than to be obliged to use a cane if it is a case of one or the other, because the former choice leaves his hand free for functional tasks, such as carrying a coffee cup or plate or something else while walking. When deciding which type of calliper or brace would be the most suitable to order for a particular patient, it is interesting to note that, during a study carried out by Ofir and Sell (1980), "the number of patients progressing in their functional ambulatory capability did not seem to change, and did not seem to be related to the kind of orthotic device or brace prescribed".

There are numerous different names and types of orthotic devices presently available, and all have certain disadvantages, a common one being that they hold the foot in a fixed position, often against considerable muscle forces. Those less rigid to allow some degree of mobility tend to stimulate even more hypertonus in the plantar flexors due to the springy resistance with which they oppose these muscles.

However, two types of support correct the position of the foot adequately without blocking the required movements and appear to be less prejudicial.

■ **A Plastic Ankle Brace.** A small, light brace, originally intended for orthopaedic patients with injuries to the ligaments of the ankle, counteracts supination of the hemiplegic foot and assists dorsal flexion. Not only is the ankle orthosis cosmetically pleasing for the patients, as it fits easily into a normal shoe, but it also allows free movements of the forefoot. The orthosis, which is far less expensive than other types, comes in different sizes, for left or right feet, and can be quickly and easily adjusted for the individual patient. The ankle fits snugly into the brace and is held securely in place by straps with Velcro fasteners (**Fig. 9.24 a**) It is easy to put on and fasten with one hand, and the foot anterior to the heel is not immobilised (**Fig. 9.24 b**). The brace is ideal for a patient who can walk without an orthosis but who has to walk slowly and carefully because of the supination and inadequate dorsiflexion of his foot (**Fig. 9.25 a**). While carrying out routine activities in daily life or when walking outdoors he is in constant danger of spraining his ankle or catching his toes on an uneven surface and falling. With the brace, his foot clears the ground easily during the swing phase and supination is prevented, allowing weight to be transferred safely over the hemiplegic leg at the beginning of the stance phase (**Fig. 9.25 b**). Because movements of the forefoot are not impeded by the brace, the heel is able to leave the floor behind when the foot plantar flexes before initiation of the next swing phase (**Fig. 9.25 c**).

The therapist can keep examples of these inexpensive and readily available braces on hand to try out with suitable patients. They can also be used as a provisional support to protect the patient's ankle when he first starts to walk and active control is still being retrained. The brace can provide temporary protection for the ankle when walking at increased speed is being facilitated or when objects to stimulate rhythm and independent head movements are introduced.

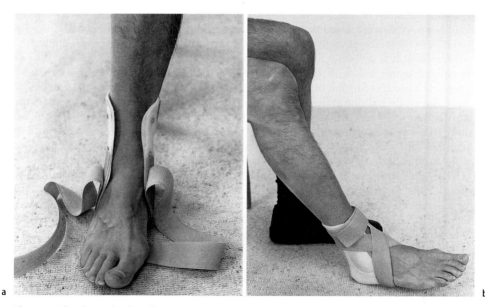

a   b

Fig. 9.24 a, b. The Arthrofix ankle and tarsus orthesis. **a** Light and easy to put on with one hand. **b** The forefoot is not immobilised

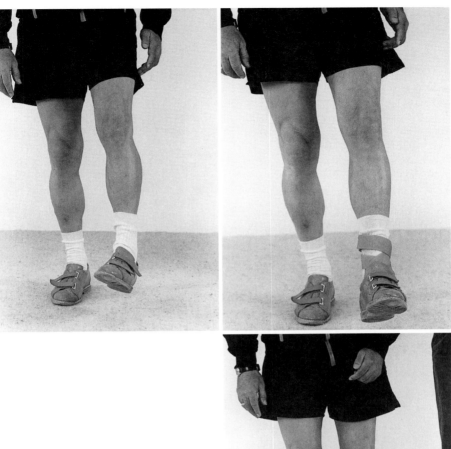

a

b

Fig. 9.25 a–c. Type of walking difficulty correctable with the ankle brace. **a** Patient walks carefully because of supinating foot. **b** With the brace the foot swings forward easily without supination. **c** Plantar flexion of the foot is possible for initiation of the swing phase

c

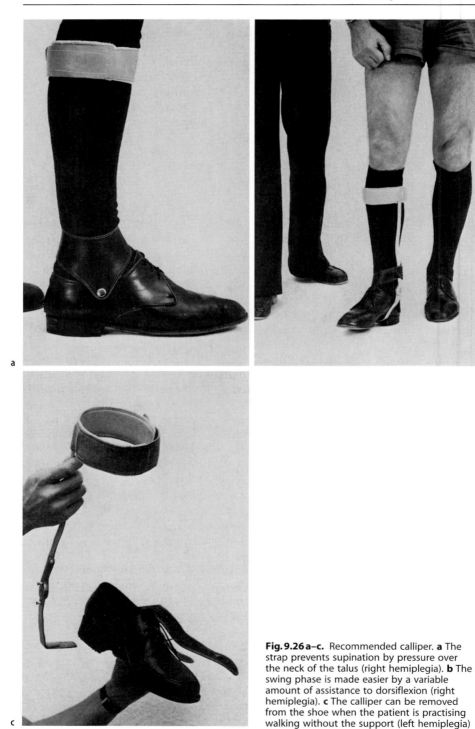

Fig. 9.26 a–c. Recommended calliper. **a** The strap prevents supination by pressure over the neck of the talus (right hemiplegia). **b** The swing phase is made easier by a variable amount of assistance to dorsiflexion (right hemiplegia). **c** The calliper can be removed from the shoe when the patient is practising walking without the support (left hemiplegia)

■ **A Calliper to Prevent Supination and Assist Dorsal Flexion.** If the plastic brace does not correct the position of the patient's foot or offer enough assistance to dorsal flexion it may be necessary for him to have a calliper, which is more stable. Many types of calliper have been described and are available, but the design based on the original English inside-iron and outside-T-strap type and later developed in Switzerland is recommended (**Fig. 9.26 a, b**). This calliper has the advantage of preventing supination through direct pressure over the talocrural and subtalar joints. Other forms of calliper tend to increase hypertonus in the muscles of plantar flexion and inversion because they all act primarily on the sole of the foot, through either the shoe itself or an insole. They also fail to control marked supination unless the patient wears a boot.

The recommended calliper, named the "Valens" calliper after the rehabilitation clinic where it was developed, is cosmetically pleasing, particularly for patients wearing trousers, when only a fraction of the medial, metal strut is visible.

The ankle joint of the calliper does not block plantar flexion and has a useful mechanism whereby tightening or loosening a small screw varies the amount of assistance given to dorsal flexion of the foot. The amount can be varied from total support to no assistance, which is important, because for many patients help is required only to prevent the foot from supinating, and a total support of dorsiflexion at the ankle would eliminate the demand for active muscle contraction.

The calliper is easy to put on with one hand and can be removed from the shoe and fitted to the patient's other shoes as well (**Fig. 9.26 c**). Because the calliper is removable, gait training can be continued without the calliper but with the patient still wearing the same shoes.

Going Up and Down Stairs

Practising the stairs has a beneficial effect on the gait, and walking cannot be truly functional if the patient is not able to manage stairs. Once he leaves the protected environment of the hospital or rehabilitation centre or later the confines of his own home he is constantly confronted by steps when entering theatres, restaurants, toilets and older public buildings, and even when crossing the road he will have to mount the pavement. When entering or leaving a building he will often find no handrail (**Fig. 9.27**).

If stairs are included at an early stage in the rehabilitation, the patient will have little difficulty in learning the activity, and he will achieve independent walking more quickly as a result. From the first attempt onwards, the patient is taught to go up and down stairs in a normal way, i. e. one foot after the other on alternate steps. At first, sufficient support is given by the therapist, so that the movement occurs smoothly and rhythmically and the patient is not afraid (see Chap. 7) As his confidence grows, the patient gradually depends less and less on the handrail and the therapist reduces the help she has been giving him.

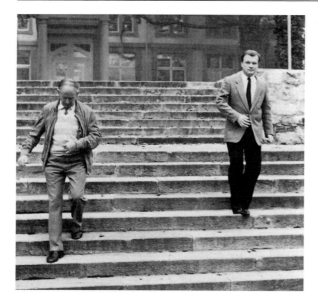

Fig. 9.27. Two patients leaving an old public building, managing the steps with no handrail available (left hemiplegia and right hemiplegia)

Using a Walking-stick or Cane

It should not be assumed that giving the patient a cane for support will enable him to walk safely. The hemiplegic patient invariably falls towards his hemiplegic side or backwards, when the cane would be of little help to save him. It is therefore useful for the therapist to apply the somewhat paradoxical rule, "a patient should be given a cane only when he can already walk without one". This means that the patient should not lean on a cane during early walking training, but should rather be taught how to maintain his balance in other ways. If the patient uses a cane too soon, he may well find it difficult to manage without it later and thus be unable to carry something while walking or to perform tasks in an upright position because his sound hand is required for balance. When the patient is able to walk in the sheltered environment of the hospital or his home without a cane, the therapist can decide whether or not he really needs the additional support.

Many patients, particularly older ones, like to have a walking stick with them when they venture out on the street. They feel that other people will then recognise that they have balance problems and be more considerate. If it is at all possible, even these problems should be overcome through further practice and experience in the actual situations. However, the fact that the patient feels confident and is prepared to go out on his own is of prime importance, and taking the cane with him is far better than his sitting indoors. The presence of a walking stick can also be a help for relatives who are afraid that the patient will overbalance towards his sound side and are in this way encouraged to walk on his affected side. It must always be remembered, though, that if a person has a support in one hand he will lean towards that side, and that the other arm tends to be in an adducted position as a result.

The ordinary wooden walking stick is the type that is recommended, if one is to be used at all. It is cosmetically more acceptable, can in fact be elegant, and does not immediately draw attention to the person as an invalid. The adjustable metal walking stick should be used only to select the correct height for the individual patient. Sometimes, using a cane that is somewhat longer than the recommended height of trochanter level may help the patient to avoid leaning on it so heavily.

Some therapists feel that a Canadian elbow crutch should not be used because it would encourage the patient to support himself even more or cause a greater degree of asymmetry. In fact, the crutch offers the hemiplegic patient no extra security, and there is no reason why he should lean more towards it than he does with a cane. Some patients prefer an elbow crutch to a walking stick because it looks less geriatric, and being available in attractive modern colours as they now are makes them cosmetically more acceptable.

Quadripods or tripods should never be used, as they are cumbersome to manoeuvre and do not offer increased support unless the weight is transferred directly over them, that is, away from the hemiplegic side. The metallic appearance is definitely associated with hospitals and disability, and changes the attitude of other people towards the patient. Any such type of manual support causes the centre of gravity to be more over the sound side and emphasises the retraction of the affected side. In some cases, the patient will be walking almost sideways and the side of the body which is constantly behind him will tend to be more and more neglected.

If the patient is still using either a cane or an elbow crutch he should nevertheless try to maintain certain normal patterns of movement. For example, when standing up from sitting the patient should push the end of the cane or crutch along the floor in front of

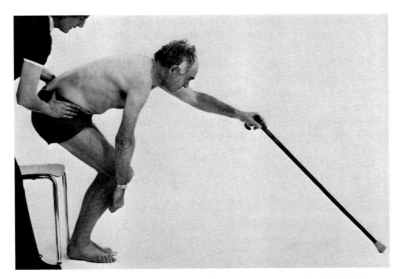

Fig. 9.28. Despite the walking-stick, the patient stands up in a normal pattern

him as far as he can, with the hemiplegic arm remaining forward in extension. In this way, his head is brought forward well over his feet, which will help him to stand up in a normal pattern of movement (**Fig. 9.28**). The same principle applies when he sits down again. With his feet parallel, the patient slides the tip of the cane well forwards before lowering himself onto the chair. A patient who stands up by pushing down on a support with his sound hand immediately takes all the weight over to that side and will assume a starting position for walking that is already asymmetrical. Often the hemiplegic foot, without any weight being taken through it, will even lift off the floor.

Considerations

Walking is a natural and enjoyable activity for human beings and enhances the quality of our lives. Every patient is eager to learn to walk again and will be more than ready to work hard to achieve this goal because it is one which he can really understand. When walking training commences he feels that he is making progress and his morale improves considerably. Seeing him on his feet again encourages not only the patient's relatives but the staff caring for him as well. For the doctor who is responsible for the continuation of treatment, walking constitutes an objective improvement, one which is measurable and observable and thus more helpful than the therapist reporting on the ward round, for example, that muscle tone or balance is "a little better this week". From a physical point of view, the erect position improves circulation, muscle extensibility and activity, as well as other vital bodily functions.

A patient who is already walking when he arrives for further treatment should not be put back in a wheelchair, even if his gait is far from ideal, because it is terribly demoralising and long periods of sitting will not improve the walking pattern or reduce hypertonicity. Instead, the patient continues to walk during the day, and the therapist analyses the difficulties and works on those components which are causing them, helping the patient to change some habitual, abnormal feature little by little and day by day.

Patients who do not achieve completely independent walking will nevertheless benefit from being in the upright position and from the activity it demands. Even if a patient can walk only with the help of another person, many aspects of his daily life will be easier and more enjoyable. Being able to walk at all provides access to places where a wheelchair would be impossible, and the patient therefore has a greater freedom of choice. Patients who walk functionally will achieve greater independence and be better able to maintain their mobility and level of achievement when treatment is discontinued.

10 Some Activities of Daily Living

Rehabilitation aims at the highest possible level of independence in daily life for the patient with hemiplegia. For the adult patient, being independent is the first vital step to being able to return to his former life style. Independence means no longer being an invalid, dependent on help from others for all everyday activities. Being independent enables the patient to choose where, when and with whom he would like to be at any given time, and even allows him the choice to be on his own. The fact that he knows he can manage is important for the patient, but a little help can often go a long way and should not be rigidly withheld.

Therapeutic Considerations

- How the patient carries out the routine activities in his daily life will affect not only the quality of his overall movement but also the maintenance of the standard he ultimately achieves. The importance of the 24-hour way of life has already been discussed (Chap. 5). It is self-defeating if, after a concentrated treatment with full inhibition of spasticity, the patient then struggles to dress himself incorrectly and marked associated reactions occur.
  All activities of daily living should be performed in such a way that associated reactions are avoided. The movements should be as economic and normal as possible, and the correct postures encouraged. Careful and repeated training, with sufficient guidance, will often be needed before the sequences are automatically carried out correctly in a therapeutic way. They must become a part of the patient's repertoire through repeated experience, so that he reproduces them in any situation when they are required, and not only in the presence of the therapist.
- Because the activities take place regularly, they can be a valuable recurring therapy and later form an integral part of any home programme for the patient. For the same reason, if they are performed incorrectly the detrimental effects are considerable.
- The patient will learn more easily in familiar everyday situations, and the retrieval of previously stored functions is facilitated during actual events (Chap. 1). In daily-life activities the patient can learn to plan, move and perceive. Activities such as washing and dressing help to overcome the neglect of the hemiplegic side.
- Balance reactions are considerably improved by standing and walking during those activities which would normally be carried out in an upright position.

Every patient will have different wishes and expectations for his life. A few activities which are common to most people have been chosen, and the same principles can then be applied to individual requirements such as working conditions and hobbies. It is never too early to start incorporating the activities in the treatment programme, as long as the therapist guides the patient adequately to avoid frustration or failure (Chap. 1).

Personal Hygiene

Washing

The patient sits at the washbasin, preferably on a stool or an upright chair. When he has filled the basin and checked the water temperature, he places his hemiplegic arm in the basin. The downward pull of the side is inhibited, and a symmetrical upright posture achieved. Washing the arm and the axilla is also easier in this position (**Fig. 10.1**).

To wash the sound arm, the patient fixes the soapy face flannel over the edge of the basin and rubs his arm and hand over it (**Fig. 10.2**). To dry the sound arm, he places the towel over one of his legs and moves his arm over the towel (**Fig. 10.3**). A nailbrush with suction caps attached enables the patient to clean his fingernails (**Fig. 10.4**).

Cutting or clipping fingernails is possible for only a very few patients. A nailfile attached to a small strip of wood can be held in place on a supporting surface by two suction caps and enables the patient to file his nails (**Fig. 10.5**).

To dry his back, the patient tosses the towel over one shoulder and then reaches behind him, grasps the other end and pulls the towel down across his back. He repeats the procedure over the other shoulder. The same procedure can be used after bathing or showering, or in fact whenever the patient needs to dry his back (**Fig. 10.6**).

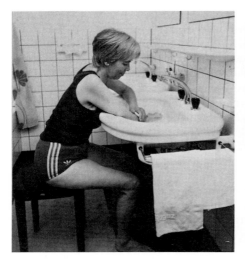

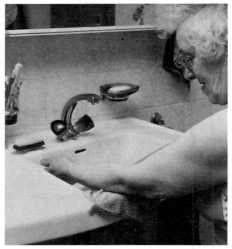

Fig. 10.1. Position at the washbasin (right hemiplegia)

Fig. 10.2. Washing the sound arm (right hemiplegia)

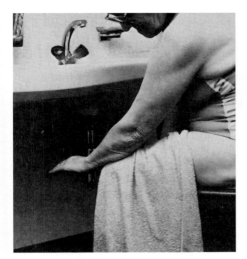

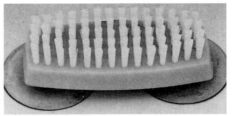

Fig. 10.4. Nailbrush adaptation, for cleaning nails or false teeth

◁
Fig. 10.3. Drying the sound arm (right hemiplegia)

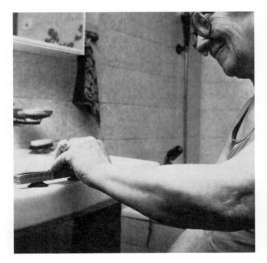

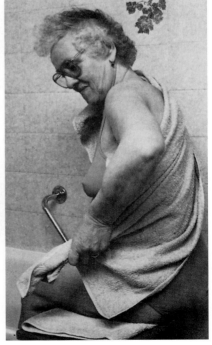

Fig. 10.5. Adapted nailfile (right hemiplegia)

Fig. 10.6. Drying the back by pulling the towel with the sound hand after tossing it over the other shoulder (right hemiplegia)   ▷

Brushing Teeth

At first in sitting, the patient rests his affected arm along the edge of the basin if the space is sufficient. Even with very little return of active movement, the hemiplegic hand can be used to hold the toothbrush while the toothpaste is applied instead of balancing it on the basin. As soon as it becomes possible, the patient stands to brush his teeth. When sufficient activity has returned he can hold the side of the basin, but otherwise he can leave his arm forward in an inhibited position.

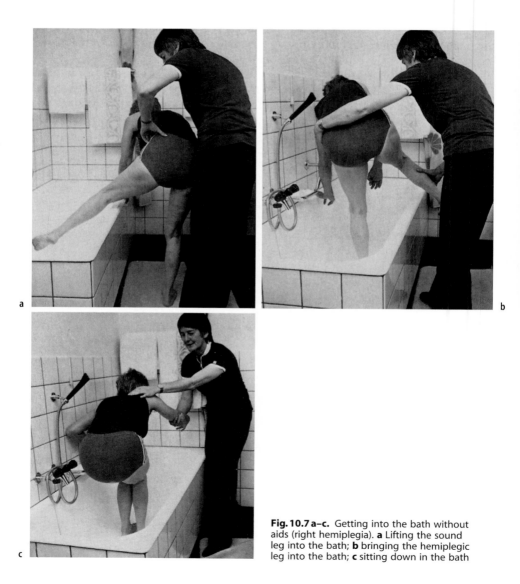

a

b

c

Fig. 10.7 a–c. Getting into the bath without aids (right hemiplegia). **a** Lifting the sound leg into the bath; **b** bringing the hemiplegic leg into the bath; **c** sitting down in the bath

Having a Bath

Not only for hygienic reasons, but also for his enjoyment, it is important to teach the patient how to get in and out of the bath safely and easily, preferably without aids. Most patients who can walk unaided will be able to manage the following method. The patient requires help from the therapist to learn the movement sequence, which often seems difficult when attempted for the first time. The method was worked out by patients themselves and is worth practising, as it does not require a special bath or handrails.

Getting into the bath:
(**Fig. 10.7 a**) The patient stands with his sound side to the bath, irrespective of at which end the taps and plug are situated. The water, at the correct temperature, is already in the bath. He lifts his sound leg into the bath while holding on to the side nearest to him. The therapist assists by holding both sides of his pelvis.

(**Fig. 10.7 b**) The patient moves his sound hand to the other edge of the bath and lifts his hemiplegic leg forwards and upwards into the bath. The therapist helps him to bring the knee and hip into sufficient flexion. It is almost always impossible for the patient to lift his leg behind him into the bath, as the movement is too selective, i.e. active knee flexion with hip extension.

(**Fig. 10.7 c**) The patient holds the side of the bath, or the tap, and lowers himself down into the sitting position. The buoyancy afforded by the water assists him. The therapist, her hand placed over his scapula, leans away so that her body weight counteracts his descending movement. With her other hand she eases his arm forwards to prevent an associated reaction in flexion.

(**Fig. 10.8**) The patient washes himself, a bar of soap on a string around his neck facilitating the manipulation of the soap onto a flannel or his sound hand.

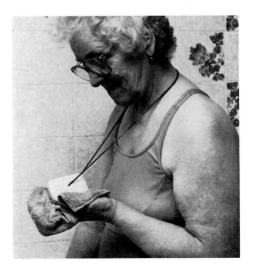

Fig. 10.8. Soap on a string (right hemiplegia)

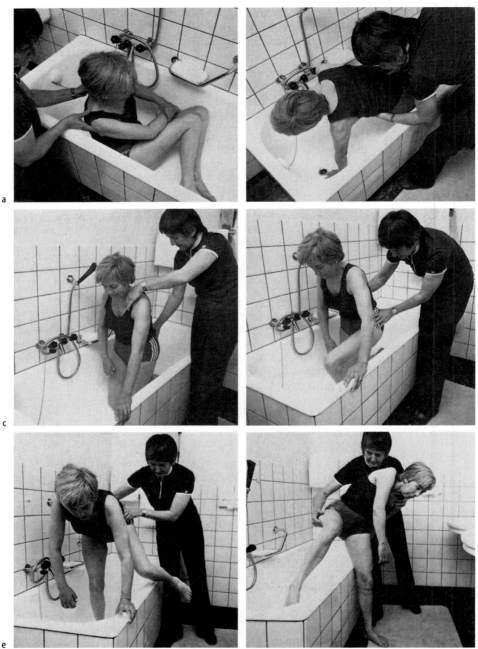

Fig. 10.9 a–f. Getting out of the bath without aids (right hemiplegia). **a** Preparing to turn around onto the knees; **b** turning onto the knees, with the therapist assisting from the pelvis; **c** coming to an upright kneel-standing position; **d** half-kneel-standing on the hemiplegic knee; **e** standing and lifting the sound leg out of the bath; **f** turning and lifting the hemiplegic leg out of the bath

Getting out of the bath:
(**Fig. 10.9 a**) When the washing is completed, he removes the plug and then prepares to get out of the bath by drawing his legs up into as much flexion as possible. The patient uses his sound hand to turn both knees to that side, the feet placed as far as possible to the opposite side of the bath. With his sound hand he draws his hemiplegic arm forwards across his body and as far round towards the sound side as he can, so that his shoulder is well forward and trunk rotation achieved.

(**Fig. 10.9 b**) He then places his sound hand behind him for support, either on the bottom of the bath or up on the end, and lifts his buttocks as he turns himself around completely to take his weight on both knees. The therapist holds both sides of his pelvis to facilitate the lifting and turning movement.

(**Fig. 10.9 c**) He then kneels upright with his hips well forward in extension.

(**Fig. 10.9 d**) Holding the side of the bath, the patient brings one foot forward (preferably the sound leg) to come to a half-kneeling position.

(**Fig. 10.9 e**) Bringing his weight forward over the foot in front, he rises to a standing position, but with his hand still holding the side of the bath, and then lifts his sound leg out of the bath.

(**Fig. 10.9 f**) He keeps his hand in place as he places his foot on the floor with outward rotation of the hip. The patient reaches back behind him, turns his hand around to grasp the side of the bath on his sound side, and lifts his hemiplegic leg up and out through flexion.

For patients who cannot yet manage to get in and out of the bath in this way, two intermediate stages can be of help:

1. For the patient who is still using a wheelchair and has difficulty coming from sitting to standing, a board is placed over the end of the bath. The board is held firmly in place by rubber knobs screwed on underneath it (**Fig. 10.10a**). The patient transfers from his chair, with assistance, towards his hemiplegic side on to the board (**Fig. 10.10 b**) and lifts his hemiplegic leg into the bath with his clasped hands (**Fig. 10.10 c**). He then lifts his sound leg actively into the bath. A towel placed on the board helps the patient to slide to the middle. He then takes a shower and washes himself while sitting on the board. A shower curtain tucked in beneath his sound buttock will prevent water from running on to the floor (**Fig. 10.10 d**). He dries himself and is helped to transfer back into his chair.

2. A lower bath stool is placed below the board and the bath is filled with water. The patient is transferred or sits down first on to the board as in stage 1. He then leans well forwards and lifts his buttocks from the board to enable the helper to remove it and guide him down to sit on the bath stool (**Fig. 10.11 a**). In this position he washes and dries himself, allowing the water to run out of the bath when he has finished. He then lifts his seat from the stool and the helper replaces the board on which he can sit again. Because the seat is so low, the patient may need to reach forwards and hold on to the side of the bath for support instead of clasping his hands together (**Fig. 10.11 b**). He transfers with assistance back into his chair.

Fig. 10.10a–d. Getting into the bath with assistance (right hemiplegia). **a** A board is placed over the bath; **b** transferring towards the hemiplegic side from the wheelchair to sit on the board; **c** lifting the hemiplegic leg into the bath; **d** sitting on the board: the shower curtain is tucked under one buttock before showering

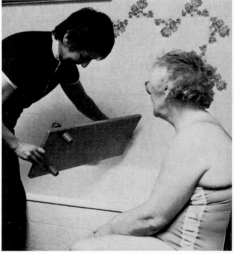

a

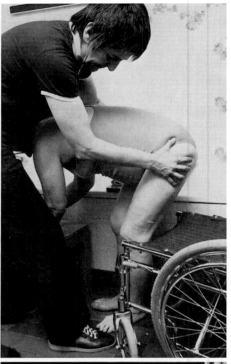

b

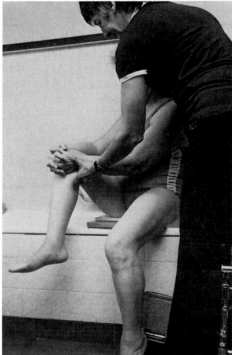

c

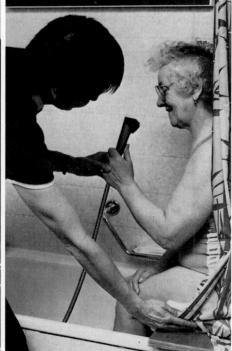

d

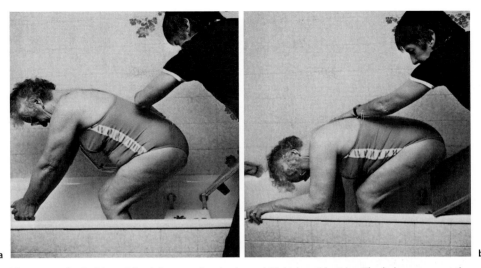

a
b

Fig. 10.11 a, b. Bathing while sitting on a low bath stool (right hemiplegia). **a** The helper removes the board and the patient sits down on a bath stool. **b** After bathing, the patient lifts her buttocks so that the helper can replace the board

Having a Shower

Some patients may prefer or find it easier to take a shower. A seat must be provided so that the patient can sit while he washes himself. In a separate shower the seat can be of the folding type, attached to the wall, or a bathroom stool can be placed in the shower, in a corner for additional support (**Fig. 10.12**). Where the shower is over the bath, the patient must first climb into the bath as already described and have some sort of seat in or attached to the bath. The cake of soap with a string attached is once again most useful.

Dressing

It must not be forgotten that getting dressed also necessitates deciding what to put on and fetching the clothes from the wardrobe (**Fig. 10.13**). The patient should sit on an upright chair with his feet flat on the floor, and not on the edge of his bed. The mattress is unsteady and would entail his struggling to maintain his balance, and the height of the bed itself is often unsuitable. Patients should eventually be able to put on the clothes of their choice, but loose, simple clothing enables them to learn the sequence and arrangement more easily and rapidly at first (Leviton-Rheingold et al. 1980).

When the clothes are arranged in front of the patient, i.e. within his field of vision and in the correct order, the task becomes far simpler for him, being then on the recog-

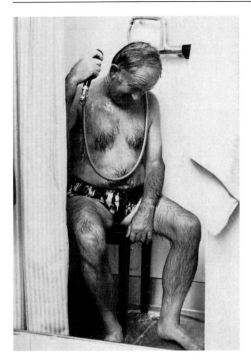

Fig. 10.12. Taking a shower while seated on a stool (left hemiplegia)

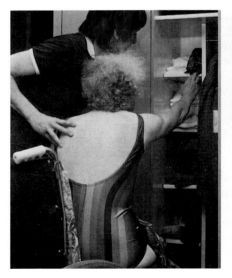

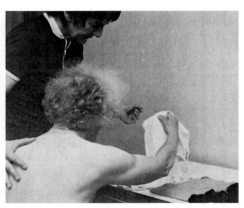

Fig. 10.14. Clothes arranged in the correct order in front of the patient simplify the task (left hemiplegia)

Fig. 10.13. Choosing what to wear and fetching the clothes from the wardrobe (left hemiplegia)

nition level (**Fig. 10.14**). Later, the clothes should be placed ready at his hemiplegic side so that he turns towards that side as he reaches for each garment.

When the patient first starts learning how to dress himself, he need not put on all the clothes himself. This could take far too long if he has marked perceptual difficulties. Instead, the therapist or nurse goes through the routine with him and he helps, with guidance, to put on one or two articles of clothing. What is important is that from the start, each person who assists the patient should follow the same routine so that he can learn the sequence for getting dressed.

There are many different methods of putting on clothing with one hand, but here the decision rests with the individual therapist. What is important is that the patient should succeed, without undue effort and without associated reactions appearing. The following method is recommended for the majority of patients. A simple rule is to start each sequence by first dressing the hemiplegic limb.

Underwear

With the clothes placed on a chair at his hemiplegic side, the patient first puts on his underwear. He puts on his underpants in the same way as he does his trousers, first crossing his hemiplegic knee over the other to enable him to draw the garment over his foot (see **Fig. 10.16 a**).

Socks

To put on his socks, the patient first crosses his hemiplegic leg over the other leg. If he is unable to do so actively, he uses his clasped hands to lift it (**Fig. 10.15 a**). He should never grasp his leg with his sound hand and struggle to pull it into position, as this will cause the hemiplegic side to retract strongly in an unwanted spastic pattern. He then opens the sock, using his thumb and first fingers, and leans well forwards to pull it over his foot. Before doing so, he brings his hemiplegic arm forwards with the shoulder protracted and the elbow extended (**Fig. 10.15 b**). He should put on the other sock in exactly the same way, so that his weight is then over the hemiplegic side and associated reactions in the arm and leg are prevented (**Fig. 10.15 c, d**).

Trousers

To put on his trousers, the patient first crosses his affected leg over the other one and pulls the trouser leg up as far as possible over his knee (**Fig. 10.16 a**). When he has placed the affected foot back flat on the floor, he steps into the other trouser leg. The hemiplegic arm remains well forward all the time.

Taking weight on both feet, he lifts his buttocks off the chair and pulls the trousers up to his waist (**Fig. 10.16 b**) before fastening them, either while standing or after sitting down again. His hand needs to be guided at first to ensure that the hemiplegic side is not neglected, leaving the trousers pulled down on that side. If the patient has difficulty in maintaining his balance while standing, a table in front of him is a great help. It provides security and also orientation (**Fig. 10.16 c**).

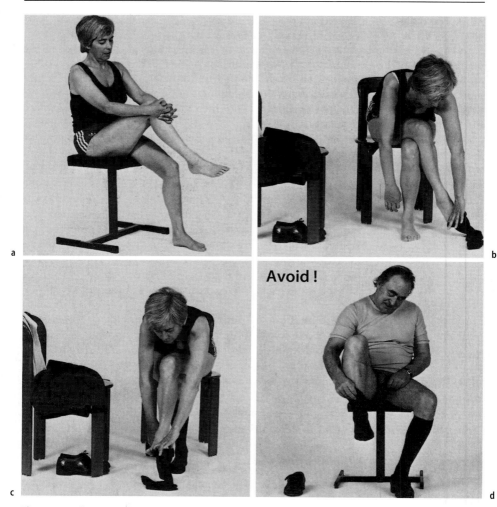

Fig. 10.15 a–d. Putting on socks (right hemiplegia). **a** Crossing the hemiplegic leg over the other leg.
b Putting the sock on the hemiplegic foot. The arm remains forward. **c** Putting the sock on the sound
foot with the leg crossed over. **d** Associated reactions occur when the sound leg is not crossed over
the other one (left hemiplegia)

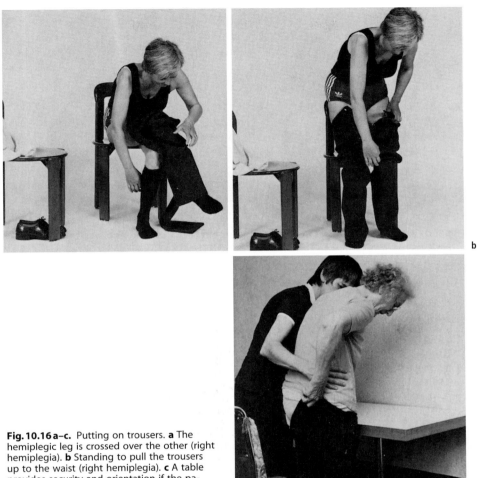

Fig. 10.16a–c. Putting on trousers. **a** The hemiplegic leg is crossed over the other (right hemiplegia). **b** Standing to pull the trousers up to the waist (right hemiplegia). **c** A table provides security and orientation if the patient has poor balance (left hemiplegia)

A Shirt or Jacket

To put on a shirt, cardigan or jacket, the patient arranges the garment across his knees in such a way that the sleeve hangs free between his knees, creating an easy passage through which he pushes his hemiplegic hand (**Fig. 10.17a**). He then pulls the sleeve well up the arm, to the shoulder (**Fig. 10.17b**). With his arm well forward, the elbow will remain extended due to the protraction of the scapula. The patient then reaches round to grasp the jacket and pulls it towards the other side until he can place his sound arm in the sleeve. Some patients with good standing balance may find it easier to put on a shirt while standing.

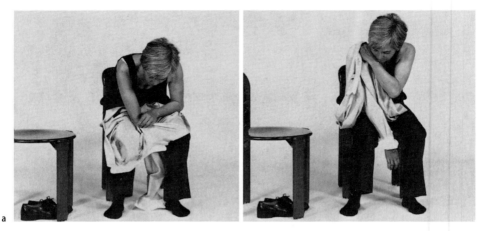

a   b

Fig. 10.17 a, b. Putting on a shirt or blouse (right hemiplegia). **a** The hemiplegic arm is pushed through the carefully arranged sleeve. **b** Pulling the sleeve well up to the shoulder

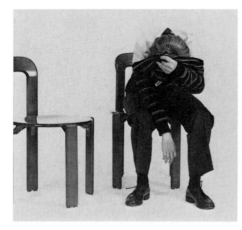
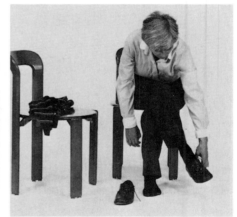

Fig. 10.18. Putting on a pullover (right hemiple-   **Fig. 10.19.** Putting the shoe on the hemiplegic
gia)   foot (right hemiplegia)

The problem of fastening the button at the cuff of the sound arm is solved by sewing it on with an elastic thread. He leaves the button fastened but is able to push his arm through the end of the sleeve.

A Pullover or T-shirt

To put on a pullover or T-shirt, the patient arranges the garment across his knees with the collar furthest away from him and the label at the neck uppermost. The sleeve for the affected arm is once again arranged so that it hangs down open between his knees. Having placed his arm through the sleeve with the help of the sound hand, he draws it right up to his shoulder before slipping the sound hand through the other sleeve. Grasping the back of the pullover, he then places it over his head, still leaning well forwards so that his arm remains extended (**Fig. 10.18**).

Shoes

The patient puts on his shoes as he does his socks (**Fig. 10.19**) but can fasten them when the feet are flat on the floor. If the patient is wearing lace-up shoes the lace should be threaded in such a way that he can fasten it using one hand if need be (**Fig. 10.20 a–c**).

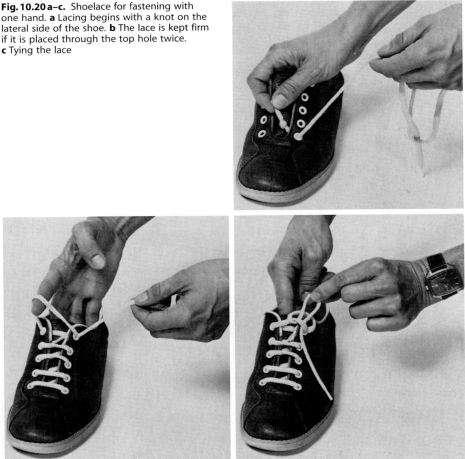

Fig. 10.20 a–c. Shoelace for fastening with one hand. **a** Lacing begins with a knot on the lateral side of the shoe. **b** The lace is kept firm if it is placed through the top hole twice. **c** Tying the lace

Moccasin-type shoes can look smart and avoid the necessity for coping with shoelaces, and nevertheless give good support (**Fig. 10.21 a**). Some patients find a half-boot with a zip fastener easy to put on and welcome the added support at the ankle. Some shoes or half-boots are available with Velcro fasteners, or the patient can have Velcro straps fitted on his own shoes by the local shoemaker (**Fig. 10.21 b**).

An Outdoor Coat

An outdoor coat is best put on when the patient is standing, and he puts it on as he does a cardigan. If the hemiplegic arm is very spastic or the garment rather heavy he may need to arrange the coat on a table, so that he can place the hand in the sleeve with the help of his sound hand.

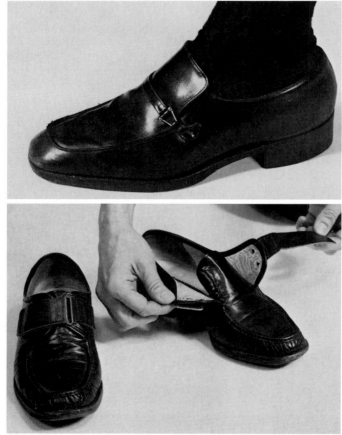

Fig. 10.21 a, b. Avoiding shoelaces. **a** A moccasin-type shoe giving firm support. **b** Leather straps with a Velcro fastening sewn onto the patient's shoes can replace the original laces

Putting on a Brassiere

How to put on a "bra" with one hand warrants a separate section because previous solutions to the problem have proved to be unsatisfactory, if not impossible, for the majority of female patients. Many modern women, by choice, no longer wear a brassiere, but those patients who wore one before they became hemiplegic should not be obliged to relinquish their preference merely because they are unable to put on the support alone. Older patients indeed feel very uncomfortable without a bra. There is, in addition, another reason for the patient to wear one, particularly for those who have fuller, somewhat heavier breasts. Maintaining extension of the thoracic spine when walking has been shown to be a common problem in hemiplegia (Davies 1990), and the weight of the unsupported breasts can add to the difficulty considerably. A lady who herself suffered a hemiplegia years ago has discovered an easy and efficient way to put on a bra with one hand, and since then many others have learned to do so using the same method.

For a patient with a left hemiplegia:

- The patient places the bra on her left thigh, close to her body, in such a way that the inside of the right cup is uppermost and the shoulder strap on that side points towards her knee.
- With her sound hand she hooks the right shoulder strap over her left thumb and pulls the bra towards her until the strap presses against the web between her thumb and index finger. She makes sure that the end of the bra is lying flat on her thigh with its hook(s) facing upwards (**Fig. 10.22 a**).
- She then reaches across the front of her body and places the other end of the bra as far round behind her as she can.
- Her sound hand moves back behind her right buttock to feel for and grasp the waiting end of the bra, which she pulls round to the front of her body to where the other end is lying with its hooks facing upwards (**Fig. 10.22 b**). Despite the elastic pull, the end is held in place by the shoulder strap pressing against the web of her hemiplegic hand.
- Holding the end of the bra with her sound hand so that its eyes are facing downward, she brings it into place and presses downwards and to the right to catch the eyes over the hooks (**Fig. 10.22 c**).
- Removing the shoulder strap from her hemiplegic thumb, she then pulls the bra sufficiently round to the left, until the other shoulder strap is sufficiently far forward to allow her to place her left hand into its free loop with her sound hand (**Fig. 10.22 d**).
- Still using her sound hand she pulls the strap up over her left shoulder and draws the bra a bit further round and then upwards, so that her left breast fits exactly into its cup (**Fig. 10.22 e**).
- Slipping her right hand through the other shoulder strap (**Fig. 10.22 f**), she brings it into position on her shoulder and then draws the cup up over her right breast and adjusts the rest of the bra to lie comfortably (**Fig. 10.22 g**).

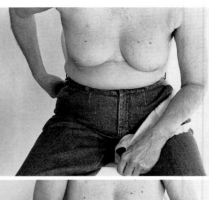

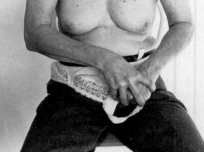

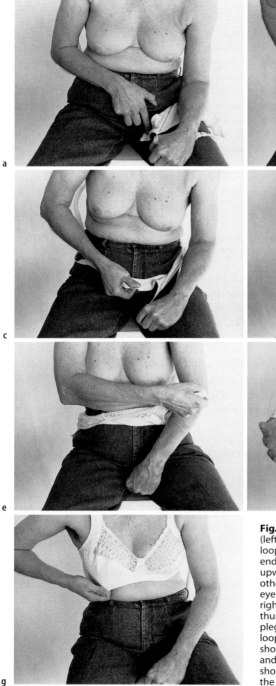

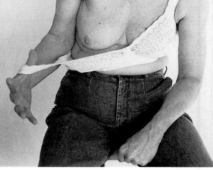

a

b

c

d

e

f

g

Fig. 10.22 a–g. Putting on a bra with one hand (left hemiplegia) **a** The right shoulder strap looped over the patient's left thumb keeps the end of the bra in place with the hooks facing upwards. **b** Reaching round behind to grasp the other end and pull it to the front. **c** Pressing the eyes down over the waiting hooks. **d** After the right shoulder strap has been released from the thumb, the bra is pulled round so that the hemiplegic hand can be placed into the left strap loop. **e** Drawing the shoulder strap up to the shoulder. **f** Using the web between index finger and thumb on the sound side to lift the right shoulder strap up to the shoulder. **g** Adjusting the position of the bra with the sound hand

For a patient with a right hemiplegia, the procedure is the same, but naturally with the sides reversed. The main difference is that with the right hand holding the left shoulder strap in position, the end of the bra with the eyes on it will be lying on the patient's thigh, and the eyes will be facing downwards. She will therefore have to turn them over before she brings the end with the hooks round to the front to fasten the bra.

- The patient places the bra on her right thigh, close to her body, in such a way that the inside of the left cup is uppermost and the shoulder strap on that side points towards her knee.
- With her sound hand she hooks the left shoulder strap over her right thumb, and draws the bra towards her until the strap is pressed against the web between her thumb and index finger. She makes sure that the end of the bra is lying flat on her thigh with the hook(s) facing upwards.
- She then reaches across the front of her body and places the other end of the bra as far round behind her as she can.
- Her sound hand moves back behind her left buttock to feel for and grasp the waiting end of the bra, which she pulls round to the front of her body to where the other end is lying with its eyes facing upwards. Despite the elastic pull, the end is held in place by the shoulder strap pressing against the web of her hemiplegic hand.
- Holding the end of the bra with her sound hand so that the hooks are facing downwards, she brings it into place and presses downwards and to the right to fasten the hooks into the eyes. Should the eyes move out of position as she pulls the other end round to the front, she can correct their position just before pressing the hooks down, using the fingers of her sound hand while still holding the end with the hooks between her thumb and index finger.
- Removing the shoulder strap from her hemiplegic thumb, she then pulls the bra sufficiently round to the right, until the other shoulder strap is sufficiently far forward to allow her to place her right hand into its free loop with her sound hand.
- Still using her sound hand, she pulls the strap up over her right shoulder and draws the bra a bit further round and then upwards so that her right breast fits exactly into its cup.
- Slipping her left hand through the other shoulder strap she brings it into position on her shoulder and then draws the cup up over her left breast and adjusts the rest of the bra to lie comfortably.

Taking off a Brassiere

Undoing the bra with one hand usually does not present a problem for the patient, particularly for those with a right hemiplegia. With her left hand she reaches up behind her back and undoes the hooks, before removing first the sound arm and then the affected one from the shoulder straps. Should it be difficult for the patient to reach the fastening behind her, she first takes her sound arm and then the hemiplegic one out of the straps and then turns the fastening round to the front to undo it.

Undressing

Undressing is simpler than dressing because the patient recognises each step which has to be taken (recognition level; Affolter 1981). The movements are carried out in the same sequence and pattern as for dressing, i.e. crossing the legs, keeping the hemiplegic arm forward in extension, etc. However, the patient must now undress the sound limbs first, to enable him to free the garment from the hemiplegic side. In normal life, putting our clothes away or in some order after undressing is a part of the routine and should be included in the sequence for the patient.

Eating

The problems experienced by patients when eating are fully discussed in Chap. 13. It is important, in addition, that the patient be taught how to sit down and move his chair near enough to the dining-room table. He walks to the table and moves the chair sufficiently away to enable him to sit down. When seated he grasps the front of the chair between his thighs, leans forwards enough to be able to raise his seat and draws the chair nearer to the table (**Fig. 10.23 a**). The patient places his hemiplegic arm forward on the table, adjacent to his place setting. The correct position of the arm will help him to maintain an upright symmetrical posture while eating (**Fig. 10.23 b**). When some active

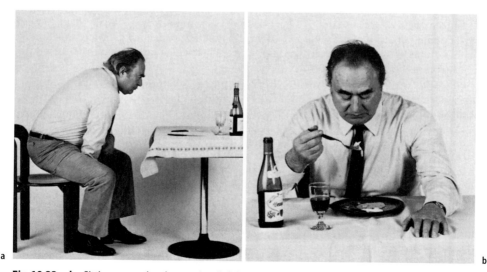

a   b

Fig. 10.23 a, b. Sitting correctly when eating (left hemiplegia). **a** Bringing the chair near enough to the table. **b** An upright symmetrical posture with the hemiplegic arm supported on the table

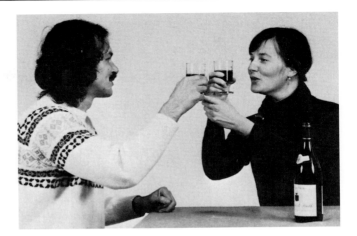

Fig. 10.24. Drinking from a glass with the hemiplegic hand (right hemiplegia)

movement returns to the hemiplegic arm the patient can use his affected hand to bring food to his mouth (such food as we normally eat with our hands). Manipulating a fork or spoon requires far finer movement and control. Fruit, toast and biscuits are some of the easiest things for the patient to manage at first. Drinking from a glass requires only a little active movement, and the patient can even assist the activity by using his sound hand to steady the other one (**Fig. 10.24**). As soon as it is feasible, the patient should be encouraged to use both hands for eating with a knife and fork, even though he may have become adept at managing with the sound hand alone.

Driving a Car

Being able to drive again brings added freedom and independence for the patient and enhances the quality of his life. The possibility should be considered whenever a patient has progressed sufficiently. The legal requirements of the relevant country should be investigated so that the patient may drive safely, legally and competently.

The conversion of the car for a hemiplegic driver is relatively simple and has been greatly improved by recent developments in electronic technology. For one-car families, the fact that the adaptations can be changed within minutes to allow nondisabled partners to drive as usual is important.

Basic criteria are the following:

- The car must have an automatic gearbox.
- Driving is much easier with power steering, and a knob attached to the steering wheel enables the wheel to be turned easily with one hand.
- The accelerator and brake must be operated with the unaffected leg, which means that for a patient with a right hemiplegia, the accelerator pedal must be moved or have an additional extension to the other side (**Fig. 10.25 a**).

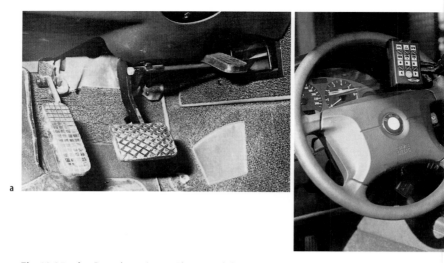

Fig. 10.25 a, b. Car adaptation. **a** The sound foot operates the accelerator and brake pedals (right hemiplegia). **b** The sound hand can control headlights, indicators and windscreen wipers without releasing the steering-wheel knob (left hemiplegia)

- Headlights and windscreen wipers must be operable without the sound hand having to move from the steering wheel **(Fig. 10.25 b)**.
- An arm rest to support the hemiplegic arm helps to maintain a symmetrical posture while the patient is driving.

Considerations

Naturally, the patient's ability to stand up, walk and negotiate stairs freely and easily will add considerably both to his independence in daily life and to his enjoyment. Good balance is essential for carrying out all everyday activities easily and safely. Although helping the patient to become independent is one of the main aims of rehabilitation, it should always be an independence which is at the same time therapeutic, so that he can continue to make further progress even after discharge from treatment. The question to be considered is therefore not only, for example, whether he can get dressed alone, but also how he does so. Repeated use of effortful and abnormal movements during daily tasks will increase hypertonus and, once habituated, they are difficult to change later. Care must be taken that certain repeated postures do not lead to a further loss of symmetry. For example, most patients carry a sling bag to enable them to manage more easily with only one functioning hand. If the bag is carried over the sound shoulder, the patient holds that shoulder in a constant elevation to prevent the strap from slipping. The elevation of the unaffected shoulder emphasises the shortening of the affected side. When the bag is worn differently the posture is immediately improved. Such observations, and finding alternative solutions, can play an important role in maintaining the patient's level of achievement, both cosmetic and functional.

Teamwork is therefore of the utmost importance during all stages of rehabilitation. During the period when the patient is learning how to perform the activities of daily living in a therapeutic way, all who assist him should follow the same procedures and principles of treatment. It is confusing when different members of the team give conflicting assistance or advice. For example, even if the patient is being helped to dress hurriedly to be on time for an appointment, the person helping him should use the same sequence that he has been learning for dressing himself. The patient's relatives are valuable members of the team, and with careful instruction they too will be able to help him correctly and enable him to make further progress.

11 Mat Activities

Activities on a mat on the floor play an important role in the treatment of the hemiplegic patient. On the mat he learns to move his body again, feeling it in contact with the firm surface as he changes from one position to another. Patients with disturbed sensation have difficulty when exercising in free space, where they are completely dependent upon their own feedback systems to inform them if a movement is correct or not. The mat provides an absolute resistance, and the patient is better able to orientate himself because he feels the changing resistance against different parts of his body as he moves. The patient can move freely in a situation where he is not afraid of falling. Patients who are afraid to walk or move in the open can be helped to overcome their fear by working on the mat and learning to stand up from the floor. Often the fear diminishes on its own when the patient becomes familiar with the distance down to the floor and knows that he would be able to stand up again should he fall. No patient is completely independent unless he can get up from the floor in some way. Many patients have fallen when alone and have had to lie sometimes for hours, even though unhurt, until someone has found them.

Helping the patient to move on the mat should, however, not be considered only as a means to teach him how to stand up again should he have fallen. Activities on the mat can be used therapeutically in many other ways as well. They provide opportunities where distal spasticity can be remarkably reduced by moving the body proximally against the limbs, and for regaining selective movements of the trunk and limbs. Patients of all ages enjoy the experience (**Fig. 11.1**) and benefit from it as long as they are

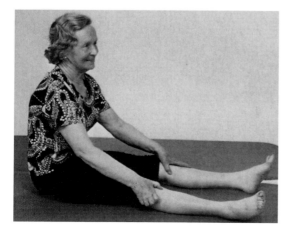

Fig. 11.1. Even an 80-year-old patient enjoys her mat programme (right hemiplegia)

appropriately supported and the facilitation is adequate, particularly when they are first attempting the various activities. Gradual progression is essential, and if patient and therapist at first feel unsure about going right down onto the floor and standing up again afterwards, the different movement sequences can be practised on a high mat until they have gained sufficient confidence.

Going Down Onto the Mat

The aim is for the patient to learn to kneel down on the mat, through half-kneeling on the hemiplegic leg, and then to sit down to one side. From side-sitting he can either lie down or sit with his legs out in front of him. If he feels unsure at first, or if the therapist is not certain that he will be able to support himself in kneeling, the patient can be asked to go down onto the floor in any way he chooses with the necessary amount of help. The easiest way is usually with the therapist standing behind him and supporting him firmly as he puts his sound hand down on the mat, slowly bends his knees and sits down (**Fig. 11.2**). How he gets down on to the mat is not important at this stage, as long as it is achieved quickly, safely and smoothly. Once the patient is down on the mat the individual components of a more therapeutic normal movement sequence can be practised.

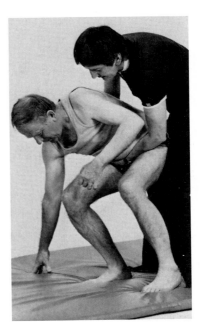

Fig. 11.2. Helping a nervous patient safely down onto the mat before he has learned the correct method (left hemiplegia)

The correct sequence is facilitated as follows:

- The patient walks to the centre of the mat and takes a step forwards with his sound foot, in preparation for kneeling down on the hemiplegic knee (**Fig 11.3a**). Stepping forwards with the sound leg is usually necessary because. most patients are unable to move their affected leg back in flexion in the normal way prior to kneeling down. Such a movement is very selective, requiring flexion of the knee while the hip is extending actively and the foot plantar-flexing.
- The therapist, who has been assisting the patient with her hands on his hips, places her hands over the top of his shoulders and stands close behind him. She facilitates flexion of his knee by easing it forwards with her knee on that side (**Fig. 11.3 b**).
- As the patient moves slowly towards the mat, the therapist takes some of his weight by letting his hip slide down over her thigh and controls the speed of the movement to prevent its being too rapid (**Fig. 11.3 c**).
- As the patient's knee reaches the ground, she presses her knee firmly against his hip from behind to prevent it from collapsing into flexion and guides his pelvis and trunk forwards over the supporting leg (**Fig. 11.3 d**). Her hands in front of his shoulders help him to extend his trunk and correct the position of the weight-bearing hip. Once his position in half-kneel-standing has been adjusted, he places his sound knee back beside the other to kneel on both knees.

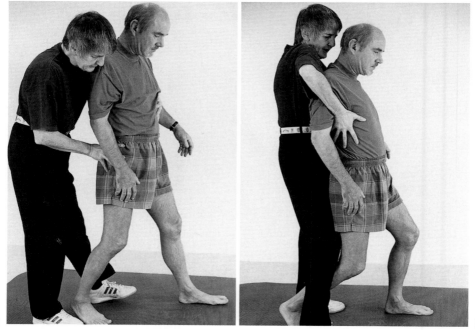

a   b

Fig. 11.3 a–e. Facilitation when teaching the patient how to get down on the mat in a more normal and therapeutic way (right hemiplegia). **a** The therapist assists hip extension as the patient steps forward with his sound foot. **b** She initiates flexion of his hemiplegic knee by guiding it gently forward with her knee

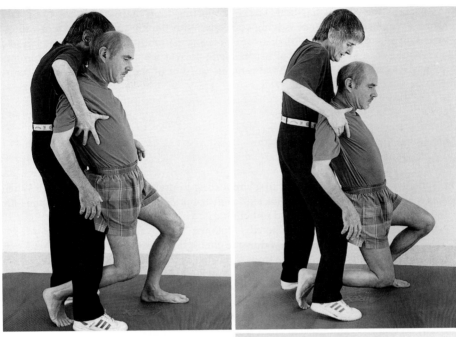

c

d

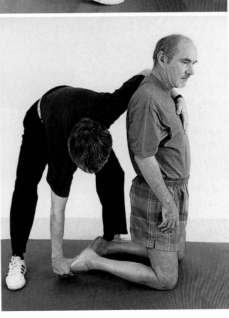

Fig. 11.3 c–e. c Standing close behind the patient, she regulates the speed of the movement as he slides down over her knee. **d** The therapist presses her knee firmly against his hip extensors to prevent the hip from flexing when his knee reaches the ground. **e** As soon as the patient is kneeling on both knees, the therapist corrects the position of his hemiplegic foot

e

- As soon as the patient has both knees supporting him, the therapist checks to see whether his hemiplegic foot is lying correctly. With the knee flexed, the foot will often pull into supination, with his toes pressing painfully against the mat. Should this be the case, she uses one of her hands to correct the position of the foot immediately (Fig. 11.3 e). Her other hand remains in front of the patient's chest to ensure that he does not fall forwards.

Moving to Side-Sitting

The patient sits down on one side, first supporting himself with his sound hand. When he has learnt the movement and has sufficient trunk control, he moves from one side to the other without using his hand to help him.

The movement sequence is facilitated as follows:

- When the patient is moving to sit down to the right, the therapist stands behind him and places her left hand over the front of his left iliac crest. Her right hand helps him to bring his right shoulder forwards and elongate the side, while her left hand presses downwards and sideways to guide his right buttock down onto the floor (Fig. 11.4a).
- She moves her feet quickly so that she can support his trunk between her legs as he slowly lowers his seat to the floor. Her right leg assists the forward rotation of the trunk on that side and prevents him from falling sideways and backwards, as he will tend to do at first (Fig. 11.4b). If the head does not right itself automatically, the therapist can assist the reaction.

To move so that he sits on the other side, the patient brings his knees up together in front of him (Fig. 11.4c) and turns them until he is sitting on his left buttock, the underneath leg flat on the floor and his knees together.

The therapist helps by using one hand to assist the hemiplegic knee to move appropriately; she changes the position of her feet while he moves, so that she is correctly placed to support the opposite side of his trunk with the inside of her left leg (Fig. 11.4d). Due to the loss of trunk rotation and appropriate lengthening and shortening of the side flexors, the movement may be difficult and even uncomfortable at first. If the patient's knees are moved gently and slowly from one side to the other, without necessarily reaching the final position immediately, the movement becomes easier and easier as tension in the trunk is gradually reduced and he can eventually sit fully on one side or the other.

Side-sitting on the hemiplegic side inhibits any hypertonicity in the trunk and frees the scapula as a result. The effect can be increased by elevating the patient's arm fully in outward rotation and asking him to move his weight towards the hemiplegic side and then away from it. In the same position the therapist can place the patient's hand at his side, with the elbow extended, to practise supporting his weight through his arm and extending his elbow actively (Fig. 11.5).

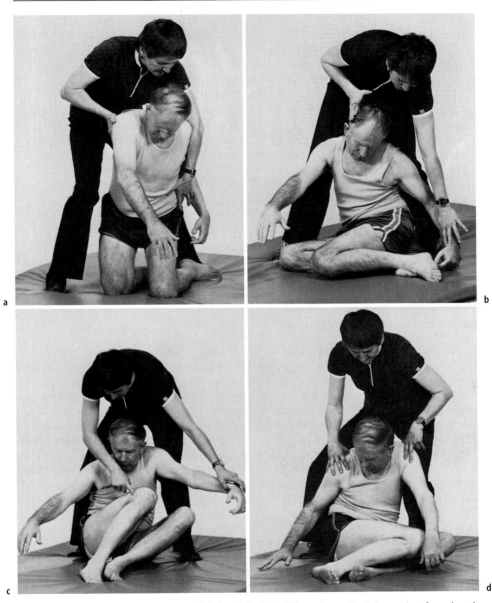

Fig. 11.4 a–d. Side-sitting on the mat (left hemiplegia). **a** When the patient is moving from kneel-standing to side-sitting on the sound side, the therapist facilitates trunk rotation and moves her feet so that she is ready to support his trunk with the inside of her right leg. **b** The patient tries to maintain the corrected position without using his sound hand. **c** Moving to sit on the hemiplegic side. **d** The therapist supports the patient's trunk with her legs

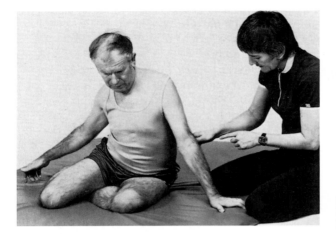

Fig. 11.5. Side-sitting with selective extension of the hemiplegic arm

Activities in Long-Sitting

From side-sitting, the patient straightens his legs out in front of him and places his hands forward on his legs. Keeping his knees as straight as possible, he slides his hands gently along his legs towards his feet. The therapist kneels in front of the patient and guides his hemiplegic arm so that the movement is performed without effort. When she feels that the whole arm is no longer pulling back from the scapula, she asks him to leave his hands resting on his legs (**Fig. 11.6 a**). If necessary, she holds his foot in dorsiflexion. When the patient places his hemiplegic hand on the opposite leg, protraction of the scapula is achieved and rotation of the upper trunk. He is assisted by the sensation in the sound leg as he learns to inhibit the retraction of his scapula, and in fact the whole pattern of flexor spasticity in the arm and hand. While moving his sound hand actively, he tries to let his hemiplegic hand remain in place (**Fig. 11.6 b**).

With his hands placed on the mat behind him, he supports his weight through his outwardly rotated, extended arms. With the therapist helping to maintain extension at the elbow, the patient transfers his weight from one side to the other, so that the scapula moves freely over the chest wall. The balls of both his hands should remain flat on the floor. Flexor spasticity is inhibited and at the same time extensor activity is stimulated. The patient can also inhibit the spasticity around the scapula by rounding his thoracic spine, while his hands remain in the same position, both scapulae being fully protracted as a result (**Fig. 11.7 a**). He then extends his spine again as fully as possible, inhibiting the hypertonus in the arm and shoulder as he moves his trunk against his fixed arms (**Fig. 11.7 b**).

The same activities can also be performed in standing and sitting positions with the hands supported on the plinth as described in Chap. 8. The patient places his hands flat on the floor between his legs in front of him and the therapist inhibits the retraction

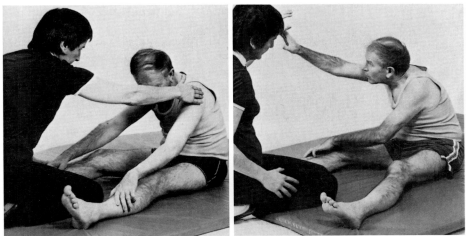

Fig. 11.6 a, b. Long-sitting with inhibition of flexor hypertonus in the whole arm (left hemiplegia). **a** The patient leaves his hands resting on his legs, as close to his feet as possible. **b** His hemiplegic hand remains in place on the sound leg when he moves his sound arm actively

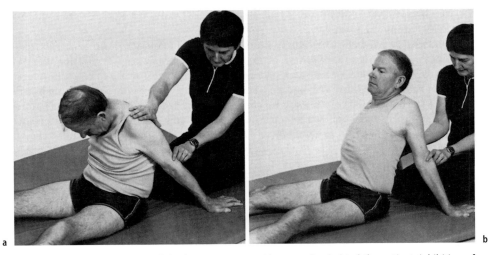

Fig. 11.7 a, b. In long-sitting with both arms supported in extension behind the patient, inhibition of distal hypertonicity by moving the trunk proximally: **a** into flexion; **b** into extension (left hemiplegia)

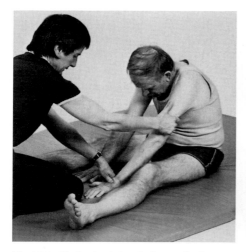

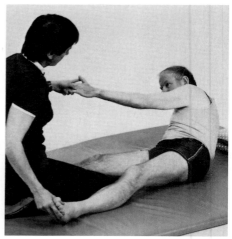

Fig. 11.8. Placing both hands flat on the floor to inhibit retraction of the scapula

Fig. 11.9. Lying down and sitting up with trunk rotation emphasised (left hemiplegia)

and depression of the scapula **(Fig. 11.8)**. When she feels that the hypertonus is inhibited she asks him to leave his elbow in extension. He then allows the elbows to flex slightly before extending them actively.

In order to move from long-sitting to supine lying and come back up again, with the therapist maintaining full inhibition of the arm to keep it forward in extension, the patient slowly lies down over his sound side with adequate trunk rotation. The hemiplegic shoulder remains well forward, and he tries to prevent it from pulling back as he moves **(Fig. 11.9)**. The patient comes back up to long-sitting again, over the sound side. He brings his hemiplegic shoulder forwards and the therapist keeps his arm in extension. When the patient is lying supine, the activities involving rolling follow well in a movement sequence.

Rolling

Rolling over onto the side is an easy movement for the patient and can be so facilitated that it is light and rhythmic. Whether he is rolling over to either side or turning right over to lie prone, the therapist must ensure that the normal pattern of movement is used. Often the untrained patient will use his sound leg to push off from the floor behind him or bring the sound foot onto the floor in front of him to slow the movement down. He may hold his head in too much extension or use his sound hand to support himself in front as he rolls forwards, or behind him before rolling back. The therapist adjusts her facilitation accordingly until the patient is able to roll unaided in a normal way right over into prone.

Because rolling is so beneficial it can be used in the treatment at all stages, but always with the appropriate amount of assistance and increasing exactness. Using a broad, high mat or two plinths placed together for additional width, rolling can be practised even before the patient is able to go down on the mat. It will often serve to inhibit hypertonus before active arm movements are attempted.

Rolling to the Hemiplegic Side

Turning towards the affected side is the easier movement sequence for the patient, and he can learn to do so in the normal pattern of movement from the beginning, even when he is in bed (see Chap. 5). The vulnerable shoulder must be protected in the early stages, or later if his shoulder is already painful, and the therapist therefore cradles the patient's arm between her arm and her waist, supporting his upper arm with her hand. By doing so she keeps the scapula in protraction and the shoulder forward. With her other hand she facilitates the movement of his sound leg, which he must lift up and bring forwards over the other leg, without pushing off on the plinth or mat behind him. The patient's hemiplegic leg usually fails to rotate outwards as he rolls over it, rather pulling into internal rotation as part of the spastic extension pattern. The therapist then uses her free hand placed on the patient's thigh to facilitate external rotation (see **Fig. 5.17**). She then moves the hand quickly out of the way when his sound leg is brought forwards. The patient brings his sound arm forwards freely. He rolls back again, the unaffected leg returning to a position of extension and abduction, lying flat on the mat. To ensure that the movement is performed with flexor activity in the trunk and not by the patient using a mass extension pattern, the therapist asks him to lift his head before starting to roll over, placing his head in the correct position with her fingers (**Fig. 11.10 a**). He then lifts his sound leg off the bed and rolls onto his side (**Fig. 11.10 b**).

When the movement has released the tension in the entire hemiplegic side, the therapist eases the arm further and further into abduction, until it lies flat on the mat when the patient rolls back to the supine position (**Fig. 11.10 c**). Finally, he should try to leave his arm extended and abducted with the help of the therapist, without its pulling into flexion or causing any discomfort even when his other arm is also lying fully extended in abduction on the mat (**Fig. 11.10 d**).

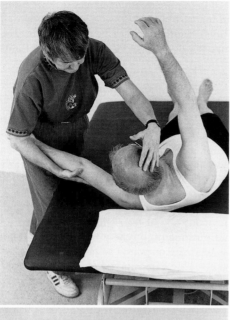

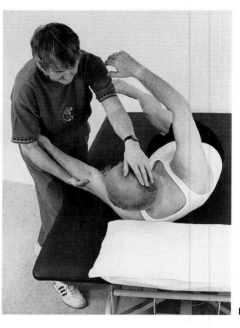

a

b

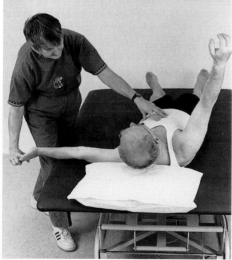

Fig. 11.10 a–d. Rolling towards the hemiplegic side and back to supine (left hemiplegia). **a** The patient first lifts his head from the pillow and the therapist protects his hemiplegic shoulder by supporting the humerus. **b** His head turns in the direction of the movement, and his sound arm and leg move through the air without pushing off against the supporting surface. **c** Returning to the supine position with the hemiplegic arm lying flat on the mat

c

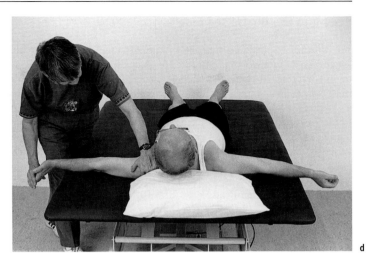

Fig. 11.10 d. Continuing the movement until both arms can lie fully extended in abduction without causing discomfort

d

For very full inhibition of the proximal spasticity, the patient rolls onto his hemiplegic side and the therapist draws his scapula into full protraction. She places her hand right over the scapula and holds its medial border forward with her fingers **(Fig. 11.11)**. Holding it firmly in the corrected position, she asks the patient to move very gently back and forth without the scapula moving at all.

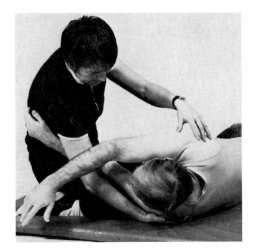

Fig. 11.11. Lying on his hemiplegic side, the patient moves gently back and forth while the therapist holds the scapula in protraction (left hemiplegia)

Rolling to the Unaffected Side

The therapist kneels on the patient's unaffected side to help him bring his hemiplegic leg forwards in a normal pattern. He clasps his hands together with his arms extended, to ensure that the affected arm is protected. The unaffected leg remains flat on the mat, rolling into external rotation as the other leg swings forwards (see **Fig. 5.18**).

When the patient is able to bring his affected leg to the front actively, the therapist holds his hemiplegic hand as he rolls back and forth with increased rotation of the trunk. With one hand she keeps his hand in dorsiflexion, while with the other she prevents his shoulder from retracting as he rolls from his side onto his back. He tries to place his affected leg far back on the supporting surface in abduction.

When the therapist feels that the hypertonus in the arm has been reduced she holds only the patient's hand and asks him to roll back without letting his shoulder go back at the same time. With her free hand she increases the amount of trunk rotation by helping him to roll his pelvis backwards (**Fig. 11.12**).

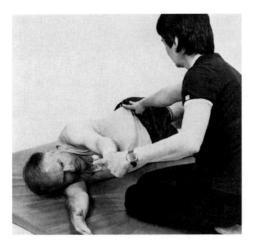

Fig. 11.12. Rolling back to supine from the sound side with increased trunk rotation (left hemiplegia)

Rolling Over to a Prone Position

Rolling to prone is somehow a very positive experience for the patient, and he feels his body from a completely different aspect, against the resistance of the mat. Care must be taken that his shoulder is protected during the roll. As he comes into the prone position there could be an increase in flexor tone (see Chap. 3), and its influence on the arm and scapula could cause pain in the shoulder. For this reason it is safer to practise the movement with the patient rolling over his unaffected side at first, as the vulnerable shoulder can be carefully supported by the therapist.

The patient rolls over the sound side to lie prone with his weight supported on his elbows, or with his arms extended in front of him. The therapist controls his hemiplegic arm throughout the movement, guiding it forwards into position without the shoulder retracting (**Fig. 11.13**).

If the shoulder is completely mobile and pain free the patient can also roll over his hemiplegic side with his affected arm in elevation (**Fig. 11.14**). He arrives in the prone position with both arms outstretched in front of him.

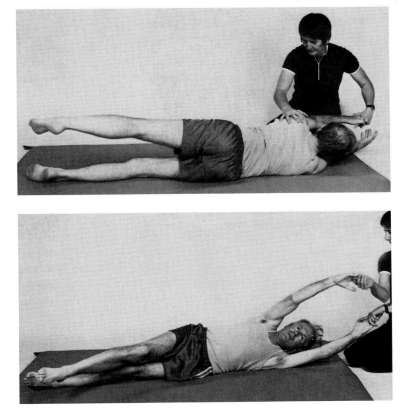

Fig. 11.13.
Rolling to prone over the sound side with the therapist guiding the hemiplegic arm forwards (left hemiplegia)

Fig. 11.14.
Rolling to prone over the hemiplegic side (left hemiplegia)

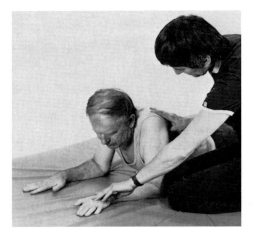

Fig. 11.15. Moving from side to side in prone lying with weight supported on the elbows (left hemiplegia)

Prone-Lying

Lying prone with the weight supported on his elbows, the patient can be helped to move in such a way that the increased tone around the scapula is reduced and selective activity stimulated. When he rounds his thoracic spine and brings his chest away from the floor, his scapulae protract, and the movement of the proximal parts against the distal inhibits the spasticity. If he transfers his weight from one side to the other, the scapula moves over the chest wall and the tone throughout the arm is reduced (**Fig. 11.15**). To inhibit hypertonus in the pronators the therapist can hold his hemiplegic arm in external rotation with the forearm supinated while the patient moves sideways.

Moving to Prone Kneeling

The patient moves from lying to prone kneeling by rolling over onto his sound side, flexing his knees and hips and pushing himself up with his arm to side-sitting, and then turning to support himself on his knees and sound hand.

If the patient still has difficulty in coming to prone kneeling, the therapist stands behind him and places one hand on either side of his pelvis. She helps him to lift his buttocks from the floor and to turn round onto his knees (**Fig. 11.16a**). Once the patient is kneeling, the therapist moves round to the front of him and places his hemiplegic hand on the mat in the correct position. When the patient is able to move into prone kneeling on his own, the therapist kneels in front of him and guides his hemiplegic arm throughout the movement sequence (**Fig. 11.16b**).

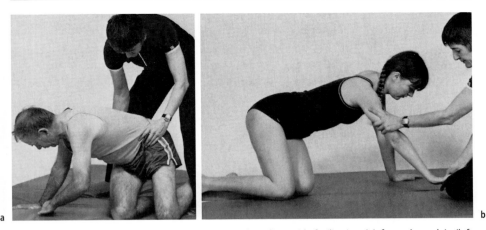

a   b

Fig. 11.16. a, b. Moving from side-sitting to prone kneeling with facilitation (**a**) from the pelvis (left hemiplegia), (**b**) from the hemiplegic arm (right hemiplegia)

Alternatively, the patient could move from kneel-standing to prone kneeling when he first goes down onto the mat. He must, however, learn the sequence of coming from lying to side-sitting to prone kneeling, so that he can stand up from the floor should he ever fall over. (Quite apart from falling over, many patients enjoy being able to sit on the grass or lie on the beach and would like to be able to stand up again easily.)

Activities in Prone Kneeling

- Kneeling beside the patient on his affected side, the therapist helps him to achieve the correct position, with his shoulders and hips in 90° flexion and his weight evenly distributed over both hands and both knees. Her thigh against his arm assists elbow extension, and with the hand nearest to him she supports his shoulder in external rotation. She places her thumb against the humeral head anteriorly while her fingers around his upper arm rotate the shoulder and help him to extend his elbow. With her free hand she encourages him to extend his spine (**Fig. 11.17 a**). Then the patient rounds his back as fully as possible, and by so doing moves the scapulae into protraction (**Fig. 11.17 b**). The therapist helps him to maintain elbow extension with his fingers remaining fully extended. The patient then hollows his back again, extending his spine, and repeats the movement. As his ability to maintain the arm in extension increases, the therapist gradually moves his hands so that the shoulder is increasingly externally rotated and the forearm supinated.
- From prone kneeling the patient sits back on his heels, leaving his hands outstretched on the mat in front of him (**Fig. 11.17 c**). With her hand still on his upper arm, the therapist helps to maintain the correct position of his hemiplegic arm, while elongat-

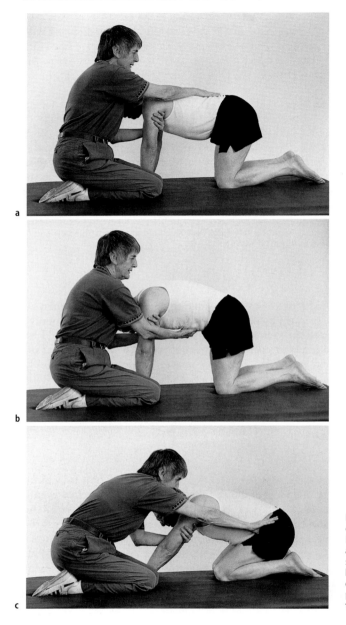

Fig. 11.17 a–c. Flexing and
extending the trunk in prone
kneeling (left hemiplegia).
a Trunk extension with the
shoulder well supported.
b Trunk flexion. **c** Sitting back
on the heels with the hemiplegic arm remaining in position

ing the side of his trunk by pressing gently back on his iliac crest. If necessary, she uses her thigh to keep his elbow extended and stabilises his shoulder forward with her hand. As a result of repeating the movement the spasticity in the entire side is inhibited and the patient can usually extend his elbow actively as he returns to the prone kneeling position. Hypertonicity in the knee extensors is also inhibited by the activity.

- Selective lateral flexion of the patient's lower trunk can be practised in prone kneeling as well, with the patient's weight equally supported on both knees and hands. The therapist extends her knees somewhat, so that she can keep his shoulder forward and maintain extension of his elbow with her leg against his arm. She places her hands on each side of his pelvis and helps him to shorten the sound side of his trunk with lateral flexion of his lumbar spine (**Fig. 11.18a**) To localise the movement the therapist stabilises the patient's thorax by holding it firmly against her body with her arm. By changing the direction of movement of her hands on his pelvis, she then facilitates the active shortening of the patient's hemiplegic side (**Fig. 11.18b**).

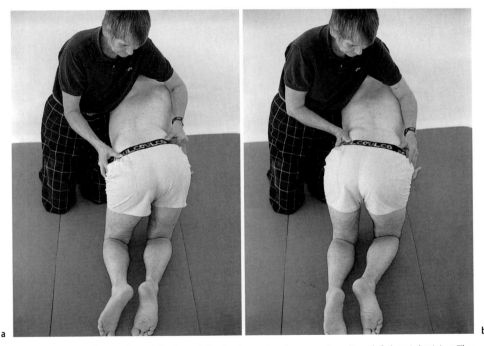

a   b

Fig. 11.18a, b. Selective lateral flexion of the lumbar spine in prone kneeling (left hemiplegia). **a** The therapist stabilises the thorax when the lower trunk shortens on the sound side. **b** With her hands on either side of the pelvis she facilitates the shortening of the hemiplegic side

Activities in Kneel-Standing

The patient comes from prone kneeling to kneel-standing, and the therapist stands up and moves into a position behind him so that she can assist hip extension with her knees. Although hip extension is often difficult in this position, it provides a useful opportunity for working on selective activity of the hip extensors. With his knee flexed, the patient is unable to use the total extension synergy, and the hip control is therefore very selective. In addition, the flexed knee may increase flexor hypertonicity throughout the limb and he will have to combat the tendency for the neighbouring joints to flex as well.

During activities in kneeling and half-kneeling the patient's hands should not be clasped together. His arms should be left free to enable him to extend his thoracic spine more easily without the additional weight. Normal balance reactions in the arm may also be stimulated. The position of the hemiplegic arm will also be a guide as to whether enough assistance is being given or whether the patient is having to struggle to perform the movements.

The patient moves his weight first over one leg and then over the other. When he moves to the hemiplegic side the whole of that side should elongate, his trochanter

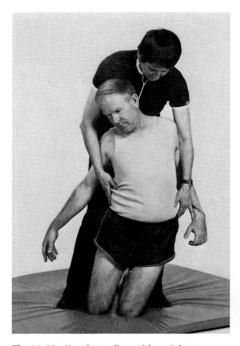

Fig. 11.19. Kneel-standing with weight transferred over the hemiplegic side (left hemiplegia)

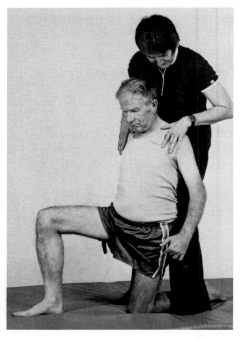

Fig. 11.20. Half-kneel-standing with the sound leg brought forward. The therapist supports the patient's hemiplegic hip with her knee (left hemiplegia)

being the most lateral point (**Fig. 11.19**). His hips must remain extended, and the therapist facilitates the extension with her knees. When she feels that the active control is improving, she asks the patient to keep his buttocks away from her knees and gradually withdraws her support. With her hands she assists the lateral movement of the pelvis. With his weight well over the hemiplegic leg, the patient brings his sound foot forwards and places it lightly on the floor in front of him (**Fig. 11.20**).

Activities in Half-Kneel-Standing

The patient practises bringing his sound leg down again to kneel-standing and then up again to half-kneel-standing, without scraping his foot on the floor as he does so. When the patient brings his sound foot forwards, his knee will tend to move medially, due to the lack of selective extension with outward rotation in the hemiplegic hip (**Fig. 11.21 a**) He is asked to keep his knee in line with the long axis of his foot while the foot itself remains flat on the floor (**Fig. 11.21 b**). The therapist continues to assist with hip extension and balance. The patient taps his sound foot lightly on the floor in front of him, and progresses until he can tap it nearer to and across the midline, and also far out to the side.

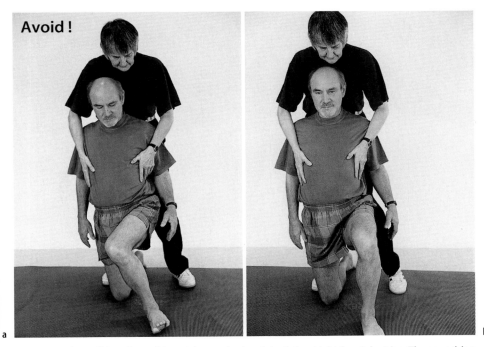

a

b

Fig. 11.21 a, b. Half-kneeling with weight on the hemiplegic leg (right hemiplegia). **a** The sound leg adducts due to lack of selective extension in the hemiplegic hip. **b** The patient holds his sound thigh in line with his foot, which remains flat on the floor

Standing up from Half-Kneeling

To stand up from the floor, the patient transfers his weight over the hemiplegic leg and brings the sound foot forwards. He pauses in half-kneel-standing and then leans his trunk forwards until his head is over the foot in front. He comes to standing and brings his hemiplegic foot forwards to the other one.

Practising the activity with the patient's hands clasped together and the arms extended will help him to bring his weight far enough forwards at first. As his ability improves, the arms can be left to swing freely when he comes to standing. The therapist facilitates the movement by placing her hands in his axillae from behind and guiding him forwards and upwards (**Fig. 11.22 a**). She can also facilitate the movement by supporting with her hands on each side of his pelvis and helping him to come upright (**Fig. 11.22 b**). If the patient or therapist is anxious about standing up at first, a chair can be placed in front of him and he supports his clasped hands on it as he comes to the upright position.

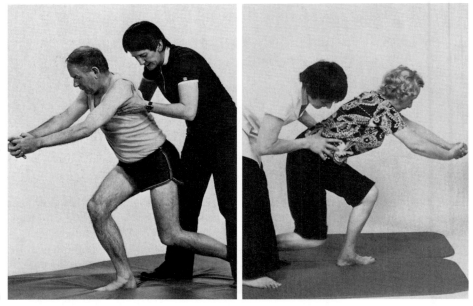

a   b

Fig. 11.22 a, b. Standing up from the floor with facilitation. **a** With her hands in the patient's axillae the therapist guides the movement forwards (left hemiplegia). **b** With her hands on either side of the pelvis she helps the patient to maintain balance and bring her weight over her sound leg (right hemiplegia)

Considerations

Exercising on the mat should be a pleasurable experience for the patient, and care must be taken that the amount of support given in the beginning is adequate. It is easy for the therapist to make the mistake of keeping him too long in kneel-standing while practising weight transference, for example. The patient's knees begin to hurt and he will be loath to go on the mat again in the future, as he will remember the unpleasant sensation. If the patient's foot pulls strongly into flexion and causes painful pressure on his toes, a small pillow can be placed beneath his foot to relieve the pressure at first. As the movements become easier, the foot ceases to pull into flexion. It would be a pity to avoid the valuable therapeutic effect of moving on the mat simply because the first attempt was unsuccessful. Moving on the floor is, after all, the way in which we all originally learn to move in early childhood in preparation for standing and walking.

Taking a patient down onto the mat is also strenuous for the therapist, and some may feel that the effort is disproportional to the benefits to be gained from the activity. Quite apart from the therapeutic effects, however, the ability to kneel or sit down on the ground and stand up again afterwards will not only further the patient's functional independence but will also open doors for him to enjoy other pleasurable activities. Functionally, he will be able to find an object which has fallen to the floor and been temporarily lost from view. He will be able to weed the garden, plant new seedlings or mop up spilt liquid from the floor. From an enjoyment point of view, he will be able to sit on the grass at a picnic, join his young grandchild on the floor for a game or lie in the sun on the warm stone beside the swimming pool.

Perhaps the most important advantage to be gained from working on the mat is that, for many patients, becoming accustomed to moving down to the ground and standing up from the floor diminishes their fear of walking independently, inside the house as well as outside.

12 Shoulder Problems Associated with Hemiplegia

The human shoulder is a very mobile joint indeed. It needs to have a vast range of movement in order to bring the hands into the right positions to perform the countless tasks of daily life and to make fine motor skills possible. Biomechanically, stability has therefore been sacrificed in favour of mobility when the shoulder is compared with the hip joint, where the opposite is the case. However, it is not the shoulder joint alone which makes movements of the arm in so many directions possible. In fact, as Cailliet (1980) explains, no fewer than seven joints must all move together in a synchronised, co-ordinated way to allow for smooth, unhampered motion and activity; the joints involved being:
1. Glenohumeral
2. Suprahumeral
3. Acromioclavicular
4. Scapulocostal
5. Sternoclavicular
6. Costosternal
7. Costovertebral

It is therefore easy to understand why patients with hemiplegia, who have a paralysis or abnormal tone in the muscles controlling their scapula and arm, may well develop problems at the shoulder if they do not have careful and informed therapy and handling, particularly during the acute phase of their illness. The most commonly described problem is that of pain and limitation of movement, a secondary complication that is preventable and should not be considered an inevitable symptom of the stroke itself.

Unfortunately, even today, in many hospitals and rehabilitation centres all over the world, hemiplegic patients still suffer from severe pain in the shoulder, and the problem is most distressing for both the patient and the staff. The pain has been described by Caldwell et al.(1969) as affecting up to 70% of the patients, while in a study involving 219 patients, 72% had shoulder pain, a disturbing figure which rose to 85% for those with spasticity (Van Ouwenaller et al. 1986). These figures are unacceptable and, as Roper (1982) writes, "the painful shoulder is a major impairment to the entire rehabilitation programme, because the patient with an adducted medially rotated shoulder makes no attempt to use the affected arm and often fails to participate in walking training." In fact, the sequelae of the pain are even more extensive:
- The patient cannot concentrate on learning new skills, because he is constantly distracted by the pain. He has difficulty in regaining independence in the activities of daily life because the pain and stiffness interfere with dressing and washing, turning over in bed etc.

- Balance reactions are impeded both in sitting and standing, and the patient is afraid to move freely to carry out the tasks required of him. His morale is drastically lowered, and like any other person with constant pain he becomes depressed. A vicious circle ensues.
- The patient is unable to sleep and then cannot co-operate fully in the therapy sessions. As a result he makes little or no progress, and with the lack of success he becomes even more depressed. "The patient who has pain when he moves will remain immobile. If he also has pain at rest he usually withdraws from any active rehabilitation programme" (Braun et al. 1971).
- Pain itself can inhibit muscle activity, and it is very difficult to stimulate the return of active movement in the hemiplegic arm while pain persists. "There are situations in which the pain is so severe that the response is a neurological inhibition of muscle activity" (Guymer 1988).

With so many adverse effects, the correct treatment of the shoulder should surely have a high priority in the overall rehabilitation. It is also most fortunate that shoulder pain can be avoided with proper early management and treatment, and should it develop or already exist it can be overcome. Having suffered a stroke with all its devastating consequences, the patient should not have to live with pain as well.

Before treatment can be carried out successfully, it is necessary to understand both the normal shoulder mechanisms and the problems that arise in association with hemiplegia. There is a tendency to use a collective term such as "painful hemiplegic shoulder" to describe any painful condition which the patient demonstrates, but in fact, the problems can be divided into three distinct categories and may be observed in isolation or as a combination of two or even all three.

1. The subluxed shoulder
2. The painful shoulder
3. The shoulder-hand syndrome

The successful treatment varies according to the problem, and it is therefore important to differentiate between them.

The Subluxed or Malaligned Shoulder

The subluxed shoulder is in itself not painful (Diethelm and Davies 1985). It is, however, extremely vulnerable and can easily be traumatised. Subluxation of the shoulder is very common, especially where there is a total paralysis of the upper limb, and has been described as occurring in up to 73%, 66% and 60% of groups of hemiplegic patients with severe paralysis of the arm (Najenson et al.1971; Najenson and Pikielni 1965; Smith et al. 1982). It is often mistakenly thought that the subluxation is the cause of the pain, this incorrect association having arisen because usually the patient's hemiplegic shoulder is X-rayed only if he complains that it is painful. When radiological examination reveals a subluxation, the finding is immediately held to be responsible for the pain, although in all probability the malalignment has been present for some time without the patient suffering any discomfort.

During investigations carried out at King's College Hospital in 1976, it was found that all hemiplegic patients with a total paralysis of the arm showed a subluxation of the shoulder when X-rayed in an upright sitting position within the first 3 weeks after onset of stroke (**Fig. 12.1 a**). Despite the usually marked subluxation, all patients had full pain-free range of motion at the shoulder joint, and it was interesting to note that when the arm was passively elevated, the head of the humerus was seen to be correctly located in the glenoid fossa (**Fig. 12.1 b**).

The patients did, however, experience a dragging discomfort or ache if the arm was left hanging at their side too long. The ache was immediately relieved if the arm was elevated passively or supported on a table in front of them. As these patients had no pain and were being positioned and carefully treated from the beginning of their illness, it could be hypothesised that subluxation occurs spontaneously when the patient starts sitting or standing up against gravity in the early stages following a stroke, and is not, as is sometimes postulated, the result of traumatic or incorrect handling.

Roper (1975) described a large series of patients with hemiplegia who were admitted to Rancho Los Amigos Hospital for surgery to relieve severe shoulder pain. None showed radiological evidence of shoulder subluxation. As these patients had had their hemiplegia for 2 years or more, it could be postulated that subluxation becomes progressively less with the passing of time, i.e. as muscle tone or activity returns, until it usually disappears altogether and "certainly is extremely rare when the patients are reviewed after neurological stabilisation has occurred" (Roper 1982).

Factors Predisposing to Subluxation

The shoulder joint is inherently unstable, to allow for the enormous range of movement required for skilled manipulations by the hand and fingers. The joint socket is relatively shallow compared with that of the hip joint, so that two thirds of the humeral head is

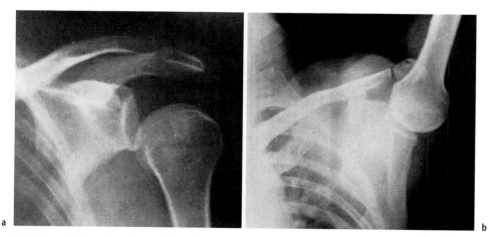

a   b

Fig. 12.1 a, b. X-rays from the patient series at King's College Hospital. **a** Subluxed shoulder; **b** position corrected when the arm is passively elevated

not covered by the glenoid fossa. Zinn (1973) describes how the loss of stability has been compensated for by a very strong surrounding musculature.

Both Basmajian (1979, 1981) and Cailliet (1980) have described fully and clearly the factors preventing downward displacement or subluxation in the normal state, as well as explaining its occurrence in hemiplegic patients. In the normal correct orientation of the scapula the glenoid fossa faces upwards as well as forwards and laterally. The upward slope of the fossa plays an important role in preventing downward dislocation because the head of the humerus would need to move laterally in order to move downwards. With the arm in an adducted position, the superior part of the capsule and the coracohumeral ligament are taut and passively prevent lateral movement of the humeral head and thus its downward displacement, which Basmajian calls the "locking mechanism of the shoulder joint" (**Fig. 12.2 a**). The supraspinatus reinforces the horizontal tension of the capsule when the arm is loaded and in some subjects even when the arm is relaxed at the side of the body.

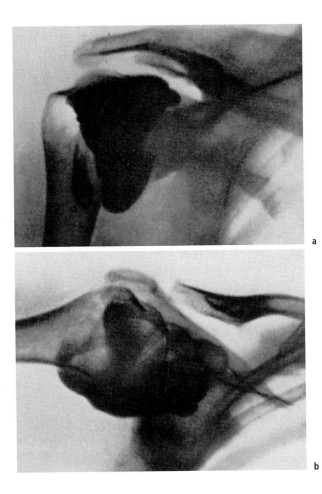

a

b

Fig. 12.2 a, b. Arthrogram: normal shoulder. **a** Arm adducted, superior portion of capsule taut; **b** arm abducted, superior portion of capsule lax

With abduction of the humerus the locking mechanism no longer operates. As the arm is lifted sideways in abduction or forwards, the superior capsule becomes lax, thus eliminating the support, and the joint stability must be provided by muscular contraction instead (**Fig. 12.2 b**). The integrity of the joint then depends almost exclusively on the rotator cuff muscles, "which should be called the guardians of the shoulder" (Basmajian 1981).

The muscles most important in preventing subluxation of the glenohumeral joint are those whose fibres run horizontally, in particular the supraspinatus, the posterior fibres of the deltoid and the infraspinatus. However, a patient who has a paralysis of the shoulder muscles following a brachial plexus lesion does not demonstrate subluxation because he is able to maintain the correct position of the scapula actively (**Fig. 12.3**). The passive locking mechanism of the shoulder joint stays intact if the glenoid fossa remains in its normal orientation and the capsule is taut.

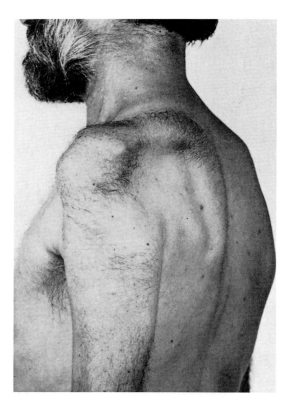

Fig. 12.3. Patient with brachial plexus lesion of 9 years' duration has no subluxation

Causes of Subluxation in Hemiplegia

Subluxation of the shoulder in hemiplegia is most commonly caused by one of the following:

Cause A

Patients who have lost not only the passive locking mechanism when the arm is hanging at their side, but also the support from reflex or voluntary activity in the relevant muscles will inevitably have a subluxation of the shoulder. A combination of the following signs is evident:

- The shoulder girdle droops with loss of tone or activity in the elevators of the scapula, particularly in their combined action with the serratus anterior to elevate the glenoid fossa with scapular rotation forwards. The fossa therefore slopes downwards (Fig. 12.4 a).
- Viewed from behind, the scapula is seen to lie closer to the vertebrae, but particularly the inferior angle is adducted, and lower than that of the scapula on the other side (Fig. 12.4 b).

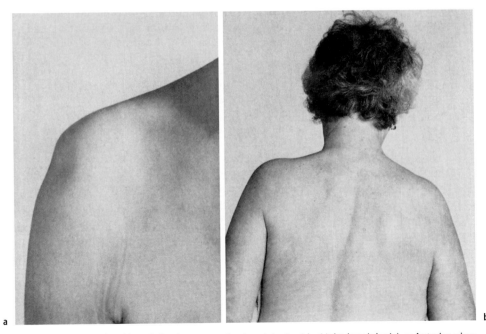

a   b

Fig. 12.4 a, b. The shoulder girdle droops on the hemiplegic side (right hemiplegia). **a** Anterior view showing typical subluxation; **b** posterior view showing position of scapula

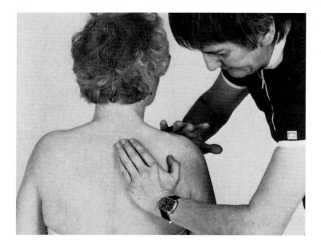

Fig. 12.5. Resistance to passive correction of the winged scapula (right hemiplegia)

- The vertebral border of the scapula is pulled away from the ribs, and, significantly, there is a resistance to passive correction of the winging **(Fig. 12.5)**. It must be assumed, therefore, that despite the apparent flaccid appearance of the upper limb, tone has increased in certain muscle groups. Even if the increase in tone is relatively slight, its effect is marked because of the hypotonus in the antagonists. The unopposed increase in tone in the pectoralis minor could be responsible for pulling the vertebral border of the scapula away from the ribs, causing the resistance to correction, and also for adding to the change in angulation of the glenoid fossa with downward rotation of the scapula. Because the scapula rotates downwards and adducts or retracts, the humerus finds itself in a position of relative abduction as the arm remains against the side of the body. The capsule is no longer taut and the head of the humerus is free to slide down in the fossa.
- The supraspinatus, infraspinatus and posterior portion of the deltoid all show marked atrophy and do not spring into activity to take over the action of the now lax capsule. Subluxation is therefore inevitable **(Fig. 12.6a)**. The effect is even more noticeable if the patient's arm is raised passively in abduction, causing further relaxation of the capsular restraint. If the position of the scapula is passively corrected by the examiner, who holds the inferior angle firmly and draws it sufficiently away from the vertebrae, the shoulder is no longer subluxed. Because the arm is once more adducted, the passive locking mechanism is re-established **(Fig. 12.6b)**.

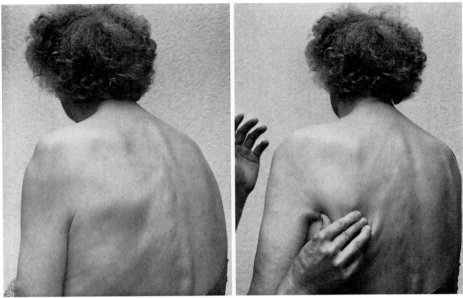

a   b

Fig. 12.6 a, b. The effect of the position of the scapula (left hemiplegia). **a** Rotated downwards with its inferior angle adducted – marked subluxation evident. **b** With the inferior angle pulled away from the vertebrae – subluxation corrected

Cause B

In recent years, clinical observations and additional scientific information have brought to light another combination of factors which lead perhaps even more frequently to subluxation of the patient's shoulder. Butler (1991) describes how increased and adverse neural tension develops following a lesion of the nervous system, and Davies (1990) explains that in hemiplegia the abdominal muscles are inactive and hypotonic.

- Increased neural tension in the cervical region elevates the clavicle and the scapula, with the flaccid trunk muscles failing to counteract the elevation of the shoulder girdle from below (**Fig. 12.7**).
- The glenoid fossa, the acromion and the clavicle are pulled upwards and away from the humeral head, whose accompanying movement is impeded by the weight of the paralysed arm.
- In addition to influencing the position of the joint, the increased neural tension can inhibit the return of tone and activity in the hypotonic muscles of the trunk and those which stabilise the shoulder. It can also lead to painful symptoms being experienced in the areas supplied by the affected nerves.

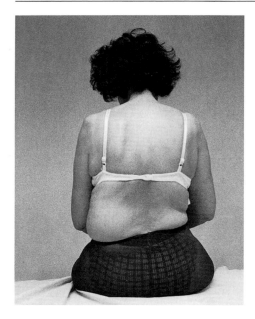

Fig. 12.7. Subluxation due to cause B: increased tension in the nervous system elevates the shoulder girdle of a patient with hypotonic abdominal muscles (left hemiplegia)

Treatment of the Subluxed Shoulder

The aims of treatment are therefore:
1. To restore the natural locking mechanism of the shoulder by correcting the position of the scapula and thus the glenoid fossa
2. To reduce the adverse tension in the nervous system so that the shoulder joint can be relocated and protective muscle activity regained
3. To stimulate activity or tone in the stabilising muscles around the shoulder
4. To maintain full pain-free range of passive movement without traumatising the joint and the structures which surround it
5. To protect the vulnerable shoulder from being injured during routine procedures

Correcting the Posture of the Scapula

After inhibition of any hypertonus which is rotating the scapula downwards and posteriorly, the patient is taught to elevate his shoulder anteriorly, in the direction of his nose (see **Fig. 8.13**). "Restoration of scapular posture to normal results in the restoration of a passive (but effective) function of the shoulder (glenohumeral) joint – the locking mechanism of the shoulder joint" (Basmajian 1979, 1981).

The therapist releases the spasticity by using those activities which move the trunk proximally against the scapula distally, e.g. rolling over the hemiplegic side, weightbearing through the arm and transferring weight sideways, moving the scapula manually in the desired direction. When moving the scapula into full elevation with protraction, the therapist needs to move both shoulders forwards at the same time. The patient's sound shoulder will otherwise rotate backwards, and the protraction of the affected side will be only apparent and not complete.

Reducing Adverse Tension in the Nervous System to Correct the Subluxation and Regain Active Muscle Control

Correcting the posture of the scapula and the position of the humeral head in the glenoid fossa requires a different approach when increased tension in the nervous system is the primary cause of the subluxation, because in such cases the shoulder girdle is already elevated with the patient's head pulled over to that side (**Fig. 12.8 a**) To overcome the problem, the therapist needs to mobilise the nervous system in a variety of starting positions, in the ways described in Chap. 15. For example, in sitting, the range of side flexion of the neck can be gradually increased, so that the neural structures responsible for the excessive elevation of the shoulder girdle regain their lengthening properties. While assisting repeated lateral flexion of the patient's neck with one hand, the therapist must use her other arm to prevent any compensatory movements from occurring simultaneously. With her hand placed over his shoulder from above, she holds the shoulder girdle down and uses the ball of her hand to keep the scapula from winging. Her forearm presses against the patient's lower ribs to stabilise the rib cage and upper trunk (**Fig. 12.8 b**). Immediately following the mobilisation, the shoulder subluxation disappears completely when the therapist helps the patient to maintain the corrected position of his shoulder girdle and to hold his ribs down and towards the midline (**Fig. 12.8 c**).

Stimulating Activity or Tone in the Stabilising Muscles Around the Shoulder

Once the contributing factors pertaining to either cause A or cause B have been overcome and the abnormal posture of the scapula been corrected, voluntary muscle control is of prime importance to maintain the integrity of the shoulder joint even when the arm moves.

All the activities described in Chap. 8 for stimulating the return of function in the arm can be used to activate the muscles which surround and stabilise the shoulder joint. Particularly useful are those where weight is taken through the affected arm, and activity is stimulated reflexly through compression of the joints of the upper limb (**Fig. 12.9**). During all weightbearing activities, the therapist must use her hands to ensure the correct alignment of the scapula, the trunk and, of course, the shoulder joint itself.

In addition, activity in the relevant muscles can be encouraged more directly by carefully graded stimulation.

- The therapist supports the patient's arm forwards, and with her other hand she taps the humerus head briskly and firmly upwards (**Fig. 12.10 a**). Tone and activity are increased in the deltoid and supraspinatus muscles by eliciting a stretch reflex from below.

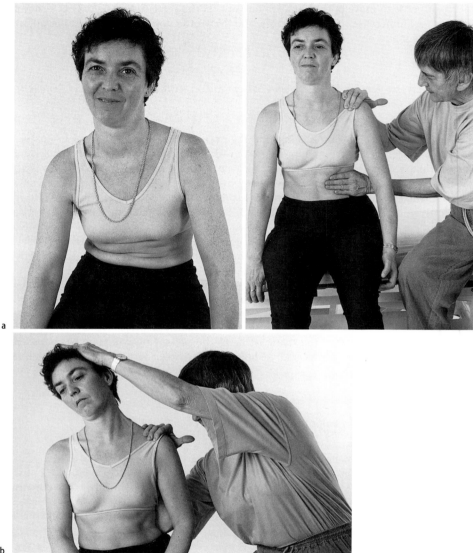

Fig. 12.8 a–c. Correction of subluxation due to increased nervous system tension (left hemiplegia). **a** Typical posture with lateral flexion of neck, elevation of shoulder girdle and the trunk elongated on the affected side. **b** Stabilising the scapula and thorax during neck side flexion to mobilise cervical nerves. Increased neural tension is clearly visible. **c** Shoulder no longer subluxed with corrected posture of ribs and shoulder girdle maintained

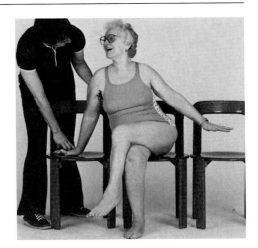

Fig. 12.9. Weightbearing through the hemiplegic arm with the shoulder supported (right hemiplegia)

- With the patient's arm held forwards, the therapist gives quick, repetitive approximation through the ball of the hand, and he is asked to keep his hand forward without letting his shoulder move backwards at all (**Fig. 12.10b**).
- With her fingers extended, the therapist strokes her hand firmly over the infraspinatus, deltoid and triceps muscles, moving quickly in the direction from proximal to distal (**Fig. 12.10c**).
- Brisk stroking with an ice cube can also help to stimulate activity in the relevant muscles when applied before an active movement is attempted.

Maintaining Full Pain-free Range of Passive Movement

The maintenance of full pain-free range of movement without traumatising the joint and the structures which surround it can be achieved by carrying out carefully and accurately the activities described in Chaps. 5 and 8. When moving the patient's arm passively, the therapist ensures that the head of the humerus is sited correctly within the glenoid fossa throughout the movement. Encircling the head of the humerus with the fingers of one of her hands, she rotates it laterally and eases it slightly downwards as the shoulder flexes. With her other hand she carefully moves the extended arm passively upwards into elevation. During the passive movement, the tips of the therapist's fingers form a cushion which prevents the humeral head from approximating with the rim of the fossa or the acromion process (**Fig. 12.11**).

At no time should pain in or around the shoulder joint be produced during therapeutic activities. Pain indicates that some structure is being compromised, and the therapist must react immediately and either decrease the range of movement or alter her support. Correcting the position of the scapula and supporting the shoulder joint adequately will usually eliminate the problem and allow a pain-free range of motion, but if not, it is far better not to move the shoulder at all than to move it and cause pain.

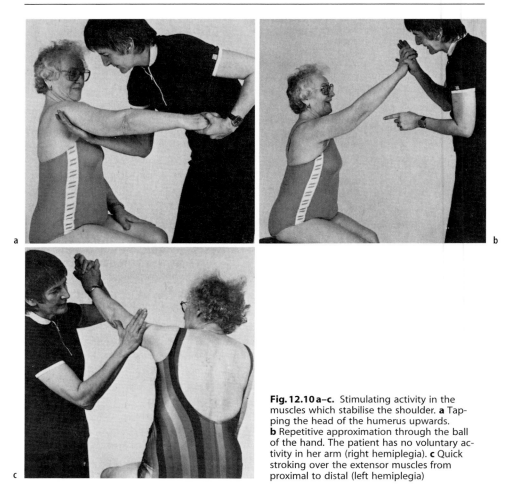

Fig. 12.10 a–c. Stimulating activity in the muscles which stabilise the shoulder. **a** Tapping the head of the humerus upwards. **b** Repetitive approximation through the ball of the hand. The patient has no voluntary activity in her arm (right hemiplegia). **c** Quick stroking over the extensor muscles from proximal to distal (left hemiplegia)

Protecting the Vulnerable Shoulder from Injury During Routine Procedures

Pain must be avoided, not only during passive movements of the arm or other therapeutic activities, but also when the patient is being helped to move in bed or to transfer into a chair. The whole team must be aware of the potential dangers and carefully instructed in how to protect the patient's shoulder when positioning and moving him or helping him with the activities of daily life. When examining the range of motion and alignment of the shoulder joint, the doctor, too, can injure sensitive structures if he lifts the arm from its distal end without supporting the scapula and humeral head proximally. Equally important are the patient's relatives, who may otherwise inadvertently traumatise the

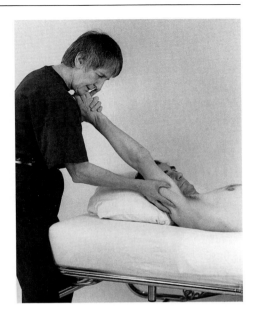

Fig. 12.11. During passive movements of the arm, the therapist's fingers align the head of the humerus in the glenoid fossa and prevent it from impinging with other bony surfaces (right hemiplegia)

shoulder when they are assisting him during the day. As Smith et al. (1982) so rightly point out, "correct handling of the patient in the early stages of a stroke is crucial in preventing the consequences of malalignment of the shoulder".

Supporting the Arm without Immobilisation

When the patient is lying in bed, the subluxation of his shoulder is automatically reduced, and no additional support is required if he is turned and positioned carefully. Correct positioning is naturally important, and the patient should sit with his arm supported forward on a table whenever he is sitting for any length of time. However, he must be encouraged to elevate the arm frequently during the day, using his sound hand to assist full elevation. When the patient is walking short distances, attending different departments for therapy or performing routine daily tasks, his arm should be left free to move and participate actively as far as is possible.

An arm sling should not be used to support the arm, as it does not reduce the subluxation and can have deleterious results (**Fig. 12.12**). In a careful study involving an albeit small group of new hemiplegic patients, Hurd et al. (1974) found no appreciable difference between the patients treated with a sling and those without, using the parameters of shoulder range of motion, shoulder pain and subluxation. Friedland (1975) agrees that "there is no need to support a pain-free shoulder in order to prevent or correct subluxation since the sling does not prevent, improve, cure or reduce such a deformity". Carr and Shepherd (1982) contend that, "There appears to be no sling which has been shown by radiographic study to be effective," an opinion confirmed by more re-

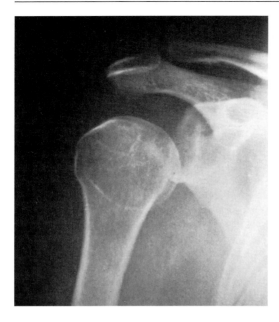

Fig. 12.12. X-ray of the shoulder with the arm in a sling shows no reduction of sub-luxation

cent radiological examinations which also revealed no satisfactory reduction of subluxation (Braus 1990).

Voss (1969) describes the consensus of a group of therapists who condemned slings for interfering with body image, immobilising the arm, reinforcing flexor tone, impairing postural support and impeding normal gait. Semans (1965) describes clearly the detrimental effects that "tying the arm against the body in a sling" can have:

- Fosters anosognosia or functional dissociation from total body movement
- Accentuates and encourages the spastic (flexor) pattern of the arm
- Prevents postural or supportive use of the arm as in turning over, rising from a chair or steadying an object for the other hand
- Prevents compensatory arm swing or guidance from the involved side during gait instruction
- Deprives patient of discriminative exteroceptive and proprioceptive input, resulting in hyperaesthesia from unbalanced spinothalamic input
- Increases the tendency to venous and lymphatic stasis resulting from immobility

Many alternative means of supporting the shoulder have been developed and advocated, but each has its disadvantage, despite claims to the contrary (Zorowitz et al. 1995). Most tend to compromise an already endangered circulation, either by compression in the axilla or by the use of a cuff-type support to take the weight of the arm. The once popular "Bobath axillary roll" was deemed inadvisable for this very reason. A prosthetic support developed in Holland and that designed by Sodring (1980) avoid compression but, like the sling, deprive the arm of input through participation and attention, which furthers neglect and can easily lead to a "learned non-use" such as that described by Taub (1980).

Observation of hundreds of patients during a 25-year period, for whom no form of support was used, indicates convincingly that careful active treatment and correct handling and positioning achieve the best results.

Conclusion

It should be remembered that subluxation of the shoulder is extremely common in the stroke population but is not the primary cause of painful conditions or limitation of range of motion. Subluxation is not painful as long as the scapula is mobile (B. Bobath 1978). The flaccid or hypotonic hanging arm will sublux, but this is not a factor to which any undue concern ought to be given (Johnstone 1978), and the subluxation is harmless as long as passive range of motion is not painful (Mossman 1976). The subluxed shoulder is in itself not painful (Davies 1980) (**Fig. 12.13 a, b**). It is, however, most important that the unprotected subluxed shoulder or malaligned shoulder does not become a painful shoulder with limitation of passive or active range of movement, the main objective being to regain motor control of an undamaged joint complex.

If subluxation is not the cause of the painful shoulder, then different aetiologies must be responsible for its occurrence according to Ring et al. (1993), who found no correlation between the degree of subluxation and the referred pain at later and even chronic stages of hemiplegia. The amount of pain was found to be unrelated to subluxation, spasticity, strength or sensation (Joynt 1992)

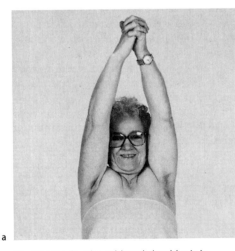

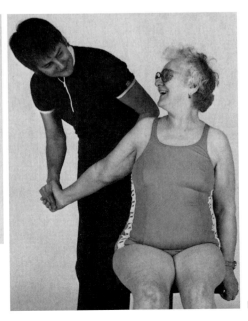

Fig. 12.13 a, b. The subluxed shoulder is in itself not painful (right hemiplegia). **a** Full self-assisted elevation is pain free. **b** No pain is elicited even in extreme positions (same patient as in Fig. 12.4)

The Painful Shoulder

A painful shoulder usually develops fairly early following a stroke, when the patient is particularly vulnerable and requires the assistance of others for every movement. Of 61 % of patients who developed diffuse shoulder pain following hemiplegia, two thirds did so within the first 4 weeks after onset and the rest in the subsequent 2 months (Braus 1990). Pain can, however, develop at a much later stage, even after several months. The upper limb may appear to be somewhat flaccid or show considerable spasticity. Subluxation may or may not be present, but as most hemiplegic patients show evidence of subluxation in the early stages of their illness, it would logically follow that many with pain in addition will also demonstrate such a malalignment. The common misconception that shoulder pain is the direct result of the subluxation has arisen because, generally, radiological investigations of the glenohumeral joint are undertaken only if the patient complains that his shoulder is hurting. The X-rays reveal a subluxation and the erroneous interpretation as to cause and effect follows automatically.

Pain at the shoulder usually develops in a typical pattern, although it can also occur suddenly as a result of a specific traumatic incident. The patient starts to complain of a sharp pain at the end of range of movement, when his arm is being moved passively during therapy or during an examination. He can point accurately to the painful localised area. If the causative factors are not eliminated, the pain increases over a period, or rapidly, and the patient describes pain on all movement, particularly elevation of the arm and abduction. He may experience pain only with the arm in certain positions or even when lying in bed at night. Severe sudden pain may occur, not only at full range of movement but also when the arm is being lowered to the side again, or at certain stages during the movements.

The patient finds it increasingly difficult to give the exact location of the pain and indicates the deltoid area by rubbing his hand over the muscle bulk. If the therapeutic approach is not altered, the patient has pain day and night and cannot tolerate his arm being moved at all. He complains of diffuse pain, in some cases involving the whole arm and the hand as well. The pain must be very intense indeed, for it can reduce proud strong men to a state of helpless weeping, begging the therapist not to move the arm or aggressively refusing to allow the arm to be touched at all. Some may try to avoid therapy altogether.

The painful condition must not be accepted as a part or symptom of the illness. It was not present at onset, so clearly something must have happened to cause it.

Possible Causes of Shoulder Pain

"The shoulder is essentially a composite of seven joints, all moving synchronously and incumbent upon each other to ensure complete pain-free movement" (Cailliet 1980). Any interruption of this co-ordinated interaction could cause pain or restriction of movements. In order to understand the disturbed mechanisms that cause pain in the shoulder following hemiplegia, the following aspects of the normal shoulder mechanism require special consideration.

1. The scapulohumeral rhythm described by Codman (1934) and Cailliet (1980) enables the arm to be lifted smoothly into full elevation **(Fig. 12.14)**. When a person is standing normally with the arm at the side of the body, the scapula and humerus can be said to be in the position of 0°. As the arm is abducted, a ratio of 2:1 exists between scapula rotation and glenohumeral movement. This would mean that when the arm is abducted to 90°, 60° of the movement take place at the glenohumeral joint and 30° are due to scapula rotation. Full elevation of the arm to 180° is performed with 120° of glenohumeral movement and 60° due to scapula rotation. The movement occurs in a smooth rhythmic pattern that the normal muscle tone allows unimpeded. The scapula rotates to change the alignment of the glenoid fossa, and without the rotation, the arm cannot fully abduct or elevate overhead.

2. External rotation of the humerus is essential for the arm to abduct fully, as it allows the greater tuberosity to pass behind the acromion process. "With the arm internally rotated the greater tuberosity impinges against the coraco-acromial arch and blocks further abduction at 60°" (Cailliet 1980).

3. A downward gliding movement of the head of the humerus in the glenoid fossa must accompany the external rotation if the greater tuberosity is to pass freely under the coraco-acromial hood.

In hemiplegia, if the patient suffers from pain and loss of range of movement at the shoulder, it is most likely that one or all of these mechanisms have been disturbed by abnormal and unbalanced muscle tone and activity. In the upper extremity, the spastic pattern of flexion predominates. Of particular relevance to the development of pain are the components of depression and retraction of the scapula and medial rotation of the humerus.

Pain arises because of injuries to the joint and/or the soft tissue structures which surround it, injuries of varying degrees of severity due to:

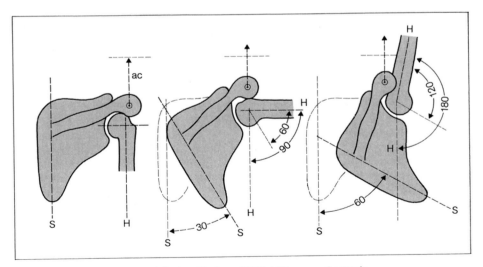

Fig. 12.14. The scapulohumeral rhythm (Codman 1934). *H* Humerus, *S* scapula

Loss of the Scapulohumeral Rhythm

When the patient's arm is lifted away from the body, there is a delay in scapula rotation. The structures located between the acromion process and the head of the humerus are mechanically squeezed between the two hard bony elements. A model of the shoulder shows clearly the pinching effect when the humerus is lifted sideways and the scapula remains fixed (**Fig. 12.15 a, b**).

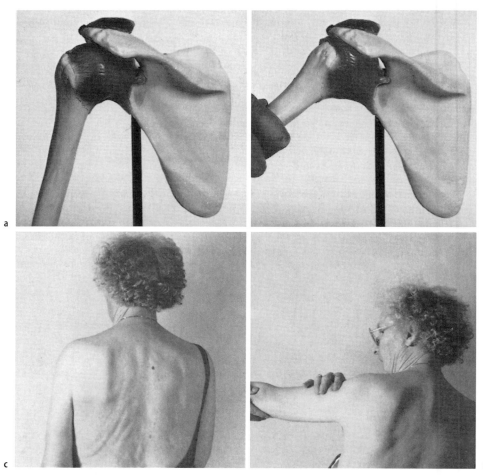

Fig. 12.15 a–d. Loss of the scapulohumeral rhythm as a cause of shoulder trauma (left hemiplegia). **a** Model of shoulder joint with humerus in a neutral position. **b** Model of shoulder joint showing mechanism of injury when the humerus is abducted. **c** Patient with her arm at her side. **d** When the arm is lifted the scapula fails to rotate and the patient experiences pain at the shoulder

Similarly, if the patient's scapula does not move sufficiently when his arm is being lifted passively, a trauma occurs and the patient experiences pain at the site of the compressed structures (**Fig. 12.15 c, d**). The same may occur if the patient performs his self-assisted arm movement incorrectly, through flexion, without sufficient protraction and rotation of the scapula (**Fig. 12.16**).

The delayed scapula rotation is due to an increase in tone in the muscles which retract and depress the scapula. The arm may appear to be flaccid, but even a slight increase in tone proximally at the scapula is sufficient to delay its simultaneous rotation. Where the tone of the muscles surrounding the scapula is the same as that of the muscles in the arm itself, the rhythm remains and both move together at the same speed, providing a natural protection.

For example, if a patient is equally spastic proximally and distally, the 'heavy' arm can be moved into abduction only slowly, which allows the scapula time to rotate slowly as well. Some patients with marked hypertonus will therefore have absolutely no pain or limitation of movement. In the same way, patients with marked hypotonus may also be pain free despite having had little or no therapy. In such cases, the flaccid arm can be lifted easily and the freely moving scapula accompanies it like a shadow. Any imbalance, with the tone around the scapula greater than that around the shoulder joint itself, will produce pain due to trauma if the patient is incorrectly handled.

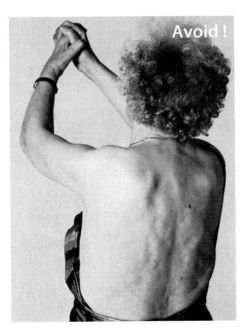

Fig. 12.16. Self-assisted arm activity performed incorrectly (left hemiplegia)

Inadequate External Rotation of the Humerus

The patient's arm fails to rotate externally, due to hypertonicity and shortening of the powerful internal rotators of the shoulder. The greater tuberosity impinges against the coraco-acromial arch during passive movement and causes pain. The patient often experiences pain and tenderness if local pressure is applied to the tuberosity. A common mechanism of rupture of the rotator cuff is a "pinching of the tuberosity cuff ligament insertion zone against the acromion which occurs when the arm is forcibly abducted without concomitant external rotation to clear the tuberosity from the acromion" (Bateman 1963).

Convincing evidence of pain being caused by insufficient external rotation of the arm during elevation, and not because of shoulder subluxation, is presented in **Fig. 12.17**. The patient illustrated in the figure had developed an extremely painful shoulder through a succession of minor injuries. The problem could have been overcome successfully by the therapeutic procedures described in this chapter, but, unfortunately, such therapy was not available to her at the time. Instead, 1 year after the onset of her illness she finally agreed to surgical intervention because the pain in her hemiplegic shoulder had become intolerable and was interfering with her quality of life. On examination, the surgeon whom she consulted noted a "very fixed internal rotation adduction shoulder contracture" (R. Dewar, personal communication).

A left Severs procedure was performed under suitable general anaesthesia, and the operation report states:

The arm was then externally rotated and the fibres of the subscapularis were identified. The fascia overlying this was bluntly retracted and the subscapularis was then divided sharply, without dividing the capsule, approximately 1.5 cm medial to its insertion on the humerus. The pectoralis major was then identified and divided approximately two inches medial to its attachment on the humerus.

The pain was relieved by releasing two muscles whose action is internal rotation and adduction of the shoulder, and possibly because the arm was immobilised postoperatively and injurious movements thus eliminated. One year after the operation the shoulder was pain free despite the fact that the subluxation was still clearly visible (**Fig. 12.17 a**) and an X-ray confirmed a gross subluxation of the hemiplegic shoulder (**Fig. 12.17 b**). Self-assisted arm activity was possible without discomfort, and external rotation of the shoulder was greater than that of the sound side during the movement (**Fig. 12.17 c**). Even when the arm was moved passively into full elevation with external rotation, no pain was elicited (**Fig. 12.17 d**).

Lack of the Downward Gliding Movement of the Head of the Humerus in the Glenoid Fossa

Less commonly, pain is experienced although the scapula is seen to be moving adequately. On palpation, the head of the humerus can be felt to be held tightly beneath the acromion process. Any attempts to abduct the arm will then cause pain, as hypertonicity prevents the normal downward movement of the head of the humerus in the fossa.

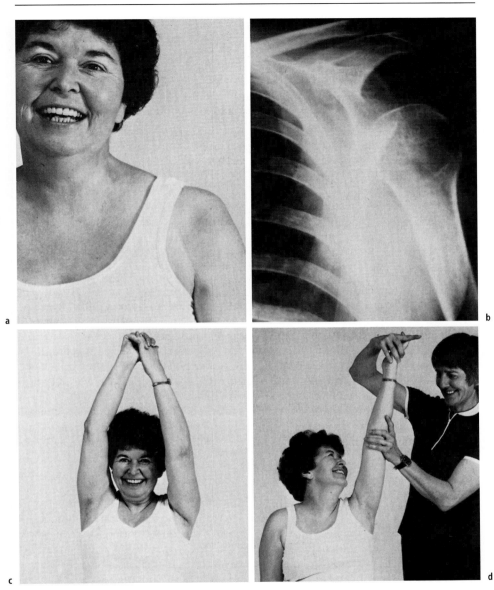

Fig. 12.17. a Patient 1 year after Sever's procedure still has a subluxed shoulder (left hemiplegia). **b** X-ray taken in the same position confirms gross subluxation (courtesy of R. Dewar). **c** Self-assisted arm elevation is pain free. **d** Despite the subluxation, full elevation with external rotation does not cause pain

Activities Which Frequently Cause Painful Trauma

- *Passive range of movement without the scapula being brought into the correct position and the humerus into external rotation.* Soft tissues are compressed if the therapist or nurse lifts the arm incorrectly from its distal end (**Fig. 12.18a**), instead of first mobilising the scapula and supporting the shoulder from below as she should (**Fig. 12.18b**). Once pain has been elicited a vicious circle follows. Pain and fear in-

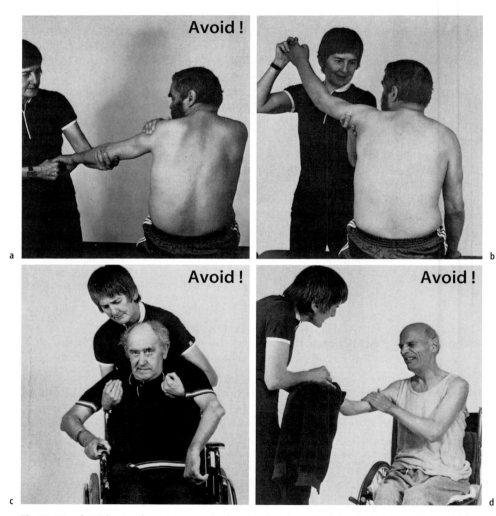

Fig. 12.18a–d. Without adequate support, the shoulder is easily injured during routine activities. **a** When lifting the arm without the scapula rotating. **b** Correct support of the shoulder and scapula rotation renders the movement pain free (left hemiplegia). **c** When lifting the patient back in the wheelchair incorrectly (left hemiplegia). **d** When putting the patient's arm in the sleeve (right hemiplegia)

crease flexor tone in man, and so the patient who has experienced pain during passive movement will have an increase in flexor tone even before the exercise is performed again. The increase in tone in the spastic pattern of flexion fixes the scapula in depression and the arm in internal rotation. Any attempt to force the elevation of the arm will result in increasingly severe trauma.

- *Assisting the patient to transfer from bed to chair by pulling on his arm.* If the nurse or therapist is assisting a patient to transfer and is holding his arm, she is unable to support the heavy trunk and, as the patient moves, the weight of his body forces abduction of the shoulder. The shoulder is easily damaged. The same can occur if the patient is being helped to walk, and assistance is given either by holding his hand and arm or by his affected arm being supported across the helper's shoulders. Any loss of balance or sudden movement immediately causes the arm to be forcibly abducted and the humerus approximates with the acromion.
- *Lifting the patient back into the wheelchair incorrectly.* The helper attempts to correct the patient's posture after he has slipped down in the chair. She stands behind him and, placing her hands under his arms, she attempts to heave him back into the chair (**Fig. 12.18 c**). The unprotected hemiplegic shoulder is forced into abduction by the weight of his body. The same thing may happen if the nurse attempts to lift the patient out of the bath when he is not yet able to assist with the movement actively.
- *Lifting the arm from the hand during nursing activities.* The shoulder is not supported adequately during procedures which involve moving the patient's arm, such as measuring blood pressure, washing the axilla, turning the patient in bed or passive dressing (**Fig. 12.18 d**).
- *Using reciprocal pulleys.* It has often been mistakenly assumed that the patient can maintain full range of motion of the shoulder on his own by working with reciprocal pulleys, because with his affected hand bound onto the handle he can pull his hemiplegic arm repeatedly up into abduction and elevation with his sound hand. On the contrary, in so doing he traumatises his shoulder by attempting to force the inwardly rotated arm upwards, with pain and decreased range of motion as a result. Najenson et al. (1971) and Irwin-Carruthers and Runnalls (1980) describe the resulting injury to the structures around the shoulder during pulley exercises. "Shoulder pulleys do not provide adequate scapular rotation and humeral external rotation and should not be used as a means of passive elevation of the affected arm" (Griffin and Reddin 1981).
- *Practising active arm elevation too vigorously.* The patient who has inadequate control of his scapula repeatedly practises lifting his arm actively, either of his own accord or at the instigation of the therapist (**Fig. 12.19**). With the failure of the scapula to provide a stable origin for the working muscles, their action results in sensitive structures being compressed between the bony surfaces above and below them.

Prevention and Treatment

When the predisposing causes of the painful shoulder are carefully avoided, the condition can be prevented altogether. Particular attention should be given to the patient's position when he is lying in bed or sitting in the chair, and to how he is assisted when he moves. All passive movements of the arm must be preceded by full mobilisation of

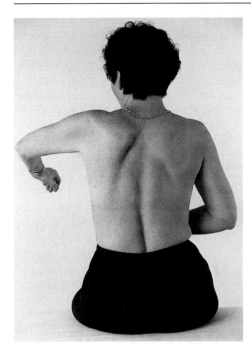

Fig. 12.19. The shoulder can be injured if the patient practises active arm movements repeatedly with insufficient scapula control (left hemiplegia)

the scapula, and then the scapula supported in such a way that the glenoid fossa continues to face upwards and forwards during movements of the arm distally.

Prevention and successful treatment of the painful shoulder are dependent upon all members of the team understanding and avoiding the possible causes. Any position or activity which causes pain must be changed immediately or carried out in such a way that the pain is eliminated. The patient must be instructed to inform the therapist immediately when any movement is hurting him, and she is guided by his feedback and can avoid damaging the sensitive structures. The patient's information about the pain is the only way she knows for certain that tissues are not being damaged, because it is usually impossible for her to feel or see the moment of injury from without. On no account should the therapist consider that a patient is making an unnecessary fuss or believe that he should tolerate a certain amount of pain "for his own good". In this respect, it is important to accept fully, the principle that only the sufferer can assess the severity of pain (Waddell et al. 1993) and that pain perception is uniquely individual and very much dependent upon the condition of different neural structures (Van Cranenburgh 1995).

Overcoming Early Signs of Pain

If a patient who has hitherto been free of pain unexpectedly complains of pain in the shoulder one day, the therapist should work to achieve full range of movement without pain on the same day. She pays special attention to mobilising the scapula and using trunk rotation to inhibit the hypertonicity before moving the arm. The patient should be encouraged to continue with his self-assisted arm exercises, and the therapist checks that he is performing them carefully and correctly without eliciting pain (**Fig. 12.20**).

The encouragement to keep moving the arm is important, because when something is painful most people will tend to hold that part still and, what is more, in flexion. For example, if someone knocks his elbow against the doorframe, he flexes his arm tightly against his body and holds the elbow with his other hand. His whole posture becomes one of flexion. If the patient has pain in his shoulder he holds it, too, in flexion and is loath to move it. Flexor hypertonus increases and fixes the scapula even more strongly in depression and retraction, and the shoulder in internal rotation. If the vicious circle is not interrupted, passive range of movement will almost certainly be more painful on the following day. It is most important to prevent repeated trauma, and particular attention should be paid to the transfers, to how the patient is helped to dress and to how he is being assisted by others when walking. His positioning in bed should be checked and he should lie as much as possible in the corrected position on the hemiplegic side, with his shoulder well forward in protraction.

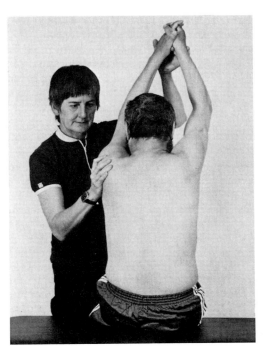

Fig. 12.20. Correcting the patient's self-assisted arm activity (left hemiplegia)

Management of the Severely Painful Shoulder

For a patient who has already developed a stiff, painful shoulder before the correct treatment programme is instituted, the approach is different. When the patient arrives for his first treatment session he will often tell the therapist immediately that his shoulder is very painful, asking her at the same time to please not move his arm. It is most important that she respect his wishes and restrain her immediate impulse to assess exactly how restricted the movement actually is. If she lifts the arm it will certainly hurt him, and the patient/therapist relationship will be off to a bad start. Inevitably, from the time the patient first complained that his shoulder was hurting him, doctors and therapists alike will have moved the arm to assess the range of movement; and each time he will have experienced pain.

■ **Relieving Anxiety.** The therapist should leave the patient's arm completely alone at first, and treat all other aspects of his disability until she has gained his full trust and confidence. To achieve this goal the patient needs to experience success, be it in balance, walking, climbing stairs or some other activity. The time required to win the patient's trust will vary, and for some it may even take weeks, but it will be time well spent. The stiff shoulder did not develop overnight, and another week or two will not be detrimental to the end result.

If the patient is afraid because he anticipates pain, the pain will be produced earlier when the arm is moved. Fear increases tone particularly in the flexor muscle groups; people tend to crouch down when afraid. The patient likewise will have increased tone in the already hypertonic flexor groups, including those which depress and retract the scapula and rotate the humerus medially. The therapist should tell the patient that she will not pull on his arm, and reassure him with conviction that the pain will be completely overcome by their work together. His expectations play a fundamental role in the successful outcome of the treatment, as do the expectations and enthusiasm of the therapist (Wall 1995) The communication is important because expectation of relief reduces anxiety. Reduced anxiety, in turn, reduces muscle tone and sympathetic outflow, and if muscle contraction or sympathetic tone are contributing to the pain the relaxation is most beneficial (Fields 1987).

■ **Positioning in Bed.** The patient with a stiff, painful shoulder has almost invariably been nursed in the supine position. The side-lying positions are essential for freeing the scapula but will need to be introduced gradually. The patient is positioned on the hemiplegic side, with perhaps only a quarter of a turn possible at first. He is asked to lie in that position for 15 minutes, or until he experiences pain, and is then helped to turn again. The time is extended over the next few days, and it is surprising how quickly the full side-lying position can be achieved. Achieving a comfortable position for the patient when he is lying on the sound side often proves more difficult. The hemiplegic arm needs to be very well supported before the shoulder remains pain free. An extra pillow placed right against his chest is usually required to prevent the arm from adducting.

■ **General Activities.** The patient who has a stiff and painful shoulder will also need to improve other movement sequences. For example, he will have difficulty in transferring weight over his hemiplegic side correctly. The therapist works on all the activities described in the previous chapters to improve his balance, gait and movement without effort.

■ **More Specific Activities.** The shoulder is moved without the arm being used as the moving lever. Particularly beneficial are those activities where the scapula and shoulder move from their proximal components, instead of the arm being lifted from the hand distally:

1. The therapist facilitates weight transference toward the hemiplegic side in sitting, emphasising the elongation of that side of the patient's trunk. She sits beside the patient and, with one hand in his axilla, asks him to bring his weight towards her. As he does so, she uses her hand to elevate the shoulder girdle. The movement is repeated rhythmically, and each time the patient attempts to move further over his affected side. The elongation of the side inhibits the hypertonicity which is preventing the scapula from moving freely. The trunk moves against the scapula. The effect is further increased if the patient's hand is placed flat on the plinth beside him, and he takes weight through his extended arm. The therapist maintains the elbow in extension for him.

2. The therapist kneels in front of the seated patient and asks him to lean to touch his feet, letting his hands hang forward. The patient concentrates on not pushing with his feet, and may be able to come only as far as the therapist's knees at first. She facilitates the movement by placing her hands over his scapulae, and by remaining close to him. When the patient can touch his toes, his shoulder will have moved to 90° without the hand having been lifted.

3. The patient, still seated, is helped to clasp his hands together and then to place them on a large ball in front of him. He leans forward, moving the ball away from his knees, and back again. The actual movement is taking place through flexion of the hips, but the shoulder is moving further into elevation at the same time. Because the hands are supported, no pain is elicited, and the patient can control the amount of movement, moving the ball back toward him if the shoulder starts to hurt.

4. Sitting with a table or the plinth in front of him, the patient places his clasped hands on a towel, which he pushes forward as far as he can. The friction-free surface facilitates an easy movement without effort, and once again the shoulder is being moved by the motion of the trunk as the hips flex (**Fig. 12.21**).

5. Rolling from supine over the hemiplegic side inhibits spasticity in the trunk and upper extremity. The therapist uses one of her hands to hold the hemiplegic shoulder well forward in protraction. With her other hand she helps the patient to roll gently and smoothly towards the affected side. The patient starts by rolling only part of the way, and then back again, to avoid hurting his shoulder. As he rolls back the therapist lifts his arm from the bed or plinth so that the fully abducted position is avoided to begin with. The patient continues to roll easily back and forth, while the therapist eases his arm into further elevation. When the activity ceases, the therapist holds his arm upwards in the newly achieved range, and the patient clasps his hands together and carries out self-assisted movements into further elevation.

6. While the patient lies supine with his hemiplegic leg flexed and leaning against the other leg, the therapist facilitates a gentle rocking motion of his pelvis (**Fig. 12.22 a**). The rhythmic rocking rotates the trunk and releases hypertonus in the whole side. The therapist holds the patient's arm in a comfortable degree of elevation with the elbow extended, and as the patient continues to rotate his pelvis she perceives a relaxa-

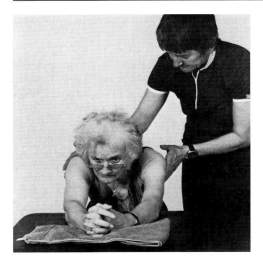

Fig. 12.21. Pushing a towel forwards with clasped hands (left hemiplegia)

tion in the muscles around the shoulder. She eases the arm into further elevation, watching the patient's face carefully as she does so. Should any tension be observed in his facial expression, she immediately brings the arm a little way out of the elevated position.

The therapist's voice is very important during the activity. With a low soothing tone she reduces the amount of effort the patient is using to rotate his pelvis, and also reduces the overall hypertonicity. An amazing amount of elevation can be achieved in this way, as long as the patient is sure that the therapist will not suddenly pull his arm into a painful range of movement.

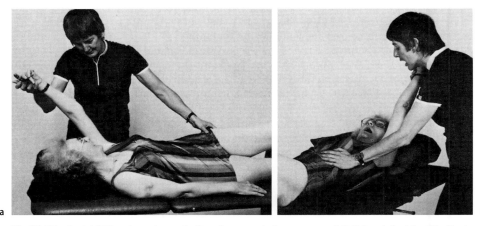

a   b

Fig. 12.22 a, b. Inhibiting hypertonus to free the scapula for movement (left hemiplegia). **a** Rhythmic rotation of the pelvis; **b** assisted expiration

7. With the hemiplegic leg lying flexed and relaxed against the other leg, the therapist assists deep expiration. Placing one hand on the patient's ribs, with her fingers pointing in the direction diagonal to the rib movement, she assists expiration by pressing downwards towards the midline as he breathes out. With her other hand she holds his laterally rotated arm in the maximum amount of painless elevation (**Fig. 12.22 b**). The assisted movement of the ribs moves the thorax against the scapula and shoulder and inhibits the spasticity surrounding them. The arm can be moved easily into further elevation thereafter. Asking the patient to produce clear, sustained vowel sounds as he breathes out not only adds interest but also helps to improve the quality of his voice and breath control at the same time.

■ **Increasing the Range of Passive Movement.** When the patient has sufficient trust in the therapist and the scapula is able to be moved easily, the arm itself can gradually be moved further into passive and, later, active elevation. It is essential that the hemiplegic side be elongated and protracted before the arm movement is attempted. The affected leg must remain flexed and leaning against the other leg, ensuring that the pelvis is forward on that side and that hypertonicity has been sufficiently inhibited in the whole of the affected side. If the leg does not remain relaxed in the inhibitory position, the therapist should on no account move the arm, as she may elicit pain in the shoulder as a result. Instead she repeats the inhibitory movements of the lower trunk and limb until the leg remains in place without being held. The therapist moves the arm carefully forwards and upwards, with the shoulder externally rotated and the elbow extended. If the patient is at all apprehensive he may be asked to move his own arm as far as he can without pain, using his sound hand to do so, with his hands clasped together. In this way, external rotation is assured, and the patient knows that he can stop the movement at any time. He is in charge of the procedure, so to speak.

The therapist then knows at what stage the patient first begins to feel discomfort. She takes over the patient's arm with one hand, maintaining the protraction and external rotation with slight traction. With her other hand she supports the head of the humerus in such a way that her fingers prevent it from impinging against the neighbouring bony prominences (**Fig. 12.23**). Her fingers ensure a normal alignment of the humeral head in the glenoid fossa as she assists its downward gliding to permit further painless elevation.

Goal-orientated movements help the patient to move without fear of pain. Because he is relaxed and concentrating on the activity, there is less flexor spasticity and he can move his arm more freely and fully. He can, for example, push a ball or hit a balloon to a partner, using his clasped hands. Either standing or sitting, he can push a ball to knock over skittles or aim at a given goal or container.

■ **Self-Assisted Arm Activity.** Finally, the patient must learn to move his own shoulder correctly, using his sound hand to move the hemiplegic arm into elevation. When not carefully instructed, many patients try to lift their arm through flexion, and in so doing traumatise their shoulder or give up after the first few painful attempts.

If the patient lifts his arm with the scapula retracted and the elbow flexed, he will reproduce the mechanism of pain (see **Fig. 12.16**) Because the arm is pulling down in flexion and adduction, it is heavy and the patient needs much effort to lift it. The effort further increases the hypertonicity. With the help of the therapist, he learns to push his arms well forward first, to ensure protraction of the scapula. Then with the elbows ex-

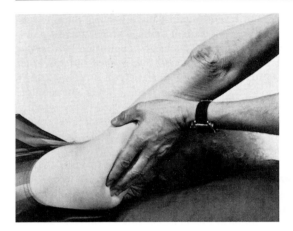

Fig. 12.23. The therapist supports the head of the humerus and facilitates the normal downward gliding movement in the glenoid fossa during elevation of the arm (left hemiplegia)

tended and the palms of the hands together, he brings his arms into as much elevation as possible. At first he may be able to lift them only a few inches from the table in front of him, but quality of movement is more important than quantity if he is to achieve success. The patient is encouraged by all members of the team, by other patients and by his family to repeat the movement correctly many times throughout the day. Once he is able to move his arm successfully himself, and does so on his own, the shoulder rapidly becomes pain free and the problem disappears.

If the programme described is carefully followed, the shoulder pain can be completely eliminated within 2–3 months, and often far sooner. It is interesting to note that the soft tissue structures surrounding the shoulder joint have not actually shortened. Full range of passive movement is rapidly regained once pain has disappeared.

However, from the time when the patient first complains that his shoulder is hurting, and certainly if the symptoms persist despite the treatment and careful handling, it is important to remember that other structures may well be responsible for causing or exacerbating the shoulder problems.

Pathological Conditions in Other Structures

The doctor and the therapist must always consider that the pain and limitation of movement may be the result of conditions other than actual trauma and injury to the shoulder or the structures in its immediate vicinity. In order to discover from where exactly the pain is originating, very careful and informed examination is necessary. Differential diagnosis is important, because failure to establish the real cause of the problems can lead to unsuccessful results of treatment and prolonged suffering for the patient. Not only can pain be referred from elsewhere in the body; other symptoms which closely mimic those associated with the hemiplegia may be present as well.

Sites which could be responsible for apparent shoulder problems include the following:

1. *The cervical spine.* Localised symptoms of pain, limitation of joint movement and muscle weakness may arise from spinal structures although these symptoms may closely resemble the clinical presentation of local disorders. "Conditions as classic as supraspinatus tendinitis and capsulitis frequently have their origin totally or in part in the cervical or uppermost thoracic spine" (Wells 1988). The author explains how a patient with a diagnosis of cervical spondylosis may present, in addition, with weakness of the muscles of the shoulder or arm, neurological deficit from nerve root irritation or compression and a tight, sore shoulder joint. Where cervical pathology exists, soft tissues involved in the structure of the glenohumeral joint may themselves be painful on palpation (Gunn and Milbrandt 1977).

   "A clinical study of conditions of painful limitation of shoulder mobility has shown that ... the limitation of mobility, in some cases, may be due to pathology involving the cervical nerve roots and/or their investing sheaths" (Elvey 1984). The author describes how other signs at the glenohumeral joint may mimic dysfunction of that joint itself when the lesion lies in the cervical spine.

   Even without any history of trauma or pre-stroke neck problems, the hemiplegic patient has predisposing factors which could easily lead to pain being referred from the cervical region. The constant extension of the neck, secondary to the kyphotic posture of the thoracic spine, is particularly common for patients who are still sitting in a wheelchair for most of the day. In addition, the neck is frequently held in lateral flexion with rotation towards the sound side. Each of these components or a combination of the three can cause pain if the posture is sustained for long periods. Older patients are more likely to suffer the effects, and a majority of patients with hemiplegia are over the age of 60.

2. *Adverse tension in the nervous system.* Because any lesion of the nervous system can lead to increased tension within the system as a whole, a patient who has a hemiplegia will invariably have such an abnormal tension with a loss of the adaptive lengthening properties of neural structures (Butler 1991).

   Movements of the shoulder girdle and joints of the upper limb require that neural tissues move, mould and extend in length (Yaxley and Jull 1991). It follows that if neural tissue has relative mobility in the dynamics of the musculoskeletal system then sensitivity of the neural tissue may well cause an impairment of articular mobility, according to Elvey (1988). The author explains how, "A sensitive cervical nerve root could possibly alter the mobility of the glenohumeral joint and shoulder as a whole, thus mimicking a true glenohumeral condition." Shoulder pain and apparent limitation may in some instances be misdiagnosed because of the area in which the pain is perceived (Elvey 1986).

3. *Abnormal rib postures and articulations.* Elevation or depression of the first rib can lead to compression or traction of the brachial plexus and cervical nerve roots and cause pain in the region of the glenohumeral joint. In hemiplegia, when the hypertonic arm moves actively, the shoulder girdle is lifted upward together with the first rib, while the passive weight of a paralysed hypotonic arm tends to drag both downwards (Rolf 1999).

   Pain in the region of the glenohumeral joint, consistent with shoulder impingement syndrome and/or partial rotator cuff tear, may be due to sprain of the second rib spinal articulation or chronic subluxation of the second rib at its vertebral articulations. With extension of a stiff upper thoracic spine the rib may be subluxed superiorly on the fixed thoracic segment, and the resultant pain and dysfunction are consistent with a false shoulder impingement. In addition, the muscles of the rotator cuff may test weak (Boyle 1999). The author describes how two patients originally diagnosed as having a shoulder impingement syndrome were completely relieved of their symptoms after treatment directed solely to the second rib. Both patients were treated with oscillatory mobilisation of the rib in a posterior-anterior direction, as described by Maitland (1986).

Additional Treatment Possibilities

There are several additional possibilities for managing the severely painful shoulder:

1. *Injection of a Local Anaesthetic With or Without a Cortisone Preparation.* Injecting the exquisitely painful shoulder may provide temporary relief for the patient, but it is clear that if the underlying cause of the pain is not corrected, the relief will be short-lived. The anaesthetic effect is undesirable when administered before attempts at passive range of movement because it robs the patient of an important protective mechanism (Diethelm and Davies 1985). As already mentioned, the only way in which the therapist can know whether she is causing trauma is by the patient informing her when something hurts. Relief of pain with improved range of motion was obtained in some cases following subacromial injection of 1 % lidocaine (Joynt 1992)

2. *The Use of Ice.* Ice has been described as a means to relieve pain and reduce spasticity (Palastanga 1988) It should be applied with wet iced towels around the whole scapula and shoulder, because melting ice cools more effectively than cold applied in other ways (McMaster et al. 1978). The time and effort involved usually do not warrant its use, because the measures described will ensure a rapid and more lasting result.

3. *Passive Mobilisation.* Some of the techniques of passive mobilisation of the shoulder as described by Maitland (1973, 1991) can be useful in gaining relief of pain and range of movement, if used in addition to the total regime. The techniques are particularly useful for the following:
   - Where pain, rather than stiffness, is the predominant feature. Passive accessory movements, i.e. those joint movements which a person cannot perform actively and selectively on his own, are the most beneficial in the treatment of pain. Irwin-Carruthers and Runnalls (1980) describe their experiences using a combined treatment of inhibition followed by mobilisation with carefully graded passive accessory movements to the shoulder joint.
   - Where pain is experienced only at the end of the full range of movement, probably because the head of the humerus fails to move downwards in the glenoid fossa.
   - Where pain is no longer present but final elevation appears to be mechanically blocked at the end of range. Once again, the head of the humerus is probably failing to glide downwards to allow the full movement.
   - Certainly where the pain is due to pathological states in the cervical spine or rib articulations, passive mobilisation of the relevant joints will be the treatment required.
   - When increased tension in the nervous system is responsible for pain and limitation of movement, the mobilisation procedures to reduce tension described in Chap. 15 are essential. In fact, whatever the actual cause of the pain may have been initially, there will invariably be a significant increase in neural tension, so that nervous system mobilisation should always be included in the treatment.

Conclusion

The therapist must remain open-minded, be on the lookout for new ideas and be prepared to seek help from therapists specialised in other treatment fields if necessary. Lack of success may otherwise result in her blaming the patient for not responding to the treatment or for not exercising enough on his own. Much depends on the patient being convinced that the pain can and will be overcome and that he must report accurately at once if he feels pain during treatment or nursing procedures. The physician must also be fully aware of all the causes, because he may otherwise inadvertently traumatise the shoulder during his repeated examinations. Avoiding repetition of the minor injuries to the shoulder joint and the soft tissues is the key to overcoming the problem of pain. The limitation of range of motion is directly related to the pain and mobility returns when pain disappears. It is therefore far better not to move the shoulder at all than to move it and cause pain.

The "Shoulder-Hand" Syndrome

The sudden development of a swollen, painful hand as a secondary complication following hemiplegia is a very disturbing and disabling condition. According to Davis et al. (1977), it affects about 12.5% of the patients and occurs most commonly between the 1st and 3rd months following onset of stroke. An even higher rate of 27% was reported by Braus (1990). The extremely painful condition interferes with the patient's overall rehabilitation, but even more seriously, if untreated leads to a permanent and irreversible, fixed deformity of the hand and fingers which precludes functional use in the future. In addition to the term SHS, many names are currently used to describe the condition, the most common being reflex sympathetic dystrophy or reflex dystrophy syndrome, algodystrophy, causalgia and Sudeck's atrophy or syndrome.

These different terms have only added to the confusion surrounding its cause and led to a rather negative attitude with regard to its prevention and treatment. The distressing condition is preventable in all but a few instances, however, and the problems can be overcome should symptoms develop.

It is important to understand the cause of the condition, because only then can appropriate preventative measures be adopted or treatment of the established condition be successful. The first step is to consider the symptoms occurring in the hand as being separate from those of the painful shoulder.

A Hand Syndrome (HS), not a Shoulder-Hand Syndrome (SHS)

If, as has been reported, between 60% and 80% of patients suffer from a painful shoulder, it becomes statistically probable that the 12%–30% who develop a swollen hand would, more often than not, have shoulder pain in addition. The reasons for the shoulder pain and limitation are those explained earlier in the chapter, and indeed, autopsy examination of the shoulder capsules of some patients diagnosed as having had a shoulder-hand syndrome showed signs of previous trauma to the affected shoulder (Braus et al. 1994).

Once it is accepted that the pain in the shoulder is the result of the mechanical factors which have been described, and is not part of a combined syndrome, effective prevention and treatment of the problems in the wrist, hand and fingers becomes possible. It is also easier to explain the findings of Moskowitz et al. (1958) when using stellate ganglion blocks and high thoracic sympathectomy in the treatment of the syndrome. The hand symptoms were relieved, but, as the authors noted, "Symptoms referable to the shoulder, including pain and limitation of motion, were not favourably affected by either the blocks or the sympathectomy." Davis et al. (1977) describe their successful treatment of 68 patients using oral steroids in addition to their rehabilitation programme and mention that: "Two patients not included in this study had signs and symptoms only in the hand and were treated successfully using the same methods . . .". If the patient's shoulder has been carefully protected and moved in the ways described earlier in the chapter, the shoulder movement remains full and painless despite the pronounced hand symptoms (**Fig. 12.24 a, b**).

The fact that the elbow is pain free and has no limitation of movement further supports the case for the shoulder and hand problems being considered separately. If the same syndrome were indeed responsible for the pain in both, it would be logical for the elbow to be involved as well, situated as it is between the two. In the literature postulating a shoulder-hand syndrome, however, no explanation is offered for the sparing of the intermediate joint.

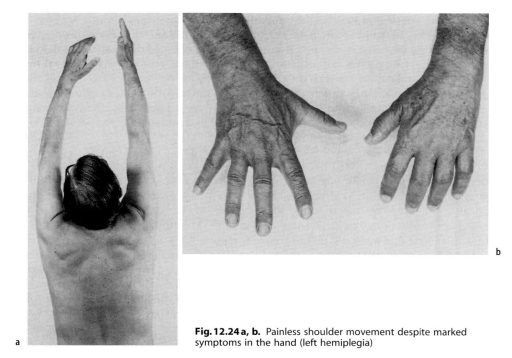

b

a

Fig. 12.24 a, b. Painless shoulder movement despite marked symptoms in the hand (left hemiplegia)

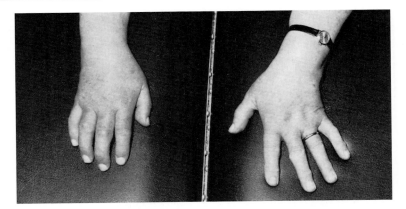

Fig. 12.25. Typical appearance of the swollen hand (right hemiplegia)

Symptoms Arising in the Hand

Early Stage

The patient's hand quite suddenly becomes swollen, and a marked loss of range of movement occurs rapidly. The oedema is predominantly apparent on the dorsum of the hand, including the metacarpophalangeal joints, and also the fingers and thumb. The skin loses its creases, particularly over the knuckles and the proximal and distal interphalangeal joints. The oedema is soft and puffy and usually ends just proximal to the wrist joint (**Fig. 12.25**). The tendons of the hand are no longer visible. The colour of the hand changes, having a pink or lilac hue, particularly noticeable if the arm is left hanging down at the patient's side. The hand feels warm and sometimes moist. The nails start to undergo changes and appear whiter or more opaque than those of the other hand.

Limitation of range of movement is noted as follows:

- Loss of passive supination with pain usually felt at the wrist (**Fig. 12.26 a**).
- Dorsal extension of the wrist is limited and pain is experienced on the dorsal aspect when an attempt is made to move passively into an increased range. The pain is also elicited during weightbearing activities in therapy, when the arm is extended and the hand supported flat on the plinth.
- There is marked loss of flexion of the metacarpophalangeal joints, with no bony prominences visible (**Fig. 12.26 b**).
- Abduction of the fingers is very restricted. For example, the patient has increasing difficulty in clasping his hands together. The fingers of the sound hand appear to be too large to fit into the spaces between the fingers of the other hand.
- The proximal interphalangeal joints are stiff and enlarged. Very little flexion is possible, and there is a loss of full extension as well. Pain is experienced when attempts are made to flex the joints passively.

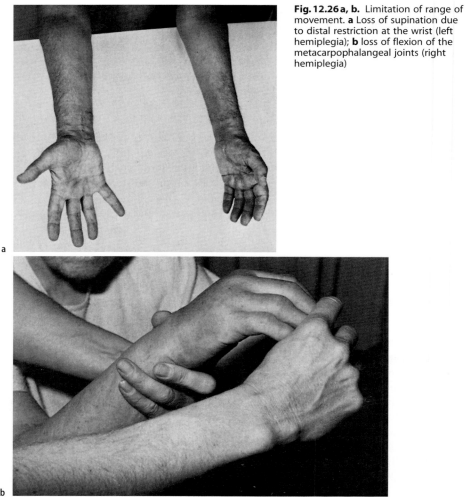

Fig. 12.26 a, b. Limitation of range of movement. **a** Loss of supination due to distal restriction at the wrist (left hemiplegia); **b** loss of flexion of the metacarpophalangeal joints (right hemiplegia)

a

b

- The distal interphalangeal joints are extended, and little or no flexion is possible. Even if these joints have stiffened in slight flexion, any attempt at passive flexion is painful and limited.

Later Stages

If the hand is not treated correctly during the early stages, the symptoms become more marked. Pain increases until the patient cannot tolerate any pressure being applied to his hand or fingers at all. A marked hard prominence appears centrally on the dorsal aspect of the intercarpal area and its junction with the metacarpals. Typical osteoporotic changes may be revealed through radiological examination, but these are not always related to the syndrome. X-rays of the hands of patients who have none of the other symptoms are rarely taken, but similar changes have been observed when the procedure was undertaken.

Final or Residual Stage

The untreated hand becomes fixed in a typical deformity. The oedema disappears completely, as does the pain, but the mobility is permanently lost.

- The wrist is flexed with ulnar deviation, and dorsal flexion is limited. The prominence over the carpal bones is solid and more obvious without the oedema (**Fig. 12.27 a**).
- Supination of the forearm is severely limited (**Fig. 12.27 b**).
- The palm of the hand is flat, with a marked atrophy of the thenar and hypothenar muscle groups.
- No flexion of the metacarpophalangeal joints is possible, and the amount of abduction is negligible (**Fig. 12.27 c**). The web space between thumb and index finger is reduced and inelastic.
- The proximal and distal interphalangeal joints are fixed in a slightly flexed position but permit no additional flexion.

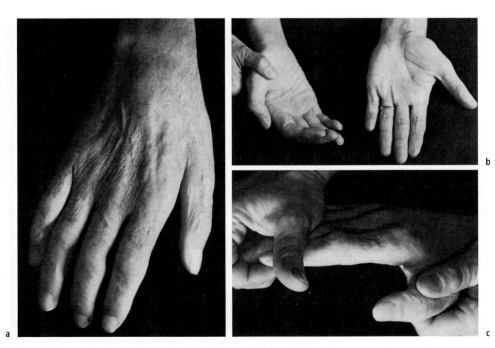

Fig. 12.27 a–c. Final or residual stage (right hemiplegia). **a** Oedema disappears; the prominence over the carpal area is solid; there is flexion of the wrist with ulnar deviation and the fingers have stiffened. **b** Gross limitation of supination. **c** No flexion of the metacarpophalangeal joints

"The oedema, containing protein, converts into a diffuse cobweb-like scar tissue that adheres to the tendons and joint capsules and prevents further movement. The joints undergo disuse atrophy of the cartilage with thickening of the capsule" (Cailliet 1980). The fibrin contained in the inflammatory exudate becomes organised into scar tissue, and in synovial joints the end result is a thickened, contracted joint capsule (Evans 1980).

Without adequate treatment to prevent the final, atrophic stage, ankylosis of the joints, particularly those of the fingers, occurs (Wilson 1989). During surgery on a hand in this stage at King's College Hospital, London, it was discovered that the ligaments of the interphalangeal joints had actually ossified, and laboratory examination revealed true bone formation.

It is therefore imperative that the swollen hand be treated in the early stages so that the final stage can be prevented at all costs. The avoidance of fixed deformities is particularly significant with regard to possible return of functional activity, because clinical observations have indicated that many patients suffering from the condition later regain selective voluntary movements in the hand and fingers (**Fig. 12.28 a, b**). Davis and co-workers (1977) support these observations, because 70.5 % of their patients had only "partial motor loss".

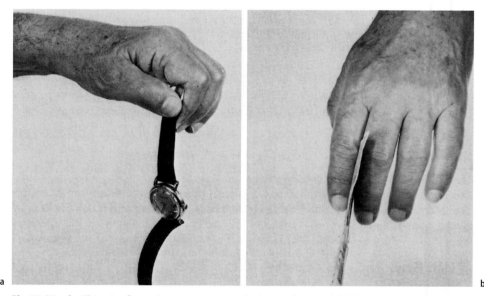

a   b

Fig. 12.28 a, b. There is often voluntary movement in the swollen hand (left hemiplegia). **a** Pinch grip; **b** selective adduction of the fingers

Causes of the Hand Syndrome in Hemiplegia

Although much has been written about the shoulder-hand syndrome in hemiplegia, very little has been convincingly postulated or proved as to its actual cause. The condition is certainly not due to a personality disorder or to the patient having a low pain tolerance, although assertions have been made about "psychological predisposition" or "causalgic personality" (Wilson 1989). Attaching a psychological cause to the problems can be most degrading for the patient and have a negative influence on the attitude of the staff towards him. Any psychological disturbances which the patient may exhibit are secondary, due to the constant pain he is experiencing. As Charlton (1991) explains, "These are the same reactive changes that may occur with any pain patient and may include anxiety, depression and hopelessness". When pain disappears with informed treatment, so do any supposed psychological disorders, and the patient's raised morale and enthusiastic co-operation are a pleasure for all who work with him.

It would be an oversimplification to attach sole blame for the swollen painful condition of the hand to the loss of motor activity or the dependent position of the arm. Were this to be the case, many more patients would then manifest this relatively infrequent complication. After remission of the symptoms following treatment, patients may continue to have a complete loss of motor activity and a dependent arm position but show no recurrence of their original symptoms of pain and oedema.

Something specific must occur which triggers off the syndrome, and such symptoms are only then perpetuated by the inactivity and the dependent position of the arm. The sudden onset of symptoms experienced by many patients who previously had no pain or limitation of movement supports this supposition. A logical hypothesis is that a mechanical happening causes a primary oedema or an oedema secondary to tissue or nerve injury with inflammation, an oedema which the inadequate muscle pump fails to resolve. A vicious cycle of oedema, pain, loss of range of movement and sympathetic nervous system involvement follows. Various causes of oedema in the hand can precipitate the development of the hand syndrome:

Sustained Plantar Flexion of the Wrist Under Pressure

The patient lies in bed or sits in his wheelchair for long periods with his arm at his side and the wrist, unnoticed, in a position of forced plantar flexion (Fig. 12.29 a, b). The plantar flexion is extreme because the antagonist muscles are hypotonic and because there is more than just the passive weight of the arm pressing on the wrist from above. Hypertonicity in the muscles which retract and depress the shoulder girdle and in those which adduct and inwardly rotate the arm add significantly to the pressure on the unprotected wrist. The effect is more pronounced when the patient is sitting in his wheelchair, as his whole body weight typically leans towards the affected side.

Venous drainage of the hand is severely compromised by forced plantar flexion of the wrist. The X-rays of a normal hand and wrist illustrate how one of the large veins is actually blocked altogether in the flexed position when a downward force is exerted by the arm. For the experiment, a contrast medium was injected into the vein distally on the dorsum of the hand. With the wrist in a neutral position the contrast medium was seen to flow freely (Fig. 12.30 a). The subject then flexed her wrist, with the metacarpal

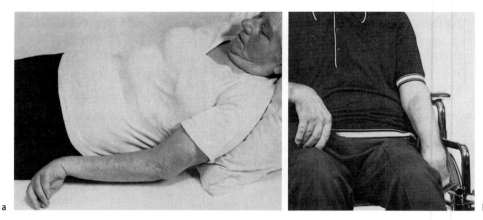

Fig. 12.29 a, b. Commonly observed positions of forced flexion of the wrist (left hemiplegia). **a** In bed; **b** in the wheelchair

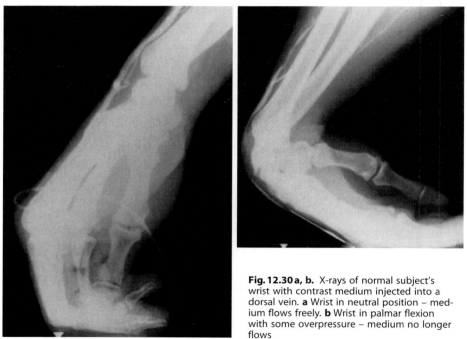

Fig. 12.30 a, b. X-rays of normal subject's wrist with contrast medium injected into a dorsal vein. **a** Wrist in neutral position – medium flows freely. **b** Wrist in palmar flexion with some overpressure – medium no longer flows

heads pressing down on the table. She exerted additional pressure by depressing her shoulder and tensing the adductors of the arm, imitating the spastic components. The flow of the contrast medium was seen to be interrupted (**Fig. 12.30 b**). Interestingly, she experienced pain on dorsal extension of the wrist after the pressure was released.

The results of the small experiment become particularly significant when the following points are considered in relation to the development of the shoulder-hand syndrome in hemiplegia.

- In the majority of cases the syndrome develops between the 1st and the 3rd month after onset of the hemiplegia. Davis et al. (1977) show a figure of 66% for that period. The patient has therefore reached the stage where he is no longer being so intensively nursed and observed as he was during the first weeks. A few hours may pass before his position in bed or sitting in the wheelchair is adjusted, or some nursing procedure needs to be carried out. The patient's hand may therefore remain for a considerable time, undetected, in a position of relatively forced flexion.
- The tone in the arm is still relatively low, even though some hypertonus may already be present in the wrist flexors and the flexor pattern at the shoulder. The wrist extensors, however, are almost certainly still hypotonic and provide no protective resistance to the wrist flexion.
- Many patients demonstrate neglect of their affected arm in the early stage of the illness and do not notice when it adopts an awkward position. Added to the neglect there can be an actual loss or disturbance of sensation: 91% of the patients examined by Davis et al. (1977) are reported as having either moderate or severe sensory loss.
- Most of the venous lymphatic drainage of the hand is located in its dorsal aspect (Cailliet 1980). The oedema is predominantly on the dorsum of the patient's hand in the early stages of the syndrome.
- The oedema is localised and usually ends just proximal to the wrist joint.
- Throughout the day and night, the patient's wrist is almost exclusively in some degree of flexion, particularly if he is not carefully positioned and supervised. The flexion is even more pronounced if he wears some form of sling, or when he is sitting with his hand in his lap.

Clinical observation has shown palmar flexion of the wrist joint interfering with venous drainage to be the most common primary cause of the hand syndrome in hemiplegia.

Overstretching of the Joints of the Hand May Produce an Inflammatory Reaction, with Oedema and Pain

The amount of movement possible in the numerous joints of the hand varies considerably from person to person. The therapist may unwittingly force the patient's hand into a range which is for him excessive, and thus traumatise the joints or structures surrounding them.

Dorsal extension of the wrist beyond its mechanical range can easily occur, for example, when the patient is being encouraged to take weight through his extended arm. The hand is placed beside him on the plinth, and the therapist holds his elbow in extension. The patient is then asked to transfer his weight to that side as far as possible. The movement of his body sideways moves the wrist into more dorsiflexion, and if this is performed in a very enthusiastic or uncontrolled way, dorsiflexion could be forced beyond

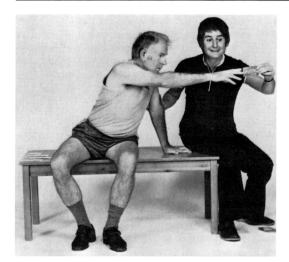

Fig. 12.31. Forced dorsiflexion of the wrist while the patient is concentrating on a task (left hemiplegia)

its normal range. If passive movements are performed too vigorously the same may take place.

A similar event may occur during occupational therapy, where the patient is carrying out tasks with his sound hand while attempting to support himself on the affected arm. While concentrating on performing the task successfully he may not notice that dorsiflexion of the wrist is being forced (**Fig. 12.31**).

Excessive dorsal flexion of the wrist is also a danger during all activities where the patient's weight is taken through his extended arm while he is in prone-kneeling, standing or sitting. If the patient is asked to practise flexing and extending his elbow while weightbearing, the wrist may inadvertently be forced too far into dorsiflexion. When exercising on the mat, particular care needs to be taken, because the degree of dorsal flexion increases as the soft surface sinks down beneath the patient's weight, causing the ball of the hand to descend further than his fingers.

Patients whose oedema is triggered off in one of these ways are often those who experience a later onset of the syndrome, or who are more active in the early stages of their illness. A typical example is the patient who has little involvement in the lower limb and can walk and exercise at a level far in advance of his upper-extremity function.

Fluid from an Infusion Escapes into the Tissues of the Hand

It is common practice to use the veins of the hemiplegic hand when repeated infusions are required, most doctors being loath to use the sound hand because the patient might then be unable to help himself at all in bed. However, if the infusion fluid leaks into the surrounding tissues, as it frequently does, a marked oedema follows.

Minor Accidents to the Hand

The patient may suffer small injuries to his hand, particularly in the presence of sensory loss or inattention. He may sustain a fall towards the hemiplegic side and compromise his hand. He may burn the hand through inadvertent contact with a hot plate, a cigarette or a hot-water bottle. The hand may be caught in the wheel of his chair, and he pushes the chair forwards without noticing what has happened. As a result of such injuries, the hand becomes oedematous.

Prevention and Treatment

Prevention

Prevention of the hand syndrome aims at avoiding all the causes of oedema in the hand. The patient is carefully positioned when in bed and when sitting in a chair, as described in Chap. 5. If he is not yet able to ensure that his wrist does not lie in full flexion or that his arm does not hang over the side of the wheelchair, a wheelchair table can prevent the danger until he has progressed sufficiently to look after his arm himself (**Fig. 12.32**).

Great care must be taken when activities which entail weightbearing through the hemiplegic arm are being practised. The therapist should help the patient to control the movement when necessary. Before such activities or any form of passive movement are undertaken, the therapist carefully establishes the patient's individual range of movement by comparing it with that of the sound side. Should the patient complain of discomfort or pain during therapy, the therapist should change the position of the hand. For example, more outward rotation of the arm at the patient's side while he is sitting will reduce the amount of dorsiflexion required, as he moves his body sideways to take weight through the extended arm. If the pain is still produced, the activity should be discontinued.

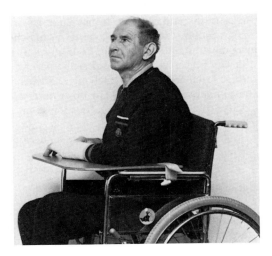

Fig. 12.32. A wheelchair table. The patient is wearing a wrist splint to support his swollen hand (left hemiplegia)

Every effort should be made to avoid using the veins of the hemiplegic hand as sites for infusions. One of the subclavicular veins may provide a satisfactory alternative and will not prevent the patient from using his sound hand.

A hot-water bottle should never be used.

All in the team, as well as the patient's relatives, can help to avoid minor injuries to the hand if they are fully informed about the risk factors. The patient's ability to take care of his own hand may easily be overestimated, especially if he has good motor activity or if he can talk well. By carefully following the criteria described above, Braus et al. (1994) were able to reduce the frequency of shoulder-hand syndrome from 27% (36/132) to 8% (6/86) in a clinically comparable series of patients.

Treatment of the Established Syndrome

The best results are achieved if the treatment is started in the early stages of the condition, as soon as the oedema, pain or loss of range of movement is observed. The treatment can also be effective, however, even after a few months, if the hand is still inflamed and if there are acute pain and oedema. Once consolidation has occurred and the hand has returned to its normal size and colour, little if anything can be done to overcome the fixed contractures. The main aim of treatment must clearly be to reduce the oedema as quickly as possible, and hence the pain and stiffness. "As disuse and loss of normal function appear to play an important role in the genesis of the clinical problem, it follows that resumption of activity is essential to sustain relief and promote ultimate resolution" (Charlton 1991). The condition of the hand must be regarded as acute and inflammatory, for which the classic trio – cooling, compression and elevation to reduce oedema – is advocated. Evans (1980) sums up the essential features of treatment for inflammatory oedema by adding an M, for gentle muscular movements, to the I for ice, C for compression and E for elevation, to form the mnemonic abbreviation "MICE".

■ **Positioning.** In bed, the positions described in Chap. 5 are continued to prevent the shoulder from becoming involved. When the patient is sitting, his arm is positioned forward on a table in elevation at all times. A pillow can be placed beneath the arm for added elevation and comfort. It may be necessary to use a wheelchair table when the patient is moving around the hospital in his chair, or to ensure that the hand does not hang down unnoticed (see **Fig. 12.32**).

It has been recommended that the patient's arm be mechanically suspended above cardiac level, both when he is lying and when he is sitting, but unfortunately such suspension is contraindicated. The downward pull of the scapula against the abducted or elevated arm inevitably traumatises the shoulder, with severe pain as a result.

■ **Avoiding Flexion of the Wrist.** Maintenance of dorsal flexion 24 hours a day is most important, to facilitate venous drainage and to prevent the sustained extension of the metacarpophalangeal joints which occurs mechanically if the hand lies in the patient's lap and even when it is supported on a table or lies flat on the bed (**Fig. 12.33**).

A small cock-up wrist splint to hold the wrist in the corrected position is advocated, in addition to careful positioning and supervision, The splint is made to fit each patient individually, out of plaster of Paris, using approximately ten layers of an 8-cm plaster bandage.

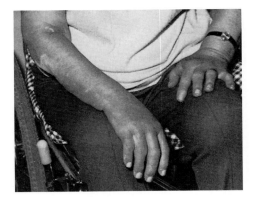

Fig. 12.33. Sustained extension of the meta-carpophalangeal joints (right hemiplegia)

While the splint is being made, the patient sits at a table with his arm supported forwards. An assistant stands next to him, keeping his shoulder forward and supporting the wrist in a comfortable amount of dorsal flexion. The therapist stands in front of the patient and positions the wet bandage carefully in place (**Fig. 12.34a**). It is essential that the distal end of the splint, when dry, does not restrict the flexion of the metacarpophalangeal joints. It should therefore not extend further than the distal crease in the palm of the hand, and should slope appropriately downwards from the first to the fifth joint. The thumb is left free (**Fig. 12.34b**). The assistant smooths the forearm portion of the plaster into place while the therapist concentrates on moulding the hand correctly. She folds the plaster back into the desired line below the metacarpophalangeal joints and then uses her thumbs to press into the palm of the patient's hand to ensure its rounded form. Her fingers on the dorsum of his hand give counterpressure to hold the wrist in dorsal flexion, in a slightly radial direction.

When the splint is dry it is bandaged in place with a small, slightly elastic bandage (**Fig. 12.34c**). The bandage is rolled on, rather than pulled tightly, because the pressure would otherwise be too painful for the patient to tolerate. Care must be taken that the wrist is correctly positioned in the splint and fixed in place. Even a few degrees of wrist flexion will push the splint distally and restrict the flexion of the metacarpophalangeal joints. The dorsum of the hand is well covered by the bandage, which starts over the knuckles and continues to the proximal end of the splint. The patient wears the splint both night and day, and it is removed only for skin checks, for washing and during therapy. Extension of the wrist is ensured at all times, no matter where he rests his hand (**Fig. 12.34d**).

The splint is worn continuously until the oedema and pain have disappeared and the colour of the hand is normal. Even while wearing the splint the patient is able to carry out the self-assisted activities which maintain full range of shoulder movement.

Where particular risk factors exist, such as large numbers of patients in acute hospital settings, older patients with severe lesions or left-sided hemiplegia with multimodal neglect, the prophylactic use of wrist splints to prevent palmar flexion and protect the vulnerable hand has been recommended (M. Brune 1998, personal communication; E. Panturin 1997, personal communication).

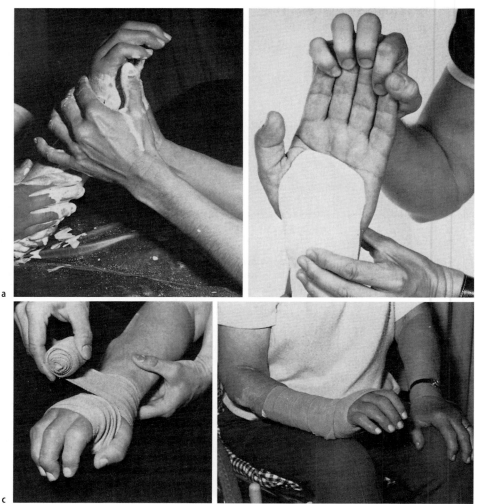

Fig. 12.34 a–d. A splint to support the wrist. **a** Placing the wet plaster of Paris bandage; **b** correct position of the splint; **c** bandaging in position; **d** flexion of the wrist prevented

■ **Compressive Centripetal Wrapping.** "Centripetal wrapping of digits or extremities has proved to be a simple, safe and dramatically effective treatment for reducing peripheral edema and its deleterious concomitants" (Cain and Liebgold 1967). Using a length of string about 12 mm in diameter, the therapist wraps the thumb and then each finger from distal to proximal. She then proceeds to wrap the hand, and continues to just above the wrist joint. Wrapping commences with a small loop made in the region of the fingernail in such a way that it does not press on the sensitive cuticle (**Fig. 12.35 a**).

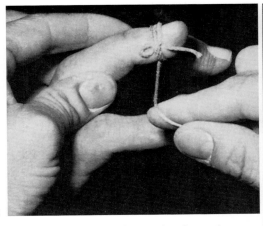
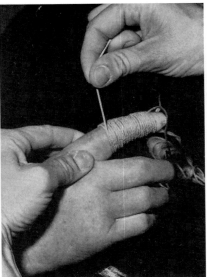

Fig. 12.35 a, b. Compressive centripetal wrapping. **a** Commencing with a small loop facilitates quick removal of the string. **b** Each finger wrapped individually from distal to proximal with no gaps between the rings of string

The therapist then wraps the finger firmly and rapidly until she reaches the hand and can go no further (**Fig. 12.35 b**). She immediately removes the string by pulling on the free end of the loop.

When each finger and the thumb have been individually wrapped, the therapist proceeds to the hand itself. Once again she commences with a small loop and wraps the string over the metacarpophalangeal joints and proceeds proximally. On reaching the base of the thumb she adducts the thumb, so that its proximal joints are included in the wrapping. The last stage in the procedure includes the wrist joint, and the therapist starts wrapping there from where she last covered the area of the hand.

The patient's relatives can soon be taught to carry out the procedure to save valuable time during therapy. The results are most gratifying and can be dramatic. "The amount of benefit has ranged from uncovering of trace motion in an apparently completely paralysed hand, to complete and lasting normal function in a hand previously swollen, painful and incapacitated" (Cain and Liebgold 1967). Certainly, the circulation is immediately improved by the reduction of the oedema, the patient feels his hand more clearly and other forms of therapy can proceed more effectively.

Fears that the wrapping could damage the soft tissues and lymph vessels have proved to be unfounded. During the past 30 years, countless patients with a painful, swollen hand have been treated successfully with centripetal wrapping in California, in the UK and in numerous centres in Europe with no evidence of such damage occurring. On the contrary, all have benefited from a dramatic reduction of their symptoms, and many have regained functional use of their hemiplegic hand with no recurrence of the original problems.

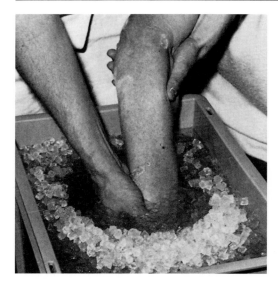

Fig. 12.36. Immersing the hand in a mixture of crushed ice and water

■ **Ice.** When crushed ice is available, the therapist immerses the patient's hand in a bucket containing a mixture of ice and water. The mixture consists ideally of approximately one-third water and two-thirds ice, so that the hand can be introduced easily, and additional cold is produced by the melting ice (**Fig. 12.36**). Empirically, the therapist should dip the patient's hand three times into the ice, with a brief pause between immersions. The sensation experienced by her own hand will guide her as to how long the cold can be tolerated.

■ **Active Movements.** Movements performed during therapy should be active whenever possible, rather than passive. Whatever active muscle function the patient has should be incorporated, even if the hand itself still has no active movement, because muscle contraction provides the best pumping action to reduce the oedema.

For example, even if the patient's arm appears to be completely paralysed, it is usually possible to stimulate some activity in the elbow extensors with the patient lying supine and his arm held in elevation (**Fig. 12.37**). Activities carried out with the arm in elevation after mobilisation of the scapula are beneficial, because the elevation in combination with muscle contractions reduces the oedema considerably.

In sitting, any activity which stimulates or facilitates voluntary movements in the hemiplegic arm can be used, particularly activities where grasping an object with flexion of the fingers is required.

● The patient grasps one end of a folded towel in his hemiplegic hand and the therapist holds the other end. The towel is rolled sufficiently so that he is able to hold it firmly despite the limitation of flexion in his fingers joints. The therapist swings the towel in different directions and the patient follows her movements lightly without releasing his grip (**Fig. 12.38**).

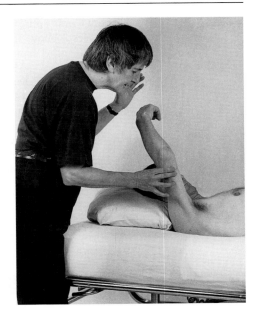

Fig. 12.37. Some active elbow extension is usually possible in supine with the arm in elevation (right hemiplegia)

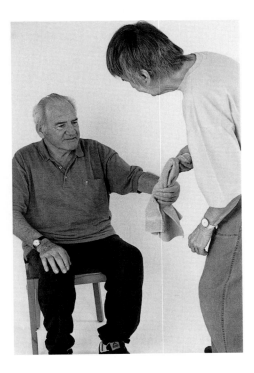

Fig. 12.38. Holding on to a rolled towel which the therapist moves freely in different directions

- The patient clasps a wooden pole approximately 2 cm in diameter in both hands. He releases one hand and places it above the other hand, holding the pole steady with his other. He then releases the other hand and takes another step upwards with it before clasping the pole again.
- Grasping and releasing a thick towel has proved to be most successful for reducing swelling and regaining passive range of movement as well as voluntary control in the hand. The towel lies flat on a table beneath the patient's hand, and he tries to pull it towards him by flexing his fingers (**Fig. 12.39 a**). The therapist helps him to keep his wrist in place as he grasps and regrasps the towel to draw it together in folds underneath his hand. The patient then lets his fingers extend again so that the towel is returned to its original position, either with active extension or by relaxing the

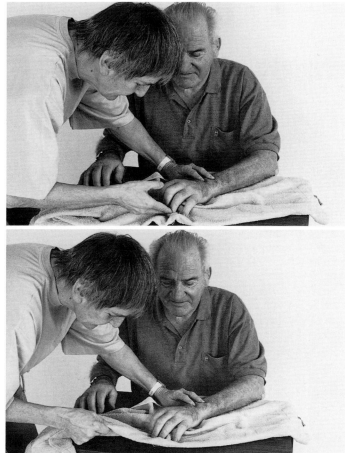

a

b

Fig. 12.39 a, b. Activating a muscle-pumping action of the hand by crumpling a towel. **a** Flexion of the fingers to crumple the towel under the hand. **b** Assisted extension of the fingers as the towel straightens out again

flexors as the therapist eases the towel away (**Fig. 12.39 b**). The patient enjoys the simple exercise, and his relatives can assist him to perform it successfully at other times during the day. Once he can flex his fingers actively without flexing his wrist, he can be encouraged to practise the activity on his own.

WARNING: Activities or exercises which entail weightbearing through the hand with the wrist dorsiflexed and the elbow extended should not be practised until all signs of pain and oedema have been eliminated. They may have been the precipitating cause of the syndrome and in any case will often cause pain and perpetuate the condition. In fact, any activity or position which elicits pain should be assiduously avoided. The same applies when passive movements are being performed by the therapist.

■ **Passive Movements.** Careful passive range of movement prevents the shoulder from becoming painful, and passive movements to the hand and fingers should be eliminated or performed very gently indeed, so as not to produce any pain. The therapist should never try to flex the fingers with the wrist in palmar flexion, because with the oedema elevating the extensor tendons on the dorsum of the hand the movement is mechanically blocked. Use of any degree of force would lead to a flare-up of the inflammatory condition. The loss of supination which accompanies the problems in the wrist and carpal area should not be forgotten. The therapist includes the component in the therapy by easing the forearm into as full a range of supination as is possible without pain, assisted actively by the patient. All the movements are carried out with the arm in elevation to improve venous drainage, the patient lying supine or with his arm supported on a table in front of him.

Because therapists so dread the development of contractures, they tend to be too vigorous when treating the swollen hand. In this condition, too little rather than too much is infinitely preferable.

Tempting as their use may seem, passive mobilisation techniques are also contraindicated until all signs of inflammation have disappeared, because they, too, would lead to an exacerbation of the acute condition. When the oedema resolves and the pain decreases, active range of movement is soon restored.

■ **Mobilising the Nervous System.** Despite diverse precipitating factors, the common denominator in conditions due to sympathetically maintained pain appears to be neurological damage (Wilson 1989). Following any damage to neural structures there is an increase in tension in the nervous system, according to Butler (1991), so that when symptoms are present in the hand, there is always increased tension in the nervous system as well. Clinically, for example, a marked reduction of the straight leg raise has been observed in all hemiplegic patients with a swollen hand, particularly when the sound leg is tested.

The nervous system must therefore be progressively mobilised in the treatment by both the passive and active movements described in Chap. 15. The advantage of such mobilisation is that the symptoms can be relieved considerably without the affected, painful limb being moved at all. Because the nervous system is a continuum, movements of the neck, trunk, legs and the contralateral arm frequently improve the overall condition of the hand quite dramatically.

■ **Assisted Lymph Drainage.** Lymph drainage enhancement procedures have been recommended, with reportedly good results after their inclusion in the treatment of the swollen hand syndrome. Supportive bandaging has proved to be helpful in controlling the oedema, but use of elastic gloves following massage techniques must be avoided. The gloves hold the metacarpophalangeal and interphalangeal joints of the fingers in extension, causing them to stiffen in the nonfunctional position despite the reduction of the swelling. When assisted lymph drainage procedures are used in addition, the overall principles of treatment must still be followed, particularly those of eliciting no pain during activities, positioning the limb in elevation and the wearing of a cock-up splint for the wrist.

■ **Oral Cortisone.** If the symptoms continue to be a problem despite the treatment regime having been strictly followed, they become a cause of grave concern and urgent steps should be taken to overcome them for the following reasons:
- If the patient has some return of activity in the hand, as many do, future function could be jeopardised by pronounced muscle atrophy with contractures and permanent joint ankylosis, particularly digital.
- Persistent and excruciating pain may be making the patient's life intolerable and interfering with his total rehabilitation.
- The treatment of the hand may be disproportionately time consuming during therapy sessions, and the patient is unable to make progress in other areas.

The administration of an oral cortisone preparation has proved to be dramatically and lastingly effective for these cases (Davis et al.1977, Diethelm and Davies 1985, Braus et al. 1994, Christensen et al. 1982). The pain often disappears within a few days and the patient can once again participate fully in the rehabilitation programme. The medication is seldom required, but it should definitely be considered if treatment is not proving effective within a week or two. The total therapeutic regime is continued in the same way as before, but with the oral steroids being administered in addition. In spite of the rapid relief of symptoms, the medication should not be discontinued too soon. A 2–3 week period is generally necessary for lasting results, with the period needing to be repeated should the symptoms reoccur.

Considerations

Distressingly painful conditions of the hemiplegic shoulder and hand are unfortunately all too common in many hospitals and rehabilitation centres even today. The patient suffers not only from the pain but also through being unable to benefit fully from the rehabilitation programme available to him. Some of the painful stiffness may lead to permanent deformity, with limitation of function as a result. With careful supervision and treatment the painful complications can usually be avoided altogether, once the factors which cause them are understood. Should the problems arise despite the careful prophylactic measures, they can soon be overcome, particularly if detected in the early stages of their development. The whole team needs to be involved in the prevention or treatment of both the painful shoulder and the swollen hand. The patient and his relatives are an integral part of the team and need to be carefully instructed and encouraged to participate in the necessary measures for preventing or overcoming the problems. Once the pain has diminished or disappeared, the patient is able to co-operate fully, and his rapid physical progress and improved emotional state are most rewarding.

13 The Neglected Face

Many patients who have suffered a hemiplegia will have some disturbance of movement or feeling in the area of the face and mouth. No matter how slight the disorder, it will be most distressing for the patient himself. Our faces play an important role in our lives because, for each of us, it is as if we exist just behind our eyes. Unlike other parts of the body, the face is always on show and cannot be concealed or disguised by clothing. When we meet someone new, we form our first impression from his face and its expression. We say that someone has "such a friendly smile", "an intelligent face", "an intent look". From the information we receive we decide whether we would like to know the person better, and it also influences how we speak to or behave towards that person.

With the fine, richly innervated muscles of the face we are able to alter our expression by using a wide variety of very small movements. Together with movements of the head, facial expression is a prime communicator, and we use both constantly to support what we are saying or to replace speech altogether at certain times. Through minute changes we can express pleasure, disbelief, love, disapproval etc.

Getting to know someone better entails talking, and we listen not only to what is being said but also to the quality of the speaker's voice. We appreciate the sound of the voice with its melody, pitch and the way in which the words are pronounced, and while listening to someone talking we make further judgements about him or her.

When people meet and talk, usually they eat or drink something together. We eat and drink not only for nutrition but also for enjoyment and as part of our social custom. We continue to form an opinion of the other person while he eats. Any abnormality or strangeness in facial expression, voice or eating habits is immediately obvious and disturbs communication and the easy contact with others. Most of us have had the experience after a visit to the dentist which entailed an injection of local anaesthetic that caused our lip to droop, or when a small pimple has assumed the imagined proportions of a carbuncle, of feeling that everyone was staring at us.

In the total rehabilitation programme, where learning to walk and self-care are in the foreground, the problems of the face and mouth are often overlooked and not included in the treatment. The persisting difficulties will detract from the patient's quality of life and interfere with his social re-integration. He may no longer enjoy eating and drinking, either alone or with others. Other people may misjudge him or misinterpret his reactions due to inappropriate or reduced facial expression. If the patient cannot speak as he did before, he may have difficulty in establishing new relationships or in maintaining previous ones. Other people will react differently towards him, and may converse with him at an inappropriate level.

The degree and type of difficulty varies considerably, from a patient who is unable to eat at all (**Fig. 13.1**) to another whose face is not quite symmetrical (**Fig. 13.2**). When any difficulty is noticed, careful observation and investigation are necessary if the patient is

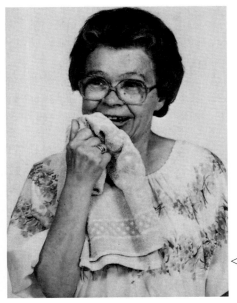

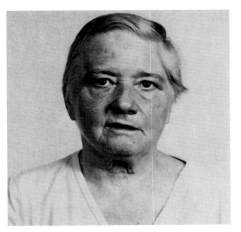

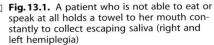

Fig. 13.2. Slight facial asymmetry (left hemiplegia)

◁ **Fig. 13.1.** A patient who is not able to eat or speak at all holds a towel to her mouth constantly to collect escaping saliva (right and left hemiplegia)

to be helped to overcome the problems. Because the therapist usually meets the patient after his stroke, she may be unaware that some of the problems exist. The patient and his relatives may be better able to offer information as to any differences they have noticed, if carefully questioned.

Important Considerations for Facilitation of the Movements of the Face and Mouth

Before she can observe, analyse and treat the problems experienced by hemiplegic patients in the area of the face and mouth, the therapist needs to understand the basic normal movements associated with communication and eating. Despite individual differences, we all have similar patterns of movement which are partly reflex and partly learnt from earliest childhood, so that we can receive adequate nutrition and at the same time be accepted by the people around us.

Movements Associated with Nonverbal Communication

Movements of the Head

The postures and movements of the head can in themselves express a wide variety of signals and emotions. We certainly use them to reinforce what we are trying to express verbally. The slight bowing and nodding movements when we meet and greet someone, the nodding and shaking of the head to express agreement, disagreement or surprise, and the aloof nose-in-the-air position are but a few examples. We turn our heads to look at someone who is talking to us and adopt a listening posture, frequently moving our head to acknowledge or emphasise what the other is saying. Turning the head away is often a negative signal.

Commonly observed difficulties include the following:

- The patient's head remains stiffly in one position, owing to the exaggerated pull of certain muscle groups. He may hold his head in a fixed position in his attempt to remain erect or to compensate for inadequate balance reactions, and thus fail to make the customary gestures which others expect.
- Due to loss or reduction of the sensory modalities on his affected side, the patient fails to turn his head to look at someone who is addressing him, particularly if she does so from the affected side (**Fig. 13.3**). Patients frequently have difficulty in making eye contact with people, particularly with those sitting or standing on their affected side.

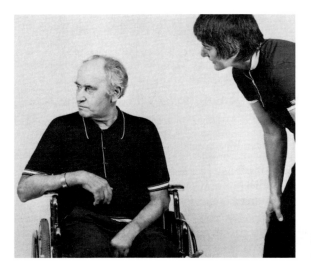

Fig. 13.3. The patient does not turn his head when someone addresses him (left hemiplegia)

Movements of the Face

The face, with its wide variety of expressions, is a prime communicator in itself, as well as reinforcing or emphasising what we are saying. We can show someone else that we are listening to him. We frown and smile, we lower or narrow our eyes, and with hundreds of such tiny movements we can reveal what we are feeling or choose to disguise our real feelings. "The muscles of facial expression endow man with extremely subtle gradations of movement for non-verbal communication skills" (Moore 1980).

When we are communicating with other people our face is constantly moving, to a greater or lesser degree. We take for granted the customary movements of the face and head, but it is most disconcerting, for example, to be introduced to a person who neither moves his head nor smiles in greeting, or to talk to someone who fails to make eye contact and whose face remains totally immobile.

Commonly observed difficulties include the following:

- The affected side of the face does not move adequately, and the asymmetry becomes more obvious when the patient is smiling, speaking or eating **(Fig. 13.4)**.
- The face assumes a constant abnormal posture, perhaps with the mouth slightly open **(Fig. 13.5)** or with the lips drawn up, away from the teeth, or held tightly down against the teeth.
- The patient's face may appear to be different from the way it was before because of changes in muscle tone and activity. For example, his profile is sometimes altered

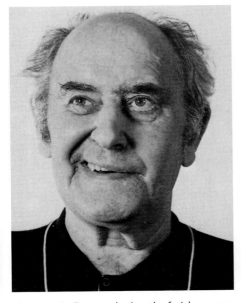

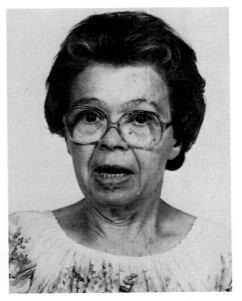

Fig. 13.4. Smiling emphasises the facial asymmetry (left hemiplegia)

Fig. 13.5. The patient is unable to close her mouth voluntarily and, because of grossly restricted tongue movements, cannot prevent dribbling (bilateral hemiplegia)

through retraction of his jaw which gives him a weak chin and protruding upper teeth.

- The whole face may be completely expressionless and immobile or show very little change of expression. In many such cases, the patient's eyebrows are constantly raised, which results in a startled or surprised expression. If his cheek muscles are hypotonic, the elevated eyebrows expose the whole iris surrounded by the white of the eye which causes the patient to look depressed even if he is not. Many patients are unable to open their eyes without raising their eyebrows simultaneously, which means that the muscles in the forehead are continuously activated throughout the day to the detriment of the antagonists. Without his eyes closing, the patient is unable to frown slightly as he would to express worry, disapproval or concerned interest, or the need for clarification on some point while looking at someone. Indeed, without specific treatment to overcome the problem, due to reciprocal inhibition, many patients are unable to frown at all.

- There may be only a stereotyped change in expression, which occurs regardless of the patient's real emotions at the time or the situation in which he finds himself. For example, a repetitive, exaggerated smile appears although the patient is in no mood to smile at all.

- The patient has difficulty in preventing dribbling (**Fig. 13.5**), particularly when he is concentrating on something else, for example putting on his shoes. He dabs constantly at his lips with a handkerchief, just in case some saliva may have escaped. Because he can only use one of his hands, it is inconvenient to hold the handkerchief at the ready all the time, and the patient is permanently distracted from other tasks by the need to put the handkerchief away somewhere or retrieve it again.

Movements Associated with Speaking

The ability to speak clearly and expressively is dependent upon many complex and co-ordinated movements. The tongue and lips are used to form the consonants, and clear articulation plays such a vital role in speaking that we are even able to understand when someone whispers, without producing any voice at all. The movements of speech have developed from those originally designed for survival, i.e. the movements of eating and drinking. For speaking they are far more rapid and co-ordinated. Agile, selective movements of the tongue are necessary to produce consonants such as "t" and "d", when the tip of the tongue has to be placed accurately behind the front teeth, and "g" and "k", where the tip of the tongue is stabilised behind the lower teeth and the middle portion of the tongue has to elevate briskly. The tongue has to move without the jaw moving simultaneously in a primitive mass synergy. Quick, accurately graded movements of the lips produce the "p" and "b" sounds. Generally, slow, slurred speech tends to be associated with fatigue, illness, the influence of alcohol or even dim-wittedness, so that a patient who has difficulty in articulating clearly may easily be misjudged by others.

Breath control is essential for voice production. Air passing through the vocal cords produces the sounds, and by altering the amount of air we change the volume of our voices. We speak more loudly or softly to emphasise, add interest or express different emotions. In order to use sentences and phrases of an adequate length we need to be able to sustain a sound effortlessly for between 15 and 20 seconds. A trained singer could perhaps manage about 1 minute.

The larynx moves up or down as we change the pitch of our voice to add quality or to express emotion. The ability is under voluntary control and is dependent upon the normal tone of the muscles of the neck and throat, and of the vocal cords themselves. The sound of the voice is clear because of the co-ordinated tension in the vocal cords. Essential for the clarity and quality of the sound is the effective action of the soft palate which, together with a constriction of the pharyngeal wall, seals off the nasal cavity completely to prevent air from escaping through the nose during vocal sounds. The soft palate must also move downwards for the required nasal sounds. The movement has to be very rapid and co-ordinated, as the position of the soft palate changes repeatedly during a sentence, or even during one word. The vowel sounds are altered by changing the shape of the mouth, by moving the lips and jaw.

Commonly observed difficulties include the following:
- The consonants are slurred or inaccurately produced and the speech may be difficult to understand as a result.
- The patient speaks slowly and carefully or even laboriously with great effort.
- The patient speaks too softly and has difficulty in making himself heard. He uses short sentences and may need to take another breath after saying only one or two words. Very often, he can maintain a sustained sound for only about 5 seconds.
- The voice is monotonous, with little or no variation in pitch. It may be lower or higher than it was previously.
- The patient sounds hoarse, as if he constantly needs to clear his throat. The voice may sound strained and effortful.
- The patient speaks nasally, or air may be heard escaping through his nose with certain sounds.
- Saliva escapes while the patient is speaking.

Movements Associated with Eating and Drinking

We eat and drink in order to survive, but also for pleasure. We are required to adhere to many learnt rules concerned with eating in order to be acceptable within our social group. Allowing for different habits and customs, the basic pattern of eating and drinking remains constant.

Most people sit in an upright position at the table to allow the head and neck to be in an optimal position for the act of eating. For this reason most societies have straight-backed dining-room chairs. In the erect position the mouth is horizontal to the food or liquid being presented, and within the mouth the movements of chewing and manipulation by the tongue are more easily carried out. The larynx can move up and down freely because the muscles surrounding it are not stretched and taut. The food is placed in the mouth from the front and in the middle, and the lips close to receive the mouthful. The swallowing programme begins with jaw closure in adults.

Solids

Chewing starts automatically, the food portion or bolus having been moved to one side and placed between the back teeth by the tongue. It is kept in the correct place by the muscle tone of the cheeks laterally and the tongue action medially. The chewing action is an asymmetrical grinding movement, and the bolus is transported by the tongue from one side of the mouth to the other at intervals. The number of chewing movements is individual and continues until the bolus is sufficiently soft and moist to allow for a comfortable swallow. Intact sensory receptors allow the strength of mastication to be appropriate and to adjust automatically as the bolus becomes softer. During the chewing cycle small amounts of acceptably prepared food are selected by the tongue and swallowed. The whole bolus is therefore not usually swallowed in one piece.

The swallowing action starts with the bolus being placed centrally on the tongue, which makes a quick wave-like movement to push the portion back into the throat. The tip of the tongue elevates first and is followed by the middle and rear thirds, moving backwards like a piston (**Fig. 13.6 a**). The soft palate elevates to seal off the nasopharynx, effectively preventing food from being pushed up into the nose (**Fig. 13.6 b**). The bolus tips the epiglottis downwards and slides over its smooth convex surface to be gui-

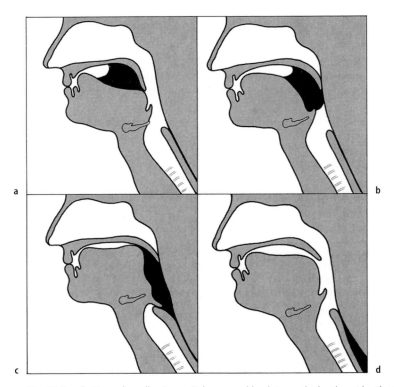

Fig. 13.6 a–d. Normal swallowing. **a** Bolus moved back towards the throat by the tongue. **b** Soft palate raised to seal off the nasal cavity. **c** The epiglottis tipped temporarily downwards to protect the larynx. **d** With the bolus safely in the oesophagus, the soft palate relaxes

ded into the oesophagus (**Fig. 13.6 c**). The larynx, which has elevated, is sealed off by the epiglottis so that the airway is protected. The vocal cords themselves provide a second safety mechanism by snapping together to expel food particles, should any accidentally enter the laryngeal airway. When the bolus is safely in the oesophagus, the epiglottis returns to its original position and the soft palate relaxes so that normal breathing can be resumed (**Fig. 13.6 d**). The swallow itself occurs reflexly.

Liquids

When a person is drinking, the fluid is placed centrally on the tongue, an active suction being used to draw it from the cup or spoon resting on the lower lip, which has come forwards to receive it. The fluid is brought to the back of the mouth for swallowing by the same wave-like movement of the tongue used to swallow solids. Normally, one large swallowing movement takes place, followed by one or two small additional swallows to clear the pharynx completely. In a relaxed situation the swallow is not audible to others and, for adults, it is possible only when the mouth is closed.

After a person eats or drinks, the teeth and mouth are immediately cleaned most thoroughly by the tongue, and also by the movement of the lips and cheeks over the teeth. The saliva also washes the mouth clean. Eating and drinking with others is an enjoyable pastime. We take solids and fluids in rapid succession, and we can converse easily, even while food is being held discreetly in the side of the mouth.

Commonly observed difficulties include the following:

- The patient is unable to achieve an upright, symmetrical posture. With the trunk flexed he is obliged to extend his neck at the back with his chin up in order to place the food in his mouth, and the muscles anteriorly are therefore stretched. The movements of the tongue and larynx are more difficult as a result.
- With the trunk and head flexed laterally towards the hemiplegic side, the central presentation of the food is a problem, and within the mouth control becomes almost impossible. Food falls between the teeth and the cheek, or escapes from the corner of the mouth, the affected side being tilted downwards.
- Pieces of food remain stuck in the mouth and may be observed long after the meal is finished. They may remain in the patient's cheek or on the roof of the mouth and can nearly always be seen on his teeth in front, or on his lips and chin. Many patients use a finger to remove pieces of food that have become lodged within their mouth.
- The patient chews only on the unaffected side and spasticity increases on the hemiplegic side. When that side is hypotonic with poor sensation, no activity is stimulated.
- The chewing is often more a "chomping" up and down action than the complex adult rotatory motion and shows no alteration as the bolus becomes softer. The patient chews toast or crème caramel with the same amount of vigour and strength.
- Because chewing is slow and ineffective, the patient chews for a much longer period and often avoids hard food sorts altogether, or takes very small pieces.
- Due to reduced sensation or abnormal tone the patient often bites his cheek accidentally, and small painful ulcerations can be felt from the inside on examination.
- Swallowing is audible and effortful, and the whole bolus is swallowed in one piece. The patient has to swallow several times before he succeeds in clearing the pharynx.
- The patient often chokes, particularly when drinking.

Owing to such problems, eating and drinking become a slow and laborious chore, and the patient has to concentrate intently. He is unable to join in the conversation at table, and often his food is cold and unappetising before he has finished.

Dentures

False teeth can be a problem for the patient both when speaking or eating. A set of teeth that previously was held in place by normal muscle activity despite an imperfect fit slips down repeatedly when the patient has altered tone and sensation. The false teeth should be worn as soon as possible and held firmly in place by a dental fixative. When the patient has progressed sufficiently to visit the dentist, the necessary alteration can be made to ensure a good fit.

The dentures should be cleaned after each meal, as pieces of food tend to become lodged between the plate and the hard palate, and the patient is not able to retrieve them with his tongue as he did before.

Appropriate Treatment for the Common Difficulties

The problems that have been described are caused by:
- *Abnormal tone.* The muscle tone of the face, mouth and neck is too high or too low.
- *Inadequate sensation.* The patient is not able to feel the side of his face adequately, or the inside of his mouth.
- *Loss of selective movement.* It is difficult or impossible for the patient to move his lips, cheeks and tongue selectively. He is able to move them only in stereotyped mass patterns.

Recognising that the problems exist and including their treatment in the rehabilitation programme is the first important step. The area of the face and mouth tends otherwise to fall into a kind of "no-man's land" and is often neglected as a result. The nurse attends to the oral hygiene and ensures that the patient has sufficient intake for his nutritional requirements. The occupational therapist enables the patient to prepare and eat the food with one hand, using aids if necessary. The physiotherapist deals with his ability to move about sufficiently to reach the dining-room table and sit correctly. In most cases the speech therapist is concerned primarily with language problems rather than with the nonverbal aspects of communication or with eating.

For the majority of patients the following treatment plan will be appropriate and helpful, and can be carried out by all those involved in caring for him. The emphasis of the treatment should be directed towards the specific difficulties which the patient has, although each difficulty will influence the other movements to a considerable extent. For more complex difficulties, specially qualified help will be necessary, but it is surprising how well the area responds to the attention it receives, even to relatively simple treatment measures.

When assessing or treating the face and mouth, two grips are particularly useful and can also be used when the patient is being helped to eat and drink or to clean his teeth.

- Grip A: Standing beside the patient, usually at his hemiplegic side, the therapist places one arm round behind his head. With the crook of her elbow and her upper arm she keeps his head in the midline and elongates the back of his neck by lifting his occiput slightly with her arm. She plantar flexes her wrist so that her thumb can rest gently against the temporomandibular joint to feel any abnormal movement or muscle tone. The therapist holds the patient's chin between her index and middle fingers to guide the appropriate movements of his jaw. With her index finger she assists lip closure and her middle finger can relax his tongue from below, or facilitate its movements (**Fig. 13.7**).

- Grip B. Sitting in front of the patient, the therapist places her thumb on his chin and her middle finger in the space between the bases of the mandibles from below. Her index finger rests on the side of his face (**Fig. 13.8**). Her thumb assists mouth closure and her middle finger can influence the tongue musculature. The index finger provides information as to lateral movement of the jaw and the tone of the cheek muscles. The grip is used when the patient has adequate head control in sitting and can inhibit the extension of his neck voluntarily. It is particularly useful when the patient has language difficulties, because he can see the therapist's face and follow what he is expected to do. For the patient who is still unable to maintain his head in the correct position, the grip can nevertheless be used if necessary, by treating him in a half-lying position in bed, with his head well supported.

When the therapist is assisting the patient with eating or drinking, the first grip is usually recommended. The patient can sit at the table in the normal way and see his food on the plate in front of him while he is being fed.. Should the patient need help

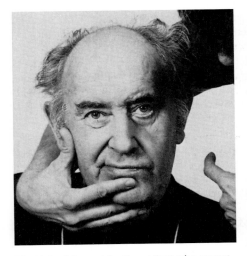

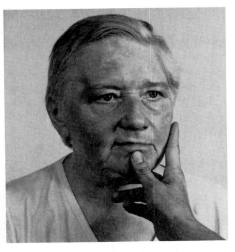

Fig. 13.7. Grip used for the patient who cannot hold his head in a normal position (left hemiplegia)

Fig. 13.8. Grip suitable for patients who can maintain a correct head position (left hemiplegia)

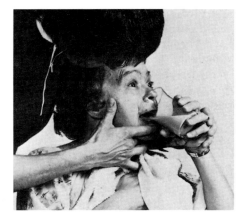

Fig. 13.9. Helping the patient with drinking (bilateral hemiplegia)

to bring the food or drinking utensil to his mouth, the therapist can guide his hand more easily, as the movement is the same one she would make herself **(Fig. 13.9)**.

For Difficulties Associated with Nonverbal Communication

Neck and Head Movements

The neck should be kept fully mobile and any hypertonus or over-activity reduced. The therapist first moves the patient's head passively, emphasising the full range of movement, and the patient tries to allow the movement without any resistance **(Fig. 13.10)**. It is often easier to regain full movement with the patient lying supine. The therapist needs to maintain the position of the patient's shoulder with one hand when moving his head into full side flexion or rotation towards the opposite side . Once the resistance has disappeared, the patient can be asked to move his head actively. All movements should also be full and free in sitting and standing positions, as these are the positions in which communication usually takes place. Group activities with music, balls or balloons can help the patient to overcome the problem of a fixed head position and the failure to make eye contact with others.

Facial Movements

Movements of the face should be facilitated from an early stage, in order to maintain mobility and to stimulate sensation.
* The therapist uses her fingertips to move the forehead into a frowning position, diagonally down towards the midline **(Fig. 13.11)**. Her fingers should not slide on the skin but instead move the muscles themselves, lying as they do just beneath the skin. The downward movement is alternated with that of raising the eyebrows to produce a look of surprise, with an upward and outward action. The patient first feels the activ-

ity and then helps actively, with the therapist assisting less and less. In most cases the downward frowning movement will need to be emphasised until the patient is able to maintain a frown with his eyes remaining open, relax the position without raising his eyebrows, and repeat small frowning movements several times in quick succession.

At first the movement may need to be a gross mass one, with the eyes closing tightly to reinforce frowning (**Fig. 13.12**) and opening wide when the eyebrows are raised. As the patient's ability increases the movements can become more selective and varied, until he can close his eyes without moving his forehead, close one eye or raise one eyebrow.

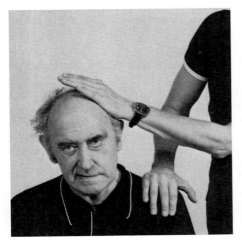

Fig. 13.10. Moving the head passively (left hemiplegia)

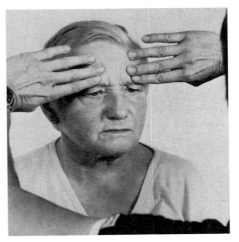

Fig. 13.11. Frowning (left hemiplegia)

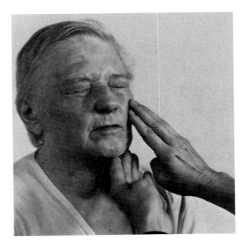

Fig. 13.12. Closing the eyes tightly (left hemiplegia)

- The patient tries to narrow his eyes as if he were looking into the far distance or as if the sun were very bright. The therapist facilitates the desired movement by placing her middle finger just below his eye and her index finger on his eyelid and then easing her fingers slightly towards each other.
- The therapist moves the patient's cheeks to normalise tone, first from the outside and then from within his mouth. She rubs her little finger along the patient's gums (**Fig. 13.13**) and then into his cheek, pulling the cheek away from his teeth at the side with a semicircular motion (**Fig. 13.14**). The stretching movement releases the spasticity but will also stimulate activity in an hypotonic cheek. The therapist can compare the tone of the muscles with those of the other cheek.
- The patient then blows air into his cheeks and keeps it there (**Fig. 13.15**). The activity requires lip seal as well as closure of the soft palate to prevent air from escaping through the nose. The patient moves the air into first one cheek and then the other, thus stimulating activity in the muscles of the cheeks and the soft palate (**Fig. 13.16**).
- The therapist facilitates a symmetrical smiling movement, followed by lip-pursing. If the sound side is too active, she uses the back of one hand to inhibit the activity, and stimulates the affected side with a quick upward brushing movement of her other hand (**Fig. 13.17**).
- The cheek and lips can be stimulated by quick stroking with ice, or by using the back of an electric toothbrush. The brush is moved from lateral to medial and the vibration increases sensation and helps to normalise tone (**Fig. 13.18 a, b**).
- The patient is asked to wrinkle his nose, as if experiencing a bad smell. The therapist places her fingertips on either side of his nose to assist the movement (**Fig. 13.19**). As the patient becomes more skilled he tries to wrinkle his nose quickly and repeatedly without moving other parts of his face at the same time.
- The patient is asked to curl his lip upwards, as if to show the therapist his top teeth and the underneath side of his lip.

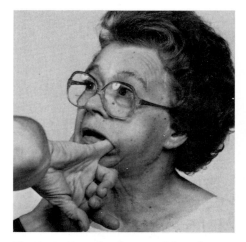

Fig. 13.13. Massaging the gums (bilateral hemiplegia)

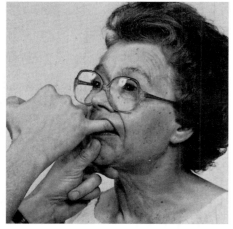

Fig. 13.14. Releasing spasticity in the cheek (bilateral hemiplegia)

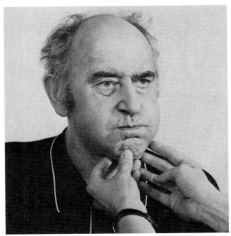

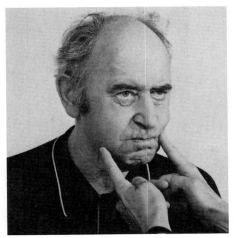

13.15

13.16

Fig. 13.15. Blowing air into the cheeks (left hemiplegia)

Fig. 13.16. Blowing air from one cheek to the other. The therapist assists the hemiplegic side (left hemiplegia)

Fig. 13.17. Facilitating symmetrical smiling (left hemiplegia)

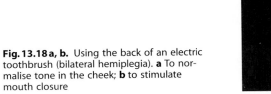

Fig. 13.18 a, b. Using the back of an electric toothbrush (bilateral hemiplegia). **a** To normalise tone in the cheek; **b** to stimulate mouth closure
▽

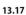

13.17

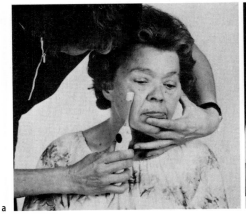

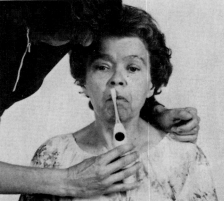

a

b

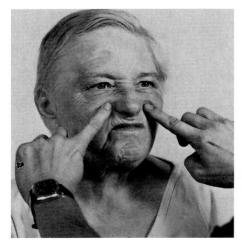

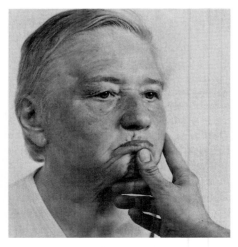

Fig. 13.19. Wrinkling the nose (left hemiplegia)

Fig. 13.20. Moving the bottom lip over the top one (left hemiplegia)

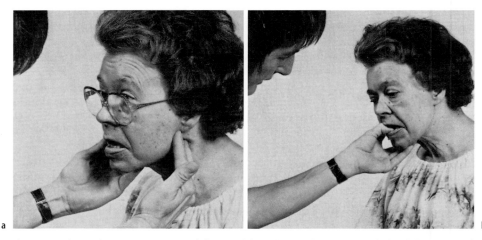

a

b

Fig. 13.21 a, b. Facilitating protraction of the jaw (bilateral hemiplegia). **a** From behind the angles of the mandible; **b** with the therapist's thumb hooked over the bottom teeth

- The patient moves his lips over each other, placing the bottom lip over the top one and vice versa **(Fig. 13.20)**.
- He can also move his bottom jaw forwards and try to place his lower teeth over the upper lip, to combat the spastic retraction of the jaw. The therapist facilitates the movement using her fingers behind the angles of the mandible **(Fig. 13.21 a)**. Because the area is sensitive to pressure, she may not be able to give sufficient help in this way. If the patient has considerable spasticity retracting his jaw, the thera-

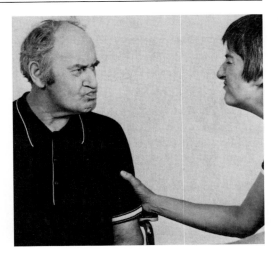

Fig. 13.22. Copying facial expressions (left hemiplegia)

pist can place her thumb behind his lower front teeth with her index finger underneath his chin **(Fig. 13.21 b)**. She then draws the jaw forward several times, and when the hypertonus has been reduced by the movement the patient takes over actively.

- The therapist helps the patient to make different facial expressions, using her fingers to move his face. He can practise copying expressions shown to him, or vary his expression to express different emotions for the therapist to interpret **(Fig. 13.22)**.

For Difficulties Associated with Speaking

Breathing is assisted, with the therapist placing her hands on both sides of the thorax to facilitate lateral costal breathing. Due to hypo- or hypertonus, the hemiplegic side often fails to move adequately. A long expiration is encouraged by her vibrating downwards over the sternum, and the patient is asked to produce a long sound without effort as he breathes out. The sound can be timed, and the patient tries to maintain the sound effortlessly for the required 15 seconds.

- The larynx is moved passively, diagonally upwards and downwards to both sides **(Fig. 13.23)**. The patient then makes sounds with a pitch change to move his larynx actively. The high and low sounds can also be practised by changing vowel sounds in combination with the changes of pitch, such as "ooh – aah" or "eeh – ooh".
- The patient licks his lips, moving his tongue right round the outside. He then moves his tongue around inside his lips, pushing them away from his teeth **(Fig. 13.24)**.
- The therapist guides him to place his tongue far back in the inside of his cheek to where her finger is indicating **(Fig. 13.25)**. He tries to stretch and massage his cheek with his tongue, moving it up and down with increasing velocity.

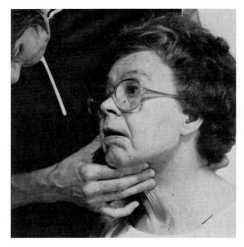

Fig. 13.23. Moving the larynx passively to normalise tone (bilateral hemiplegia)

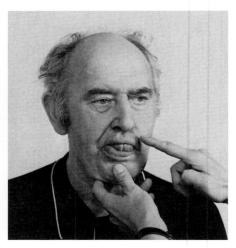

Fig. 13.24. Licking the outside of the top teeth (left hemiplegia)

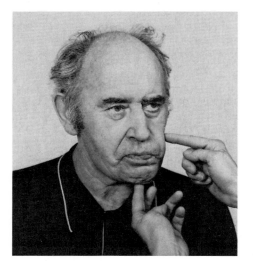

Fig. 13.25. Placing the tongue far back in the cheek (left hemiplegia)

Should tongue movements be severely reduced the therapist will have to stimulate them more directly.

- Placing her little finger in his mouth, she pushes down on the tongue and makes small steps towards the back **(Fig. 13.26 a)**. Quick strokes forwards on the tongue can activate its intrinsic muscles **(Fig. 13.26 b)**. Pushing against the lateral border of the tongue facilitates its movement sideways, and the patient can try to push his tongue against the finger actively.
- The therapist asks the patient to push his tongue against a spatula or a drinking straw, and to follow its movements both inside and outside his mouth **(Fig. 13.26 c)**.

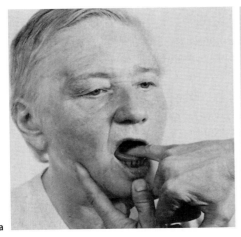

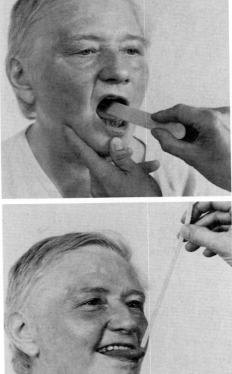

Fig. 13.26 a–c. Stimulating activity in the tongue (left hemiplegia). **a** Pressing down with small steps backwards; **b** stroking forwards along the middle of the tongue with the edge of a wooden spatula; **c** pushing the tip of the tongue against a drinking straw

Before facilitating active tongue movements the therapist should inhibit any hypertonus.

- She places her finger below the patient's jaw, in the area of soft tissue beneath the floor of the mouth. Using a semicircular movement, she presses her finger upwards and forwards to influence the tone in the muscles of the tongue and to facilitate a forward movement (**Fig. 13.27**). To facilitate the wave-like movement necessary for swallowing, the therapist assists in the same way, only in this case her finger moves upwards and backwards in its semicircular motion.
- If the patient can hardly move his tongue at all, the therapist guides its movements completely at first. Placing a piece of damp gauze around his tongue, she is able to hold it between her finger and thumb and move it in the various directions required (**Fig. 13.28**). She draws his tongue forwards, lifting it slightly upwards with her middle finger as she does so to avoid scraping it against his bottom teeth, and moves it to either side. The therapist instructs the patient to feel the movement and then try to join in actively while she is assisting him.

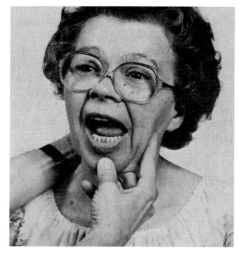

Fig. 13.27. Inhibiting tongue spasticity from below and moving the tongue forwards (bilateral hemiplegia)

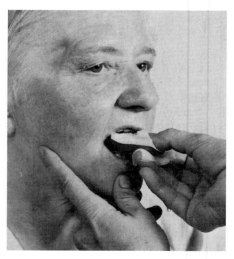

Fig. 13.28. Facilitating movements of the tongue by holding it with a piece of damp gauze and moving it in different directions (left hemiplegia)

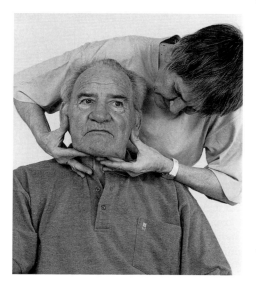

Fig. 13.29. The therapist uses her middle fingers to mobilise the tongue from below (left hemiplegia)

For a patient whose tongue is very retracted and hypertonic, the therapist will need to spend more time reducing tone before attempting to move it passively or asking him to try to move it actively. She stands behind the patient and places both her middle fingers underneath his chin in the space between his mandibles so that she can manipulate the tongue muscles directly. She then moves her fingers upwards and forwards slowly and repeatedly, thus relaxing the musculature and bringing the whole tongue to the front of the mouth (**Fig. 13.29**).

- The patient attempts to make the sounds "d" and "t" accurately, placing the tip of his tongue against the back of his front teeth. The speed is gradually increased, and he tries to make the sounds without moving his lower jaw at the same time. The sounds "g" and "k" are practised, with the tip of the tongue forward against the bottom teeth. As the patient's ability increases he alternates between the "g" and "d" sounds. These movements are those which are required for swallowing as well, i.e. the tip of the tongue first elevated for "d" or "t" and then the back of the tongue raised for "g" or "k". It may be necessary to guide the patient's tongue to the correct position at first, using a spatula to elevate its tip or point to the correct position behind the top teeth (**Fig. 13.30**). By pressing the spatula on the back of the tongue, the therapist can facilitate the upward movement required of that part for making the "g". sound. To increase the effect or to assist a patient who cannot keep his tongue forward, the therapist holds the tongue in position with a piece of gauze while at the same time stimulating the movement required for the "ga" sound by pressing down briskly with a spatula (**Fig. 13.31**). With the tongue remaining forward, outside the mouth, the activity of its posterior portion is accentuated. Soft palate closure will also be influenced positively by the movement of the back of the tongue.
- The soft palate can be stimulated actively by the patient blowing through a straw and making bubbles in a glass of coloured liquid. He tries to maintain a steady stream of bubbles for increasingly longer periods; this will improve his breath control at the same time (**Fig. 13.32**).
- If the soft palate remains inactive, a wet cotton-bud placed in the freezer compartment of the refrigerator provides a useful means of stimulating it with ice. The therapist holds the tongue down with a spatula and strokes the soft palate briskly with the iced cotton-bud, moving the iced tip upwards and laterally (**Fig. 13.33 a–c**). After the icing, the patient makes some short, sharp "ah" sounds to elevate the soft palate.
- To improve the melody and expression of the voice the patient is asked to say a short sentence in different ways, for example "What are you doing?" expressed with irritation, amazement, joy or rage.

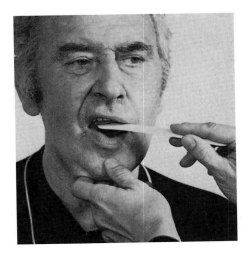

Fig. 13.30. Lifting the tip of the tongue with a spatula to touch behind the top teeth (left hemiplegia)

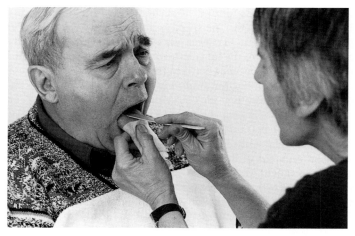

Fig. 13.31. Holding the tongue forwards with gauze and pressing down with a spatula to facilitate the movement for saying "ga" (right hemiplegia)

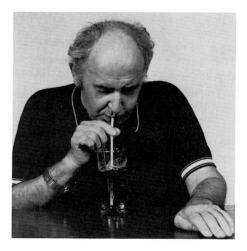

Fig. 13.32. Blowing through a straw to make a stream of bubbles

For Difficulties Associated with Eating

The activities for improving speaking will all help to improve the patient's eating pattern as well. In the same way, correct eating movements will be beneficial for speaking. Even patients who are still being tube-fed should be treated, so that they can learn to take food by mouth again more quickly. They will benefit particularly from all movements and stimulation inside the mouth. Practising good, clear phonation and changing pitch will ensure that the vocal cords and larynx are moving adequately, which will help to prevent the patient from inhaling particles of food and choking later when he starts eating and drinking.

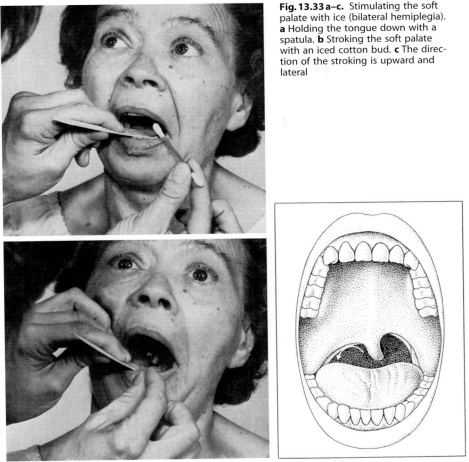

Fig. 13.33 a–c. Stimulating the soft palate with ice (bilateral hemiplegia). **a** Holding the tongue down with a spatula. **b** Stroking the soft palate with an iced cotton bud. **c** The direction of the stroking is upward and lateral

Perhaps the most important factor of all is the patient's posture when eating. If he has any problems with eating and swallowing he should never attempt to eat or drink in bed. The flexed position of the trunk and the unaccustomed presentation and manipulation of the food make the task even more difficult (**Fig. 13.34a**). Drinking in a half-lying position is almost impossible for a patient with swallowing problems. Not only will he spill much of the fluid; more importantly, he will be in grave danger of choking (**Fig. 13.34b**). Even when he is seated in a wheelchair the patient's trunk tends to be too flexed. He should therefore be transferred to an upright chair at a table, to enable an improved sitting posture to be achieved. Placing his hemiplegic arm forwards on the table assists trunk extension and prevents his affected side from pulling down into flexion, which will improve the position of his head (**Fig. 13.34c**). Should the patient have difficulty in preparing and bringing a spoonful or forkful of food to his mouth,

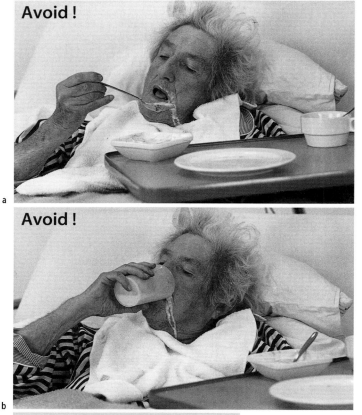

Avoid !

Avoid !

a

b

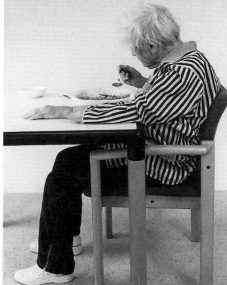

c

Fig. 13.34 a–c. A correct posture facilitates swallowing. **a** Eating in bed presents additional problems. **b** When drinking in half-lying, the fluid is difficult to control and the risk of choking increased. **c** Seated at a table in an upright chair, the same patient enjoys her meal (left hemiplegia)

the assistant should guide his hands in the way described in Chap. 1 (**Fig. 13.35a**). She helps him in the same way when he has finished eating and needs to wipe his mouth with a napkin (**Fig. 13.35b**).

Thick, slow-moving purée-type foods are the easiest to manage at first, but to stimulate chewing and sensation in the mouth the patient needs to be given crunchy food with more texture. Lightly cooked vegetables, biscuits and toast can be attempted. It is almost impossible for the therapist to facilitate chewing mechanically if the food in the patient's mouth does not require chewing.

The patient should be encouraged to chew on the hemiplegic side and place the food first to that side. If he chews only on the sound side, his face becomes more asymmetrical, and the affected side is not stimulated into activity. If chewing is inadequate or if the patient is in danger of aspirating, the crispy food can be wrapped in a piece of gauze and placed between the patient's teeth on the hemiplegic side (**Fig. 13.36**). He can then chew on something solid and at the same time savour different tastes. The chewing action will also encourage movement of the tongue and lips.

After eating, instead of dabbing at his mouth repeatedly with a napkin the patient is asked to reach for small pieces of food on his lips or chin with his tongue, or by moving one lip over the other (**Fig. 13.37**). He can also use his hand to wipe away small food particles or saliva, as is normally done.

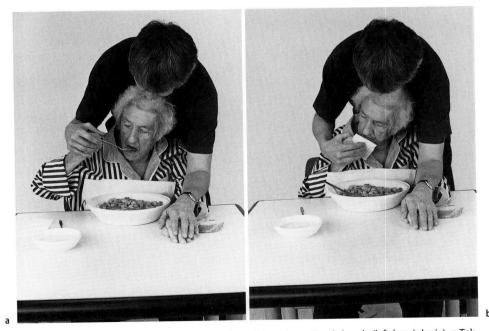

a   b

Fig. 13.35a, b. Giving assistance at mealtimes by guiding the patient's hands (left hemiplegia). **a** Taking a mouthful. **b** Wiping her mouth with a napkin

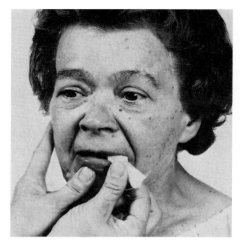

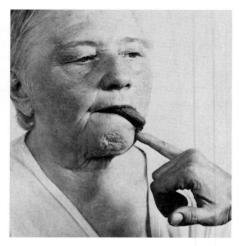

Fig. 13.36. Facilitating chewing with a piece of apple wrapped in gauze and placed between the back teeth (bilateral hemiplegia)

Fig. 13.37. The patient uses her tongue to remove a piece of biscuit from her chin (left hemiplegia)

Oral Hygiene

When tongue movements are a problem or eating is restricted to soft foods, particular attention must be paid to oral hygiene. Food remains stuck to the patient's teeth, and they deteriorate rapidly. The condition of the gums is often poor because the circulation is not stimulated by chewing solid foods and because the tooth brushing is also inadequate. It is often assumed that because the patient can use one hand he will be able to brush his own teeth properly. With poor sensation and neglect of the hemiplegic side, he often fails to brush the teeth on that side adequately, if at all. After each meal the teeth should be vigorously brushed, with the help of the therapist or nurse until the patient can manage efficiently alone (**Fig. 13.38**). An electric toothbrush is a great help because its action compensates for the loss of the skilled manipulation required when using an ordinary toothbrush. Its small brush is also more easily manipulated when the lips are paralysed or spastic, and the vibration stimulates feeling and movement within the mouth. Particular care should be taken to ensure that the inner side of the teeth is clean as well.

The patient should learn a routine whereby he brushes first the top teeth from the very back on one side to the very back on the other side, both inside and outside. The lower teeth are then done in the same way. Whether the therapist or the nurse is brushing the patient's teeth for him or guiding his sound hand to assist him, they should follow the same routine so that he learns to carry out the sequence by experiencing it. Many patients have difficulty in rinsing their mouth adequately, and particularly in spitting out the water afterwards. The therapist may need to facilitate the necessary movement, using her thumb and fingers to draw the cheeks and lips quickly forwards into

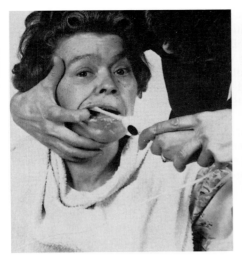

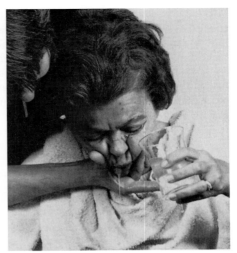

Fig. 13.38. Helping the patient to brush her teeth (bilateral hemiplegia)

Fig. 13.39. Facilitating the movements required to spit out the water after rinsing the mouth (bilateral hemiplegia)

the correct position at the right moment, giving the patient a verbal command as she does so **(Fig. 13.39)**.

If the condition of the gums is particularly poor, the therapist can massage them with her finger, or with a piece of gauze wrapped round her finger for added effect.

Brushing the teeth after every meal may be considered unnecessary and too time consuming by some because normally, the mobile tongue and lips clean the teeth so well. However, as one patient, who is a dentist himself, so pertinently pointed out, "No one would consider leaving his knife and fork unwashed after a meal, and it should be the same for our teeth, which have similar functions!" (Kasiske 1996, personal communication). For the patient who has sensory/motor problems in his mouth, this attitude holds particularly true, and despite the fact that more time is required for adequate oral hygiene three times a day, it will be time well spent. With so many advantages to be gained, finding the time to help the patient to brush his teeth more often is well worth the effort.

Considerations

The face is of such prime importance in our society, as the numerous advertisements for cosmetics surely indicate, that it seems strange that it has received so little attention in the rehabilitation literature and the various treatment programmes offered. Likewise, eating and drinking, which contribute so much to our quality of life, have seldom been emphasised apart from their nutritional aspects. Patients are most thankful for the help they receive through the treatment of their face and mouth and are always ready to cooperate fully. Certain inhibitions associated with touching another person's face or mouth may well cause members of the rehabilitation team to neglect this aspect of treatment, but once such inhibitions have been overcome the results are most rewarding. Quite astonishing improvement has frequently been observed after the activities described in this chapter have been incorporated in the treatment programme. Patients are more than willing to practise selected activities on their own, once they have been thoroughly taught what they can do.

The approach to the "neglected face" and the methods of assessment and treatment described in this chapter are based on the teaching of K. Coombes in personal communication, through treating patients together and during numerous courses given by her at the Postgraduate Study Centre in Bad Ragaz, Switzerland (unpublished work).

14 Out of Line (the Pusher Syndrome)

Most studies concerning the rehabilitation of patients with hemiplegia have shown that the majority are able to walk again at the end of their rehabilitation, irrespective of the quality of the gait pattern or type of walking aids required. Many patients learn to walk again even without formal rehabilitation. It is important to consider why a certain group of patients do not learn to walk if only conventional physiotherapy and rehabilitation programmes are followed and how such patients could be helped to overcome their difficulties and thus achieve the goal of walking.

Various reasons have been offered for the failure to achieve independent walking, such as old age, weakness, insufficient extensor tone, flexor spasticity in the leg and loss of sensation in the hemiplegic leg. Such hypotheses are obviously not valid and tend to oversimplify the problem. Elderly patients with marked motor loss have learned to walk again. Polio victims, young and old, walk around despite marked weakness and loss of extensor tone in the leg. Spasticity bears no relation to achieving ambulatory independence, only to the pattern and quality of the gait, and patients with grossly diminished sensation in the lower limb can walk independently even without a cane.

The problem is far more complex, and observation of patients over many years has revealed that those who have difficulty in achieving ambulatory independence also demonstrate other difficulties in common. The difficulties are so uniform that they could be classified together as a syndrome, the "pusher syndrome", the name deriving from the most striking of the symptoms. The patient pushes strongly towards his hemiplegic side in all positions and resists any attempt at passive correction of his posture, that is, correction which would bring his weight towards or over the midline of his body to the unaffected side.

In the acute phase following cerebrovascular accident, many patients pass through a transient phase of showing certain of the typical symptoms of the syndrome, but in such cases, within a short period the more classic picture of hemiplegia develops, and the patient achieves a degree of independence with only a few weeks' delay. However, if the pusher syndrome is pronounced and prolonged, without receiving specific treatment to overcome their difficulties, the patients may still be confined to a wheelchair after many months, conventional treatment in a general hospital situation having proved unsuccessful. Such patients are often considered to be unsuitable for rehabilitation and are sent instead to nursing homes or other long-term institutions, with little hope of making further progress. Sadly, it is often erroneously assumed that they were not sufficiently motivated or did not try hard enough, which is not the case at all.

The Typical Signs

Many more patients with left hemiplegia than with right suffer from the pusher syndrome. However, when the symptoms are observed in a case of right hemiplegia of long duration, the patient will have either a very severe aphasia or no problem with speech at all. The latter group may consist of those patients whose right cerebral hemisphere is dominant. The degree of difficulty will vary from patient to patient and is not always directly related to a loss of active movement. Some patients may have selective movement in the hemiplegic hand and foot, despite marked manifestations of the syndrome.

The syndrome in its most severe form, using a left hemiplegic patient as an example, is characterised by the following problems, and when one or two of the symptoms are observed, then the others will invariably be present as well, in varying degrees.

1. The head is turned to the right and is at the same time shifted laterally towards the right; that is, the distance from the point of the right shoulder to the neck is markedly shortened. When the patient is sitting, he is unable to relax his muscles in order to allow the head to be side flexed towards the hemiplegic side, although it moves freely to the sound side (Fig. 14.1 a, b). When the hemiplegia is of some months' duration the neck may be so stiff that almost no movement is possible. When the patient is lying down the neck movements are noticeably freer, particularly if he is instructed verbally to give no resistance to the passive movements. The eyes are often turned to the right as well, and the patient has difficulty in bringing them to the left and then maintaining their position.

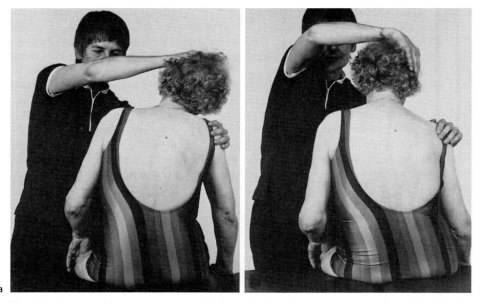

a   b

Fig. 14.1 a, b. Lateral flexion of the neck (left hemiplegia). **a** Free to the sound side; **b** limited to the hemiplegic side

2. The patient's ability to perceive incoming stimuli from his left side is reduced in all the perceptual modalities. Describing the profound contralateral neglect which he relates to parietal lobe lesions, Mountcastle (1978) writes: "Such a patient no longer has the capacity to attend to that contralateral world: for him it no longer exists."

   a) *Tactile or tactile/kinaesthetic:* The sensation may be almost absent or markedly reduced, but even if the patient appears to perform well during formal testing he neglects the hemiplegic side of his body when moving, or when he is not concentrating specifically on that side, as he is during testing. His hemiplegic arm may hang over the side of the chair, and even be caught in the wheel of the wheelchair. When being helped to clasp his hands together he may try to fold his sound hand with the therapist's hand, instead of his own. He frequently dresses or washes only the right side of his body.

   b) *Visual:* The patient does not see objects on his left side. He may have a hemianopsia, and he fails to turn his head in order to compensate for the visual field defect. Even with no demonstrable hemianopsia he neglects incoming visual stimuli and frequently pushes his wheelchair against objects in his path. Because his head is turned to the right, any visual field loss is in front of him and his field of vision is severely curtailed.

   c) *Auditory:* Because the patient does not hear when someone speaks to him from his left side he may be thought to be deaf (see Fig. 13.3). On formal testing, however, his hearing is found to be unimpaired.

3. There is a general dearth of facial expression. The face is immobile and when activated is one-sided, with overactivity on the right.

4. The voice is monotonous, with poor breath control and little volume.

5. Lying supine on a plinth or in bed, the patient shows an elongation of his hemiplegic side from head to foot (**Fig. 14.2**). Particularly noticeable is the discrepancy between the left and right side of his trunk. The right side appears to be shortened. The right hip extends actively with the knee held slightly flexed and the heel pushing down against the supporting surface. The therapist has to tell him to relax it and let it lie flat before she is able to place it on the plinth. The patient holds his head actively off the pillow until instructed verbally to relax it.

   The left side is at the same time retracted, the shoulder, thorax and pelvis lying below the level of their right equivalents. The left leg therefore lies laterally rotated and, if the patient has been nursed on his back, will frequently show pressure areas over the lateral malleolus and/or along the outside of the heel (**Fig. 14.3**).

6. Even when lying fully supported on a wide plinth or bed, the patient holds on to the edge with his sound hand and is anxious that he may fall over the side.

7. Placing does not automatically occur when the sound leg is moved by an examiner, although when told to hold that leg in a certain position the patient can do so easily (**Fig. 14.4 a, b**).

8. When both knees are flexed with the feet supported on the bed, they lean towards the left. A marked resistance is felt when the therapist tries to turn both knees to the right side, i.e. as if to lay them on the bed on that side. No resistance is met when both knees are rotated to the hemiplegic side.

9. In sitting the difficulties become more obvious. The head is held stiffly to the right side, and the right side of the trunk shortens markedly. The hemiplegic side is elongated and the navel is shifted towards the right, with hypotonus showing clearly in the muscles on the left side of the abdomen. The weight, however, remains over the

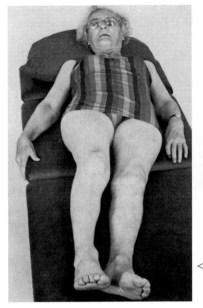

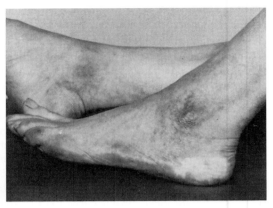

Fig. 14.3. Pressure mark on the outside of the heel after lying supine (left hemiplegia)

◁ **Fig. 14.2.** In supine the whole hemiplegic side is elongated. The head is held off the pillow, the sound foot presses down actively with the knee slightly flexed and the patient holds the side of the plinth (left hemiplegia)

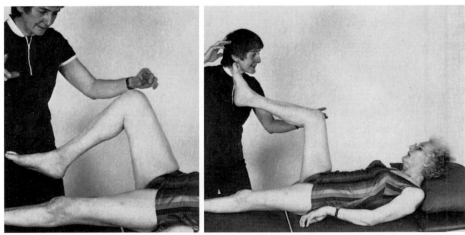

a

b

Fig. 14.4 a, b. Placing of the sound leg (left hemiplegia). **a** Fails without verbal command. **b** The patient holds her leg in the position when verbal instruction is given

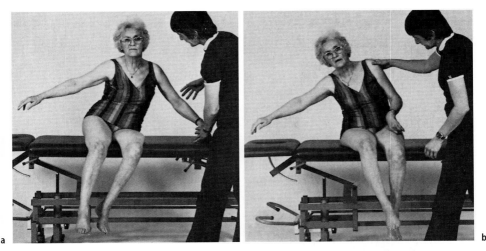

a   b

Fig. 14.5 a, b. Balance reactions when moving sideways in sitting (left hemiplegia). **a** To the hemiplegic side; the reactions of the head and trunk are almost normal. **b** To the sound side; the hemiplegic side does not react at all. The sound side shortens too actively

left side. Resistance is encountered when an attempt is made to transfer the weight over to the right side, with the patient pushing back with the help of his sound hand. He may protest, although no fear was expressed when he was overbalancing to the left.

When the patient's weight is transferred to the left, that is, towards the hemiplegic side, the balance reactions appear to be almost normal because the right side of his trunk is already shortened, but he will still fall over if not supported by the therapist **(Fig. 14.5 a)**. If the patient is asked to take his weight over the sound side, no head-righting reaction occurs. The head remains fixedly to the right, and the trunk on that side fails to elongate, shortening actively instead **(Fig. 14.5 b)**. Little or no muscle activity occurs in the left side of the trunk and the shoulder girdle elevates. The untrained patient will use his sound hand on the plinth to resist transferring his weight towards the right.

10. Transferring the patient into a chair presents difficulties, as he pushes backwards and away from the sound leg, which would otherwise support him. The transfer is particularly difficult if an attempt is made to move the patient to a chair placed on his sound side. His right hand and leg push strongly in the opposite direction to the movement.

11. Seated in the wheelchair, the patient adopts a typical posture. His trunk is flexed and shortened on the right side, his head is turned to the right and his right arm maintains constant activity, pushing down and away on the arm, the seat or the wheel of the chair **(Fig. 14.6)** Due to the overactivity on the right, the hypotonic left side of his trunk elongates further causing elevation of the shoulder girdle on the left. He sits more towards the left of the chair and strongly resists having his buttocks moved more to the right, for instance to allow someone to replace the arm of the wheelchair on that side.

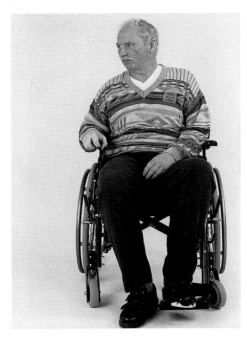

Fig. 14.6. In the wheelchair the head and trunk assume typical postures and the hemiplegic leg abducts until the thigh presses against the upright of the footrest (left hemiplegia)

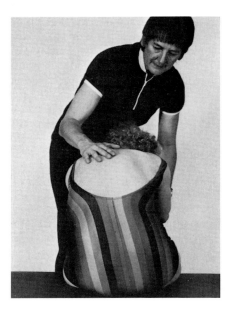

Fig. 14.7. When the patient leans forwards the hemiplegic side lengthens and there is no weight on the sound buttock (left hemiplegia)

12. When leaning forwards in order to stand up or transfer into bed, the patient pushes towards the hemiplegic side, with his trunk markedly shortened on the sound side (**Fig. 14.7**). His affected foot may slide back under the chair or show no activity at all.

13. In standing, the patient's whole centre of gravity is to the left, so that a line drawn from his sound foot to his sternum would be diagonal to the floor. Perry (1969) has also described this symptom, and relates it to the patient who "with a distorted body image has lost awareness of the involved side of his body". The patient, however, remains surprisingly unperturbed, showing no fear, even though the therapist may be experiencing difficulty in holding him upright (**Fig. 14.8 a**).

As Perry writes, "he will make no attempt to support or otherwise accommodate for the weight of that side if the lesion is complete and thus falls toward the involved side without making an effort to protect himself". He expresses alarm only when the therapist tries to achieve a vertical posture for him. Remarkably, some patients actually pivot sideways with the sound foot to avoid being brought vertically over that leg. The legs are adducted, and the hemiplegic leg flexes and takes little if any weight. The flexion increases when the feet are apart (**Fig. 14.8 b**). As the patient stands up from sitting his left leg may even flex up in the air, which it will certainly do if the therapist attempts to bring his weight over his sound leg (**Fig. 14.8 c**).

Brunnstrom (1970) has observed this symptom and writes that in "rather unusual cases the flexor synergy dominates the motor behaviour of the lower limb", sometimes to the extent that the patient is unable to lower the limb to the floor in standing.

During all standing attempts the sound leg is held constantly in exaggerated extension, and the influence of the crossed extensor reflex thus elicited further increases flexor hypertonicity in the hemiplegic leg. In addition, the fixed position of the patient's neck, with his head rotated constantly towards the sound side, will also have an adverse effect on the tone and activity in his limbs due to the influence of the asymmetrical tonic reflex (ATNR) described in Chap. 3. With insufficient extensor tone in the affected lower limb, the patient is unable to take weight on his hemiplegic leg in standing, and this adds to his difficulty in maintaining an upright posture.

14. When he is standing, the patient leans back against the therapist's supporting arm. The shortening of the sound side of the trunk becomes more marked in standing, through overactivity. The head is held fixedly, inclined laterally towards the sound side (**Fig. 14.9**). Some patients flex their trunk forwards from the hips and fail to stand fully upright at all.

15. If it is possible to walk with the patient, the hemiplegic leg adducts so strongly that it may even cross over in front of the other leg as it is brought forwards (**Fig. 14.10 a**). Brunnstrom (1970) describes how the affected limb assumes a "scissors" posture in front of the other limb when the weight is shifted towards the normal side. The patient has difficulty in taking a step with his affected leg because he is unable to transfer his weight over the sound side before doing so (**Fig. 14.10 b**). Taking a step with the sound leg is difficult due to the inadequate extensor activity in the hemiplegic limb needed to support his weight.

16. As the patient walks towards his chair or the plinth, supported by the therapist, he sits down prematurely. He grasps the arm of the chair and starts sitting down when he is still inappropriately far away, and without turning round to align himself with his back to the chair (**Fig. 14.11**). The therapist has difficulty in supporting his weight, and the patient is often unable to interrupt the movement of sitting down

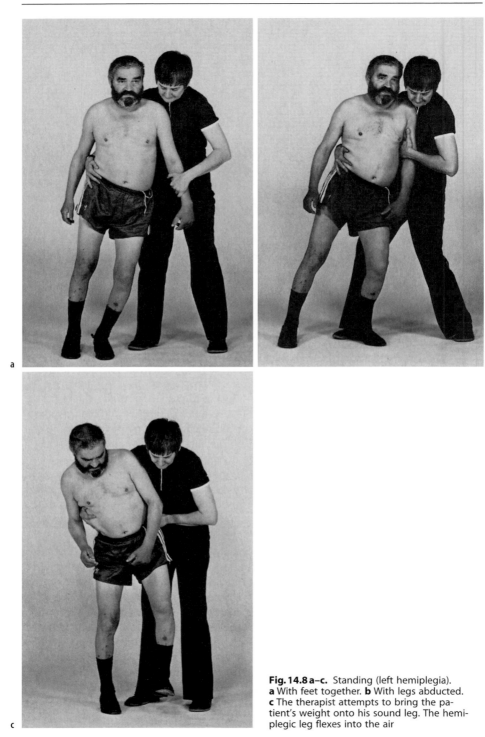

Fig. 14.8 a–c. Standing (left hemiplegia).
a With feet together. **b** With legs abducted.
c The therapist attempts to bring the patient's weight onto his sound leg. The hemiplegic leg flexes into the air

Fig. 14.9. Typical standing posture with the patient pushing strongly towards her hemiplegic side (left hemiplegia)

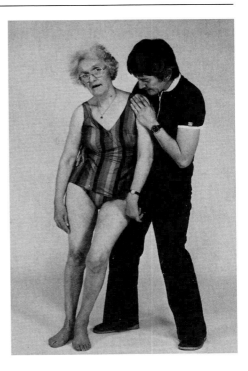

Fig. 14.10a, b. Difficulties in walking (left hemiplegia) **a** Adduction of the hemiplegic leg during the swing phase causes the foot to cross in front of the other. **b** Taking a step with the hemiplegic foot is a problem because weight cannot be transferred onto the sound side
▽

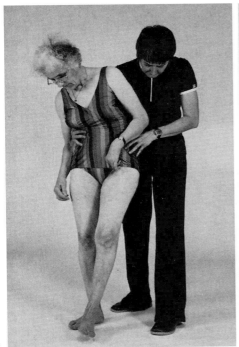

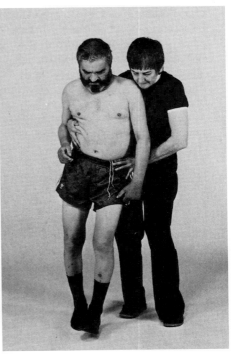

a   b

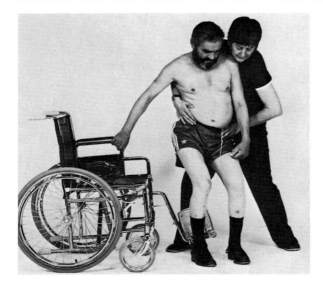

Fig. 14.11. Sitting down too soon (left hemiplegia)

in order to correct his position despite the therapist calling out to him to wait. The problem arises because the patient reacts immediately on a visual stimulus, in this case, the wheelchair. Similar difficulties are likely to occur in other situations where he sees an object and cannot stop the action from taking place at once. For example, when food or drink is placed in front of him he will immediately start eating or drinking until there is nothing left. If the therapist is practising going up stairs with the patient she needs to anticipate the problem, because the moment he sees the first step he will rapidly start climbing even before she has had time to put her hands in place to support him.

17. Those patients who have no aphasia tend to talk a great deal and offer many explanations for their failure in performance. The patient also requires constant verbal instructions from the therapist, even though the situation itself or the information provided by her hands would seem to be sufficient. For example, when the patient has taken a step forwards with his right foot and the therapist asks him to take another step, he may ask her which foot he should move.

18. The patient has considerable difficulty in learning to dress himself, and with the activities of daily living in general.

19. His sound hand appears clumsy when he tries to perform skilled tasks, even though it is often his dominant hand.

20. Many of the problems described in Chap. 1 are experienced by patients manifesting the pusher syndrome and will need to be treated accordingly.

Predisposing Factors

Despite the obvious difficulties encountered in rehabilitation, as yet no plausible explanation has been found for the occurrence of the syndrome in about 10% of patients following first stroke (Pedersen et al. 1996). Computer tomography, performed at a mean duration of 11 days in this study, revealed no specific difference in lesion side, but patients with ipsilateral pushing had more severe strokes. However, other authors found that most patients who demonstrated the typical symptoms after a period of not less than 4 weeks had marked lesions in the right parietal lobe and its connections to the lateral thalamus, and that all the lesions were in the area supplied by the medial cerebral artery (Wolff et al. 1991).

With regard to recovery from stroke, Pedersen and co-authors (1996) found that ipsilateral pushing did not affect final functional outcome per se but slowed the process of recovery considerably and prolonged the stay in hospital by 63%. Kinsella and Ford (1985) consider that "the most debilitating feature of a right hemisphere lesion is the emergence of hemi-inattention or unilateral neglect, which can be defined as the failure to report or respond to stimuli delivered to the side contralateral to the affected hemisphere. Functionally, such a patient will need supervision since he fails to integrate all sensory stimuli from the environment and is unable to deal with a dynamic environment." It has also been noted that, "poor outcomes appear to be particularly associated with right hemisphere damage (particularly when this is associated with attentional and/or proprioceptive deficits)" (Riddoch et al. 1995) The need for specific treatment to overcome such problems is obviously crucial; it must not be forgotten that "factors other than CT findings could also influence discharge Barthel index" (Saeki et al. 1994). The study by Saeki et al. also showed that only one selected location, the right parietal lobe, had a negative influence on the discharge status.

Certainly, from a clinical point of view, the fixed position of the patient's head with hyperactivity of the neck muscles unilaterally could contribute to the disturbance of subjective body orientation reported by Karnath (1994). Vibrating the posterior neck muscles on one side caused normal subjects to have a displaced subjective localisation of the body's sagittal midplane by altering the proprioceptive signals from their necks. The illusory displacement was usually in the horizontal dimension and to the side opposite to that of the vibratory stimulation (Biguer et al. 1988). Perhaps even more compelling evidence for the effects of altered muscle tone proprioception on subjective body orientation is provided by the personal experience of Kesselring (1994). During a circus performance by two roller skaters, Kesselring, himself a neurologist, was chosen by chance from the audience to participate in their act. After being spun round clockwise 15 times on a round table at a speed of 360°/s supported between the two artists, he experienced "the illusion of the ground being tilted to the right side and consequently falling of the body to the left". The artists were unable to bring him back into a vertical posture at first, so strongly did he push towards his left side, the phenomenon graphically illustrated by a photograph taken at the time. Kesselring describes the symptoms as being similar to those observed in the "pusher syndrome". Immediate neurological examination revealed slight nystagmus and definitely exaggerated reflexes in both legs, but no extensor plantar response. In conclusion, the author writes that, "The observation supports the hypothesis that vestibulogenic postural asymmetries may be an adjustment of the body[sic] long axis to align with what the nervous system erroneously computes as being vertical" (Brandt and Dietrich 1987; Gresty et al. 1992) In addition to altered neck muscle proprioception, it has been postulated that disturbed input from the vestibular system as well as disturbed central transformation of afferent information from the periphery can lead to a displaced subjective localisation of the body in space (Karnath 1994). The postural disturbances are further accentuated by the constant rotation of the head towards the sound side, because with the resultant alterations in muscle tone in the limbs and trunk, the afferent information received from them is most confusing.

Whatever factors may be involved in causing the syndrome with its disabling signs and symptoms, a specific treatment programme aimed at helping the patient to overcome the difficulties is of prime importance.

Specific Treatment

All the activities which have been described in the preceding chapters can be included in the treatment, when applicable to the patient's individual needs. Particularly important are those to enable the patient to bear weight on his hemiplegic leg, e. g. bridging, knee extension and retraining balance reactions in all positions. Correct rolling to both sides helps to re-establish head-righting reactions, and also to orientate the patient in space. As he rolls over he makes contact with the surface of the bed or mat, and the total resistance which he encounters informs him that he has completed the movement.

Guiding his hands during problem-solving tasks will help to overcome the perceptual disturbances which are always present. The therapist needs to apply the principle of providing the patient with correct tactile/kinaesthetic input for his whole body during activity. She guides his whole body during the movement sequence if necessary. The patient's position in the wheelchair is particularly important, with a firm back support to maintain extension of the trunk. He should sit with his weight inclined forward and his arms supported on a table in front of him, as the half-reclining posture seems to reinforce those symptoms which are seen when he is standing. The arm rest on his unaffected side should be removed so that he does not constantly push on it during the day.

Attention is given to restoring facial expression and to improving the quality of the patient's voice and breathing. In addition, the following specific activities should be included in the treatment programme.

Restoring Movements of the Head

It is essential to free the head from its fixed position of lateral flexion and rotation to the sound side, so that particularly side flexion toward the hemiplegic side without resistance must be maintained or regained. The therapist performs full passive range of movement of the neck, with the patient lying supine at first, because there is far less resistance to the movements in a position where the head is supported, and she can ensure that no contractures develop.

With the head of the plinth lowered, the therapist moves the patient's head right over to one side with full lateral flexion of his neck. Her hand nearest to him supports the weight of his head, with her elbow propped on her iliac crest. By transferring her weight sideways she moves the patient's head by pressing against it with the palm of her hand, instead of by pulling it over with her flexed fingers (**Fig. 14.12 a**). Her other hand is placed over his shoulder girdle to prevent its elevating when the head moves. Alternatively, the therapist can keep the patient's neck in a position of lateral flexion while with her other hand she gently moves his shoulder girdle repeatedly down towards his pelvis and back up again (**Fig. 14.12 b**) The passive movements are much more comfortable for the patient if the therapist performs them by transferring her body weight from one side to the other, rather than using the muscles of her arms for the activity, and he will therefore be better able to relax his neck muscles and not resist the motion. The movements also need to be carried out when the patient is sitting, but a gradual progression is usually necessary instead of a sudden change from lying to sitting upright. Once the range of motion is full and free to both sides when the patient is lying down, the therapist raises the head of the plinth slightly before continuing to mobilise his neck to both sides. As long as the range of lateral flexion continues to be full and without resistance, the therapist gradually raises the headrest further and further towards the upright position (**Fig. 14.12 c**). She changes her position and that of her hands each time before moving his head towards the other side (**Fig. 14.12 d**).

Once the patient is sitting fully upright and no longer requires the support of the headrest, he is better able to release the neck muscles when given tactile cues. The therapist places her hand against the side of his head and starts to move it sideways. When she encounters a resistance she asks him to relieve the pressure against her hand, and he moves his head so that the resistance against her hand decreases. The movement also becomes easier for the patient if she asks him to bring his head sideways to lean against her. The patient is then aware of achieving the correct movement when he feels his head against the therapist, which orientates him. When mobilising the neck, the therapist will need to give counter-pressure against the shoulder on the opposite side to the direction of the lateral flexion, in the same way as she did in the supine position. When the nurse or the patient's wife is talking to him, she too can encourage side flexion of his neck by standing at his hemiplegic side and helping him to lean his head against her, so that the beneficial mobilisation takes place more frequently during the day (**Fig. 14.13**).

Active movement of the neck is stimulated by using activities where the patient is required to turn his head towards the hemiplegic side in order to look at an object, e.g. to bat away a ball or balloon. When standing with the help of the therapist and with a table or plinth in front of him, turning his head towards the hemiplegic side will enhance extension in his paretic leg. If necessary, a knee extension splint can be used to support his leg (see **Figs. 14.15** and **14.16**) The therapist stands close to the patient on his hemiplegic side and uses her hip to keep his hip well forward against the plinth while he hits the ball away. To encourage activity in the hemiplegic arm at the same time, the patient can hold a short pole in both hands and use it to bat away a volley ball thrown at him by another person. The therapist places her hands over his to maintain their position on the cane and facilitate a symmetrical movement of both his arms, and the thrower moves gradually more and more to the left of the patient (**Fig. 14.14**).

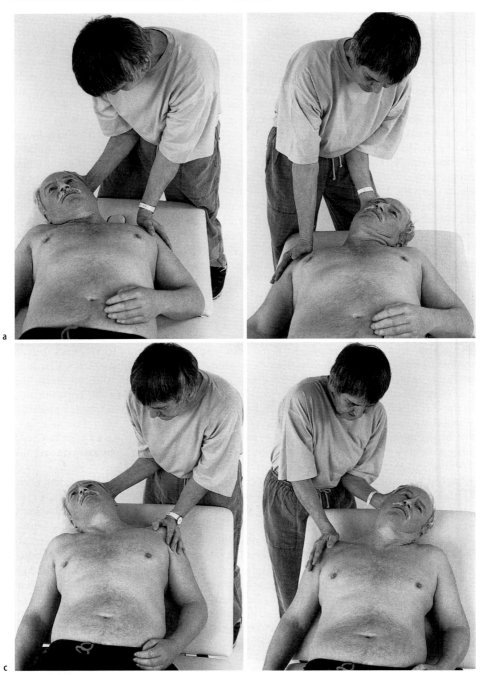

Fig. 14.12 a–d. Mobilising lateral flexion of the neck (left hemiplegia). **a** With the plinth flat, the therapist uses the palm of her hand to move the patient's head sideways. **b** Depressing the shoulder girdle with the head held to the opposite side. **c** Mobilisation continues as the head of the plinth is gradually elevated. **d** The headrest is raised as far as is possible without losing range of neck motion

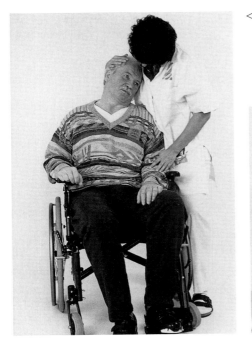

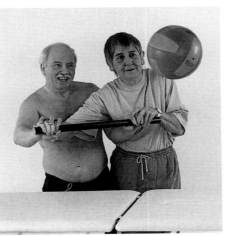

◁ **Fig. 14.13.** The nursing sister standing at the patient's hemiplegic side encourages him to rest his head on her shoulder (left hemiplegia)

Fig. 14.14. Standing with a table in front of him, the patient hits a ball with a pole held in both hands (left hemiplegia)

Stimulating Activity in the Hypotonic Trunk Side Flexors

Because of the hypotonus and inactivity of the hemiplegic side the patient has difficulty in transferring his weight towards the sound side (**Fig. 14.15 a**). For example, he cannot cross the hemiplegic leg over the other leg to put on a sock. When trying to walk, he is unable to free the hemiplegic leg to take a step forward. The hemiplegic side lengthens instead of shortening, and the sound side shortens instead of lengthening.

1. To facilitate shortening of the left side of the trunk and head-righting to the left, the patient sits with his hemiplegic leg crossed over the other one. The therapist stands in front of him, keeping his legs in place with her legs. With her left hand round behind his shoulders and her right hand under his left buttock, she helps the patient to transfer his weight over the right side. When the head fails to come to the vertical, the therapist uses her left forearm to correct its position, asking the patient not to push against her arm. He feels the pressure of his head against her arm and moves his head away to relieve the pressure, and the correct reaction is automatically achieved (see **Fig. 7.3 b**). He maintains the position when the therapist removes her supporting hands. The movement is repeated and the patient then tries to move into exactly the same position without the therapist's assistance.

2. Sitting or standing beside the patient, the therapist asks him to take his weight away from her. With one hand she presses the muscles of the side of his trunk firmly, using the web between thumb and index finger to encourage their contraction. The pres-

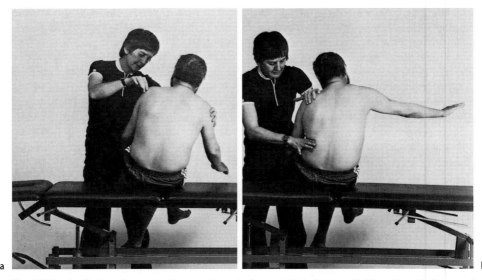

a   b

Fig. 14.15 a, b. Sitting with crossed legs and transferring weight to the sound side. **a** The side flexors of the trunk remain inactive. **b** The therapist stimulates activity in the hemiplegic side (left hemiplegia)

sure is applied intermittently. With her other hand she pushes down on the patient's shoulder to stimulate the correct righting reaction of the head, through stretch (**Fig. 14.15 b**).

3. The patient learns to lean towards the sound side, support himself on his elbow and then return to the upright position without pushing off with his hand. As he does so, the head rights automatically and the trunk side flexors are activated. The therapist facilitates the correct movement by placing one of her arms across the back of the patient's shoulders in such a way that she can control the speed of the movement and use her forearm to push down on his hemiplegic shoulder to stimulate head-righting to vertical (see **Fig. 7.1 b**). With her other hand she holds his sound hand lightly and reminds him not to use it to assist the movement. The activity is intensified by asking the patient to lean slowly to the sound side and stop before his flexed elbow touches the plinth. He can also stop and start at various stages of the movement or change directions.

Regaining the Midline in Standing

The longer the patient remains seated in a wheelchair, the more the flexion in his leg and trunk increases. It is therefore most important to start standing at an early stage. The lack of extensor activity in the leg makes the upright position difficult for the therapist to support. The more she holds the patient, the more he tends to lean or push towards her. If she tries to fix the patient's knee in extension with her knees, she has to stand so close to him that she is unable to move or support other parts of his body.

Using a back slab made of a hard material such as plaster of Paris (**Fig. 14.16**) to hold the patient's leg in extension is therefore the method of choice and changes the procedure amazingly. The use of a knee extension splint for helping the patient to stand cannot be recommended highly enough because it is a key to improving so many of his abilities. The back slab is bandaged firmly into place with at least two 12-cm crepe bandages, which must not be too elastic or else the knee will still flex forward. It is usually necessary to put on the splint with the patient in lying, because in sitting, extension of the knee is often restricted and painful. With the splint firmly in place, the therapist helps the patient to stand up in the quickest and easiest way possible, it being somewhat difficult for him to come upright because of the extended knee. Once he is standing, activities are immediately carried out which automatically elicit the desired posture and movement without the patient being dependent upon verbal instructions and feedback from the therapist.

1. The patient taps a balloon to a third person with his sound hand. The balloon is patted back to him high in the air so that he has to reach up to hit it back (**Fig. 14.17**). Immediately, his right side elongates and the standing posture is corrected.
2. The same effect can be obtained by introducing any appropriate activity which requires that he reach forwards and upwards with his sound hand. For example, play-

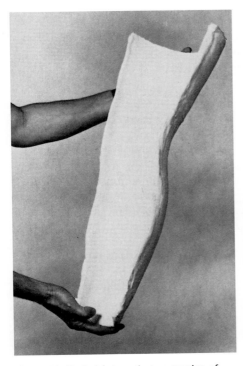

Fig. 14.16. Back slab to activate extension of the hemiplegic knee

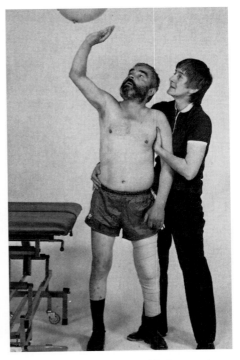

Fig. 14.17. Hitting a balloon with the sound hand elongates the side of the trunk (left hemiplegia)

ing a tambourine with different rhythms or even beating time to music will provide a good stimulus (**Fig. 14.18**). The tambourine or the balloon can be placed so that the patient needs to turn his head in different directions. He learns to turn his head to the left and make eye contact with objects on that side of him. At first, the patient may feel more secure if a high plinth is placed in front of him and he keeps his hips forward by maintaining contact with the plinth. The therapist stands on the patient's affected side and ensures that his weight is over both legs during the activity. She does not use verbal correction, as the patient is concentrating on performing the activity and should not be distracted. She simply adjusts his trunk and pelvis to achieve the desired position. If the stimulus is adequate, the patient will be able to tolerate the standing position for far longer, and extensor activity in his leg improve as a result.

3. To mobilise the trunk and improve hip extension, the patient clasps his hands together, rests his forehead on his hands and then flexes forwards until his elbows touch the plinth (**Fig. 14.19 a**) The therapist has the arm nearest to the patient around his body with her hand over his abdomen so that she can ensure symmetrical flexion of his whole trunk. Her other hand is beneath his clasped hands, to give him confidence as he bends down, and ready to assist his coming back to the upright position again. With her hip pressed against his from behind, she helps him to keep his thigh in contact with the edge of the plinth throughout the activity. By keeping his forehead

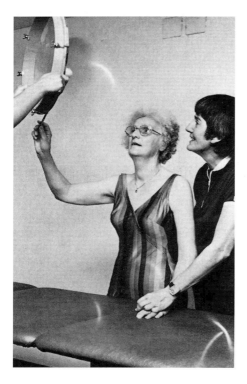

Fig. 14.18. Playing a tambourine prevents shortening of the sound side of the trunk (left hemiplegia)

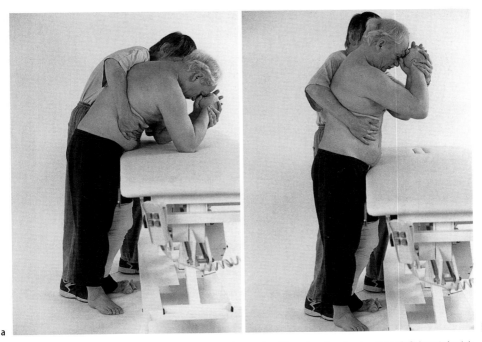

a   b

Fig. 14.19 a, b. Mobilising the trunk and improving active hip extension in standing (left hemiplegia).
a With his forehead resting on his clasped hands, the patient brings his elbows down to touch the plinth. **b** Returning to the upright position without extending his neck

on his clasped hands, the patient does not extend his neck overactively when he stands up, as he would otherwise do to compensate for the inadequate hip extension (**Fig. 14.19 b**).

4. Standing with his sound side to the plinth, the patient is asked to shift his weight until he feels his right hip touching it. At first he supports himself with his right hand on the plinth as he repeats the movement, moving his hip to the plinth and then away from it (**Fig. 14.20 a**). The therapist uses her hands to shorten the hemiplegic side of his trunk, one hand pushing down on his shoulder and the other pressing into the trunk side flexors to stimulate activity (**Fig. 14.20 b**). The activity is performed with the patient standing with his legs more and more abducted, and he tries to lift his hand from the plinth while continuing the movement.

5. The patient practises taking weight through the hemiplegic leg and can be asked to kick a football with his sound foot (**Fig. 14.21**).

6. A most effective way to help the patient regain the feeling for the midline is for him to stand in a doorway, still wearing the knee splint, and move his body to contact the door frame on either side. The therapist stands on his hemiplegic side and, without moving his feet, the patient shifts his weight right over the sound side until his hip and the side of his trunk are pressing against the hard frame (**Fig. 14.22 a**). He then transfers his weight to the hemiplegic side until his body is in contact with the

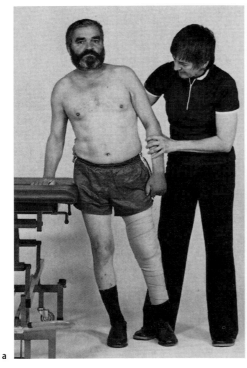 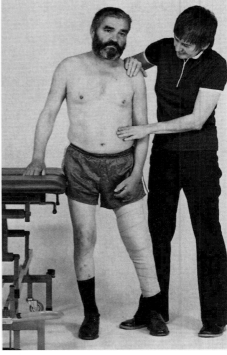

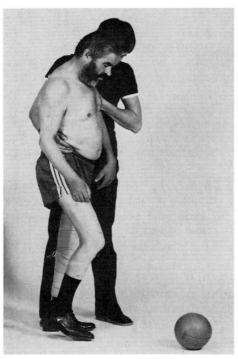

△
Fig. 14.20 a, b. Standing with the back slab, moving the weight sideways towards a plinth (left hemiplegia). **a** The patient supports too much weight with his sound hand on the plinth. **b** The therapist facilitates shortening of the hemiplegic side

Fig. 14.21. Kicking a football with the sound foot (left hemiplegia)

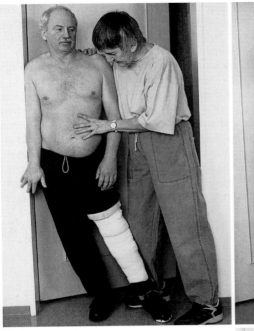

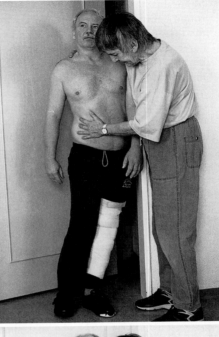

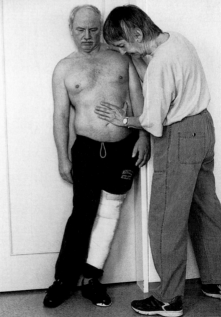

Fig. 14.22 a–c. Standing and moving sideways in a doorway with trunk activity facilitated (left hemiplegia). **a** Trunk and hip in contact with the frame on the sound side. **b** Shifting weight over the hemiplegic leg. **c** Additional support provided by the closed door

frame on that side of him (**Fig. 14.22 b**). The therapist supports him with one arm round behind his shoulders. Should the patient be very unstable in standing, either the therapist can stand behind him while he moves sideways or the door can be securely closed to prevent his falling backwards (**Fig. 14.22 c**).

7. Because the hemiplegic side is rotated backwards, the patient needs to practise bringing his left shoulder forwards in order to improve his balance. The therapist helps him to bring the whole side forwards and then he is asked to stay there, or to repeat the movement with less help. Swinging to hit a balloon with his hemiplegic arm often facilitates the correct movement. The therapist places her hands on the patient's shoulders and first rotates his left side back in readiness for the swing (**Fig. 14.23 a**). The balloon is thrown to the patient and the therapist helps him to swing his whole side forwards so that his hand hits the balloon (**Fig. 14.23 b**). Even if the arm has no active movement, the patient can hit the balloon away by swinging his hand forwards from the shoulder. He is instructed not to try to lift his arm, but rather to swing it forwards like a tennis racket.

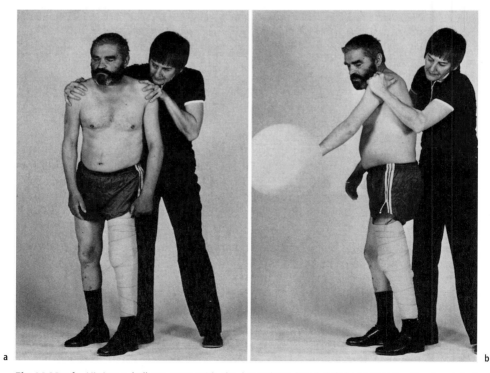

a   b

Fig. 14.23 a, b. Hitting a balloon away with the hemiplegic hand (left hemiplegia). **a** Trunk rotated back in readiness for the swing; **b** swinging forward to hit the balloon

Starting to Walk

Immediately following these activities, the therapist removes the back slab, preferably with the patient still standing, because otherwise he may lose the feeling for the midline again. The patient should not attempt to walk with the knee extension splint still on because an abnormal stiff-legged gait would then be encouraged.

He stands with his sound side against the plinth and, when the bandages have been removed, attempts to maintain the extension of his leg actively. He is asked to walk around the plinth, trying to feel his hip against it all the time (**Fig. 14.24**). The plinth gives him the orientation he requires to remain in the midline position. After walking around the plinth he may be able to continue walking away from it, with the therapist supporting him from the pelvis or thorax. It is easier for him to walk to a set goal, for example to his wheelchair placed some distance away. Parallel bars are not used, because the patient would pull himself towards the bar with his sound hand and not learn the correct mechanism of transferring his weight over the sound side. Using the flat surface of the plinth or a table provides the correct stimulus for the activity.

When kicking a football with his hemiplegic foot the patient transfers his weight spontaneously over the sound leg. Either the therapist puts his foot back in such a way as to allow him to kick with a good swing, or he can take a step forward with his sound leg (**Fig. 14.25 a, b**). The ball is placed in the correct position for the kick until the patient is sufficiently advanced and can kick a moving ball. The action of kicking the ball also facilitates the swing phase of gait, because the movement components are very similar.

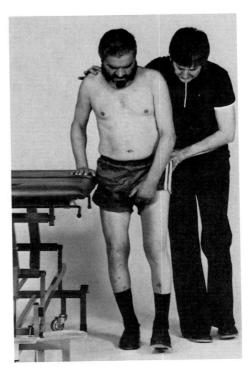

Fig. 14.24. Walking, keeping the sound hip in contact with the plinth (left hemiplegia)

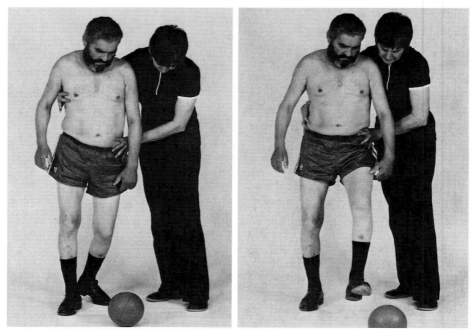

Fig. 14.25 a, b. Kicking a football with the hemiplegic foot (left hemiplegia). **a** Foot moved back in preparation for the kick. **b** Weight shifted spontaneously over the sound side for the kick

Climbing Stairs

Going up and down stairs provides the patient with an excellent stimulus. Even though he cannot balance while standing or walk without support, he can climb the stairs with facilitation from the therapist (**Fig. 14.26**). The flight of stairs offers him the information he requires to carry out the necessary movements. The therapist assists him in the way described in Chap. 7. It is often surprising how well the patient performs on the stairs, and how much better he can walk immediately afterwards.

Considerations

Patients who cannot transfer weight towards the sound side have difficulty in learning to walk and regain independence. Giving the patient a walking stick or cane does not help at all because he only uses it to push more strongly towards his affected side. Although the rehabilitation takes longer, it is well worth the effort, and the gait pattern is often surprisingly good in the end. The more the patient stands and walks, the sooner

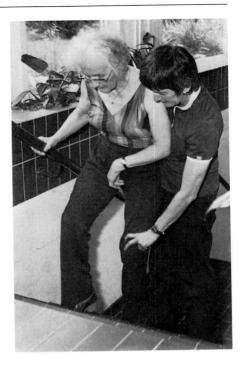

Fig. 14.26. Climbing stairs stimulates selective movement of the legs and improves midline orientation (compare Fig. 14.10 a) (left hemiplegia)

he learns to balance in the upright position. He should be helped to stand during those activities in his daily life which he normally performed in the standing position, for example combing his hair or shaving in the morning (**Fig. 14.27**). The firm surface of the basin in front of him helps his orientation, and because he is moving his head freely his vertical posture is automatically corrected.

During therapy the patient should be given as much tactile information as possible from his environment, as his own internal feedback system is disturbed. He needs the information from his surroundings in order to orientate himself in space and to learn to move again. When the patient is leaning towards his hemiplegic side and he is told by a helper to move his weight to the other side, or to the right, he is entirely dependent on the information he receives from his own sensation, which is disturbed. He is therefore unable to respond correctly. In the same way, he will probably not be able to react to a purely verbal instruction from the therapist, such as "put your hip forward" or "stand with more weight on your right leg".

Placing a fixed resistance beside or in front of him will enable him to carry out the movement if he is asked to move his weight until he feels the stable surface with his hip. The therapist can use her own body or her hand to provide the patient with a control point. She asks him to move his hip away from her hip or his head to or away from her hand. He feels the pressure or the resistance, and can then move so that he no longer feels it.

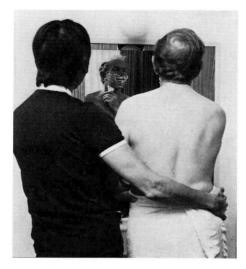

Fig. 14.27. Standing at the washbasin while shaving (left hemiplegia)

The principle is applied throughout the treatment and in the patient's daily life. When the patient is being assisted to transfer, it helps if he puts his hands forwards onto a stool placed in front of him, rather than just forwards in space. As his ability to feel improves, the patient will require less and less information from his surroundings. He will have learnt the movements. Patients with the problems described respond far better to walking and climbing stairs than to trying to learn to stand. Standing balance improves as a result of walking and carrying out actual tasks while standing. Both the patient and the therapist become frustrated and resigned if standing is practised unsuccessfully in isolation, as a prerequisite for walking.

15 Including Nervous System Mobilisation in the Treatment

Any action, reaction or interaction with the environment is possible only if a muscle contracts. It has in fact been said that, "To move is all mankind can do and for such the sole executant is muscle, whether in whispering a syllable or in felling a forest" (Sherrington 1947). However, it must not be overlooked that every movement entails accommodation on the part of the nervous system through an adaptive lengthening or shortening of nerves and neural structures, and that every muscle contraction is the result of an impulse transported by nerves. It is as if the motor systems were "servants" to the rest of the nervous system, in that they can only respond or not respond, depending upon the integrity of the different sensory systems and the integrative action of the system as a whole (Tuchmann-Duplessis et al. 1975). In addition to being the "master" of movement, the nervous system is also essential for respiratory function, heart rate, and circulation, and all perceptual modalities are dependent upon the information it transports to and from the brain.

The main function of the nervous system is to generate and transport nerve impulses, which it has to do without interruption in a great variety of movements and postures. To make this function possible, the nervous system has the property of adaptive lengthening. The term 'neurodynamics' is used by Shacklock (1995) to encompass the close interactions between mechanical and physiological functions in the system. The entire nervous system is a continuum and has roughly the shape of an H on its side when the arms and legs are abducted (Butler 1991). The H form can be visualised in Leonardo da Vinci's famous drawing from 1492, depicting the proportions of the human body (Fig. 15.1).

The peripheral and central nervous systems should be considered as one system because they form a continuous tissue tract of nervous and supporting tissues with horizontal and vertical connections. The spinal cord is continuous with the brain stem above and with the cauda equina, nerve roots and peripheral nerves below (Massey 1986).

The nervous system is a continuum in three ways (Butler 1991):

1. The connective tissues are continuous, although in different formats, and a single axon can be associated with a number of the connective tissues.
2. The neurons are interconnected electrically to allow even an impulse generated in the foot to be received by the brain.
3. The system is continuous chemically through the flow of cytoplasm in the axons, with the same neurotransmitters centrally and peripherally.

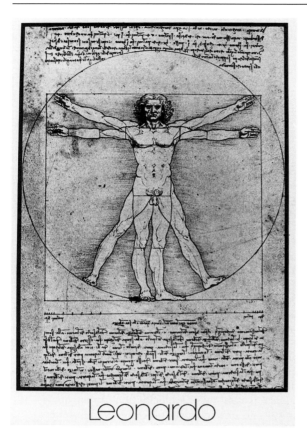

Leonardo

Fig. 15.1. With the arms and legs abducted, the nervous system has approximately the shape of an "H" on its side, as can be visualised in Leonardo da Vinci's famous drawing, "Le proporzioni del corpo umano" (1452)

Adaptation of the Nervous System to Movement

Every movement of the body, no matter how slight, results in some movement of the nervous system with an adjustment in the length and breadth of the nerves and neural tissues. For unimpeded movement of the neck, trunk and limbs adaptive lengthening of the nervous system, sometimes to a surprising extent, is essential.

Elongation of the Neural Canal

Within the neural canal, the neuraxis or spinal cord extends from the medulla oblongata right down to the filum terminale and has therefore to lengthen considerably during movements of the trunk. For example, when the trunk flexes forward from full extension the spinal canal has to elongate by 6–9 cm, and lateral flexion of the spine from one side to the other alters its length by 15 % (Breig 1978; Louis 1981). With the spine extended, the neural canal shortens. Because the nervous system is a continuous tissue tract, even without the trunk itself moving, structures within the neural canal will also be lengthened by movements of the limbs. The traction on the peripheral nerves tenses the nerve roots and hence the cord. For example, with the hip flexed and the knee extended, the addition of dorsiflexion of the foot adds further stretch to the cord via the posterior tibial and sciatic nerves, the effect reaching as far as the brain (Breig and Troup 1979). Likewise, when the neck is flexed passively, the neuraxis and the meninges in the lumbar spine and in part of the sciatic tract are moved and tensioned as well (Breig and Marions 1963)

Elongation of Peripheral Nerves

The peripheral nerves run in much the same direction as the muscles that move the limbs and therefore need to adapt their length in relation to the action of the muscles. For example, when the elbow and wrist are extended, the median nerve is 20 % longer than it is when they are in flexion (Millesi 1986).

Elongation of the Autonomic Nervous System

"Often overlooked is the fact that the autonomic nervous system (ANS) must also adapt to body movements if it is to function correctly" (Butler 1991). The autonomic fibres in the neuraxis and in peripheral nerves have to adapt in the same way as do the motor and sensory fibres. Because of its location, the sympathetic chain lengthens and shows changes in tension during movements of the vertebral column and the ribs.

Lengthening Mechanisms

Although nerves themselves are inelastic, the nervous system is able to lengthen adaptively to accommodate for body movements and postures and also to provide protection against injury through traction. The term 'neurodynamics' has been suggested to describe the close interactions between mechanical and physiological functions of the nervous system. Various mechanisms make the changes in length possible:
1. *Unfolding, untwisting and unwinding of neural structures.* Nerve roots have an inbuilt mechanism in that they lie in undulations that can unfold. The axons or nerve fibres, both centrally and peripherally, follow an undulatory course and can therefore lengthen by straightening out the corrugations (Butler 1991). Likewise, the dura has collagenous fibres which are wavy when not stretched and straight when stretched and thus allow lengthening (Massey 1986). In addition, the dura accommodates to changes in length by an axial shift, with two thirds of the movement being through dural shift and one third due to unfolding, according to Adams and Logue (1971).
2. *Sliding and gliding movements of neural structures.* Both peripherally and centrally, nerves move in relation to the tissues which surround them, and neural tissue elements move in relation to connective tissue. "The body is the container of the nervous system. Within the body, the musculoskeletal system is the mechanical inter-

face" (Shacklock 1995). Butler (1989) describes the interfacing tissues as being those against which the nervous system moves, and defines the mechanical interface as "that tissue or material adjacent to the nervous system that can move independently to the system". He describes the interface as being either intraneural, within the system itself, or extraneural, that is "outside" the nervous system. The mechanical interface may consist of muscle, bone, joint, fibro-osseous tunnels, fascial sheets or blood vessels, while a pathological interface could be an osteophyte, a swelling or fascial scarring.

Intraneural movement refers to movements of neural tissue elements in relation to the connective tissue interfaces within the system. With normal neurodynamics, there is free movement of connective tissue within the nerves; these are free to glide smoothly within their sheaths, or their bundles of fascicles can slide smoothly in relation to each other (McKibbin 1995). Similarly, the spinal cord can move easily in relation to the dura mater.

Extraneural movements are those where the nervous system moves in relation to the interface which surrounds it from without. Although the normal nervous system is able to move freely to adapt to different postures and motions, at certain sites within the system there is no movement or only minimal movement in relation to surrounding structures when a part of the body moves or is moved. The neural structures can only move together with the interface. Examples of these sites, which Butler (1989) terms "tension points", are the areas of C-6 and T-6, the posterior knee region and the anterior aspect of the elbow. Normally, the tension points do not interfere with the adaptation of the nervous system to elongation, but in the presence of pathologically increased tension, they may cause symptoms such as pain, stiffness or dysfunction to spread to other areas, particularly in the limbs.

3. *Development of tension or increased pressure in the neural structures and tissues and changes in their shape or form.* When nerves elongate the pressure within them increases and they become narrower with a smaller lumen, in the same way as a rubber tube does when it is stretched. For instance, changes in tension in the spinal cord are revealed by alterations in its shape during flexion of the trunk in addition to its adaptive movement. Angulations and compressions of neural tissues occur as well, because the pressure develops in all tissues and fluids.

Loss of Nervous System Mobility Following a Lesion

Following any lesion of the nervous system, be it central or peripheral, an abnormal increase in tension develops which interferes with its mobility and thus with its normal functioning Adaptive lengthening is impeded by the increased tension and, because the nervous system is a continuum of interrelated nerves and neural tissues, it is easy to understand that abnormal tension in any area will affect other parts of the system adversely as well (**Fig. 15.2**).

Clinical experience has revealed that the neuraxis is always involved following a brain lesion, and its lost mobility gives rise to significant problems. Prolonged abnormal pos-

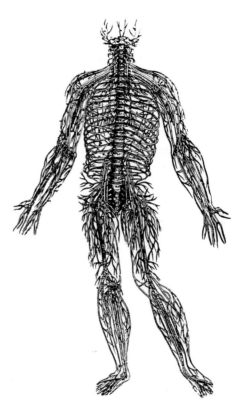

Fig. 15.2. The nervous system is a continuous tissue tract with horizontal and vertical connections

tures and the immobility due to paralysis or muscle weakness so often associated with lesions of the central nervous system tend to enhance and sustain the increased tension, causing further resistance to free movement. For example, sitting with a thoracic kyphosis – the lumbar spine flexed and the neck in extension with the chin poked forward – places undue tension on the sympathetic nervous system, and the sustained thoracic kyphosis increases tension. Such a posture is typical for patients who are still in a wheelchair throughout the day if their position is not adjusted and too little support is provided for their trunk and limbs.

"The term 'pathodynamics' may be used to describe the combination of pathomechanical and pathophysiological events in disorders" (Shacklock 1995). With regard to the treatment of patients with lesions of the central nervous system, Rolf (1999b) uses the term 'patho-neurodynamics' to encompass fully the complex disturbances occurring in the entire system and to differentiate between pathological processes affecting the system itself and those affecting target tissues.

Effect on Target Tissues

Not only does the nervous system suffer as a result of loss of mobility; its target tissues are affected as well. All structures and tissues within the body which are directly or indirectly innervated are, in effect, target tissues of the nervous system. These include muscles, joint complexes and their connective tissues, blood vessels and organs.

Conversely, the nervous system suffers from malfunctioning of the target tissues because it needs movement and mobility to remain healthy or to recover from injury or disease. Ironically, the nervous system is in effect its own target tissue because its connective tissues are innervated.

Problems Associated with Abnormal Tension and Loss of Mobility

In hemiplegia, increased adverse tension leading to loss of neural mobility is associated not only with symptoms of pain but also with many of the other commonly encountered problems. Pathoneurodynamics are certainly closely linked to most of the typical movement disorders and to the development of unpleasant symptoms, either as cause or effect. If left untreated, pathoneurodynamics will enhance and perpetuate the difficulties experienced by patients who have any of the following problems, and in their assessment, significantly increased tension will invariably be demonstrated.

Typical problems include the following

- *Abnormal Tone, either Hypertonus or Hypotonus*
Muscle tone throughout the body may be altered if neural tension is abnormally raised and is particularly noticeable in the distal segments of the limbs. With their rich innervation, the hand and foot often reveal a marked increase in tone which can lead to clonus at the ankle and even at the wrist. Because of the anatomical arrangement of nerves and muscles in the extremities, the directions in which the increased tension pulls the limbs closely resemble those of the so-called spastic patterns. Somewhat unexpectedly, also those patients whose muscles are very flaccid usually have a marked increase in nervous system tension, particularly if the hypotonicity persists. It could well be that the tension impedes or interrupts impulse conduction to the hypotonic muscles.

- *Abnormal Postures and Malalignments of the Body Segments and Limbs*
The patient may lie, sit or stand in abnormal postures, due to the forceful pull of the tense neural structures, and be unable to correct the deviations voluntarily. It is not unusual for the whole body to be pulled out of shape from head to toe. Interestingly, the abnormal or antalgic posture of a patient with increased tension resulting from a disc lesion, illustrated in Butler (1991), closely resembles the posture which has been described as being typical for hemiplegia. The alignment of different body segments may

be distorted, such as the pelvis being laterally shifted or the spine scoliosed or kyphosed. Frequently, the extremities adopt sustained, stereotypical positions, dependent upon where and to what extent neural tension is abnormally raised. For example, the shoulder is adducted and medially rotated with tension in the cervical and brachial plexuses, and the lower limb can be held constantly in abduction and lateral rotation by tension in the lumbar plexus.

- *Limitation of Range of Movement*

Any loss of range of motion in joints or soft tissues will always include a loss of nervous system mobility as well, either as cause or effect. The contractures may develop because of increased tension or the relevant nerves and neural tissue may become shortened through not being moved sufficiently. Whichever is the case, the condition will be self-reinforcing if steps are not taken to regain and maintain the full mobility of all the involved structures.

- *Loss of Selective Activity with Movements Possible Only in Mass Synergies*

Selective movements of the arms, legs and trunk are dependent upon the nervous system being able to move freely and fully. In addition, abnormal tension hampers or prevents the impulse conduction necessary for the complex control of selective movement. The loss of adaptive lengthening of the nerves and neural tissue restricts or prevents combined movements of the limbs such as elbow extension with the arm abducted, or knee extension when the hip is flexed. Without selective activity and mobility sufficient to allow combined movements, functional use of the arm is difficult, if not impossible to regain. Many of the commonly observed abnormalities in the stance and swing phase of gait are due to total mass synergies of movement and loss of nervous system mobility.

Tension in the neuraxis and other canal structures holds the vertebral column in extension, which impedes the return of tone and activity in the hypotonic abdominal muscles. The loss of abdominal muscle activity has grave consequences for the patient, because balance reactions and selective movements of the arms and legs are dependent upon selective trunk activity.

- *Inability to Feel Parts of the Body, with Sensation Decreased or Distorted*

Increased tension interferes with afferent and efferent nerve impulse transport, and the patient may have a loss of sensation or some of its modalities. Often the patient feels his limbs, but for him it is as though they are some distance away. Strange sensations experienced by patients with sensory disturbances have been described as being like "ants crawling" or "electrical shocks", while others suffer from a constant hyperaesthesia which makes even the touch of their clothes or another person unpleasant.

- *Persistent Pain of Undiagnosed Origin*

Abnormal tension in the nervous system can cause pain in bizarre distribution, which does not seem to fit in with any known diagnosis. Previously, such pain was usually erroneously termed "thalamic pain", or the patient was described as having a "thalamic pain syndrome". In actual fact, "lesions of the central nervous system rarely cause pain in previously pain-free individuals" (Fields 1987), and approximately half the patients diagnosed as having thalamic pain following a cerebrovascular lesion do not have lesions involving the thalamus at all (Boivie and Leijon 1991). Describing the difficulties involved in finding a satisfactory explanation for neuropathic pain, Wall (1991) warns, "In addition we are faced with a similarly challenging fact that chronic pain is never present in 100% of the cases with the pathology to which the pain is attributed". Certainly, "the cortex is not the pain center and neither is the thalamus. The areas of the brain involved in pain experience and behaviour are very extensive" (Melzack 1991). Because of the uncertainty regarding the cause of the pain suffered by some patients with hemiplegia, it has been more appropriately named "central post stroke pain" (CPSP) (Bowsher 1991) and described as "sympathetically maintained pain" by McMahon (1991). Regardless of which name is preferred or which hypothesis as to its cause is accepted, the fact remains that all patients with such pain have abnormally raised tension in the nervous system. Headaches and facial neuralgia are not uncommon, and usually increased neural tension is responsible for their development as well.

- *Shoulder Pain and the Shoulder-Hand Syndrome*
The relationship between increased neural tension and the problems of pain in the shoulder and the development of the swollen, painful hand are explained in Chap. 12. Whichever mechanism is originally responsible for any painful condition of the upper limb, increased tension in the nervous system is always present and is a contributory factor with regard to both the degree and the duration of the pain. Significant from a diagnostic and treatment point of view is the fact that the tension is found to be increased in the contralateral arm, the legs and the trunk, and not only during tests involving the affected upper limb itself.

- *Autonomic Nervous System Disturbances*
Circulatory disturbances are relatively common, and the patient's hand and foot feel cold and have a bluish colour. Increased sweating in the affected limbs can also be a problem. Some patients feel dizzy, and others may vomit when they move against gravity as a result of distorted and confusing impulses causing a "neural mismatch" (Reason 1978).

The Tension Tests for Assessment and Treatment

Tests of tension and restriction of movement in the nervous system have been considered important for many years, in addition to those procedures generally used in the assessment of musculoskeletal disorders. Different tests have been described and recommended by well-known experts in the field of manual therapy such as Cyriax (1942, 1978), Elvey (1979, 1984, 1986b), Grieve (1970) and Maitland (1979, 1985, 1986), to name but a few. More recently, in his book and during courses on his concept, David Butler recommends specific tests for the examination and treatment of orthopaedic patients and also for implementation as treatment techniques. Some of the tests have been taken from others, some adapted and some newly devised. Certain tests have been described as being particularly useful for the differentiation and alleviation of symptoms related to abnormal tension in the nervous system caused by brain lesions (Davies 1994). In this chapter, ways in which the tests, according to Butler (1991), can and should be included in the assessment and treatment of patients with hemiplegia are described. The way in which the tests are carried out and some of their components have been changed slightly in some cases or adapted to meet the needs and difficulties of patients with hemiplegia, both for assessment purposes and when the tests are being used as treatment techniques.

The Tension Tests

For each test the starting position, the method of handling, the components of the end position and sensitising additions are described. The patient's position should be standardised and noted during the first assessment so that a comparison with the results of later tests is valid and useful.

Upper Limb Tension Test 1 (ULTT1)

Starting position: The patient lies supine with his head on a pillow and somewhat closer to one side of the bed.
- The therapist stands beside the patient and takes his hand in one of hers, supporting his upper arm on her thigh as she moves his shoulder gradually into abduction (**Fig. 15.3 a**).
- Lateral rotation of the shoulder is then normally added, but for patients with hemiplegia the addition is usually considerably limited due to the abnormal position of the scapula, the malalignment of the glenohumeral joint and adaptive shortening of soft tissues, rather than by increased neural tension. The therapist therefore holds the arm in the fullest range of rotation which is possible for the patient and continues with the subsequent test components. (The problem of the limited range of lateral flexion will need to be accurately assessed and overcome during treatment.)
- Watching his face attentively for any signs of discomfort, the therapist carefully extends the patient's elbow in some degree of supination. Her other hand presses down against the plinth to prevent the shoulder girdle from being pulled into elevation as the neural structures elongate. When the elbow is extended, she adds the component of wrist dorsiflexion (**Fig. 15.3 b**). If there is hypertonicity in the flexors of the hand, it will be easier for the therapist to dorsiflex the wrist with the elbow in some degree of flexion, and then slowly straighten the arm after the correct position of the wrist has been achieved.
- If elbow extension is full and pain free with the patient's wrist dorsiflexed, the therapist supinates his forearm and then extends and abducts his fingers and thumb as well.
- By lowering her supporting thigh she increases extension of his shoulder.

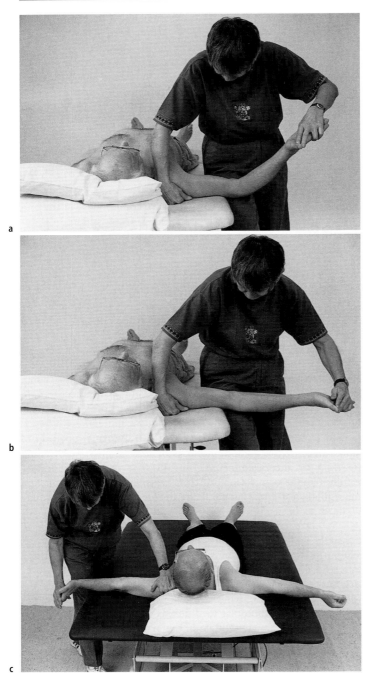

a

b

c

Fig. 15.3 a–c. Upper Limb Tension Test 1 (ULTT1). **a** Abduction of the shoulder with the arm supported on the therapist's thigh (right hemiplegia). **b** dorsal flexion of the wrist added when elbow extension is possible. **c** The goal of full abduction and extension of both arms without discomfort (left hemiplegia)

- Finally, the arm should remain abducted and extended even when the contralateral arm is placed in the same position on his other side, which further tensions the horizontal nerve connections (**Fig. 15.3 c**).

Sensitising additions:
1. Lateral flexion of the neck towards the contralateral side increases tension to a marked degree. The therapist moves the patient's head on the pillow away from her.
2. Depression of the shoulder girdle increases the amount of tension further. In addition, with the shoulder girdle depressed, full abduction of the arm is mechanically no longer possible.

Upper Limb Tension Test 2 (ULTT2) with Radial Nerve Bias

Starting position: The patient lies supine, with his head and shoulders more over to one side of the plinth or bed and his head on a pillow.
- The therapist stands beside him, facing towards his feet. The therapist supports the patient's flexed elbow with one of her hands while with her other she gently flexes his wrist (**Fig. 15.4 a**).
- She gradually extends his elbow with pronation of the forearm, keeping her thigh firmly against his shoulder girdle to prevent it from elevating (**Fig. 15.4 b**). Once again, her thigh supports his upper arm from below and adjusts the amount of shoulder extension.
- The therapist rotates the patient's shoulder medially, extends his elbow fully and adds flexion of his wrist and fingers.
- If the test components are all full and pain free, the therapist moves the patient's arm away from his body to add the component of shoulder abduction (**Fig. 15.4 c**).

Sensitising additions: Abduction of the shoulder; protraction of the shoulder girdle with the therapist's thigh tightens up the suprascapular nerve. Turning the patient's head away from the therapist and, as before, shoulder girdle depression add tension.

Upper Limb Tension Test 2 (ULTT2) with Median Nerve Bias

Starting position: The patient lies supine with his head on a pillow, with his shoulders and head nearer to the therapist than his pelvis.
- Again the therapist supports the patient's flexed elbow on her thigh, but this time with his forearm supinated and the wrist dorsiflexed (**Fig. 15.5 a**).
- Rotating his shoulder laterally, she slowly extends his elbow and extends his fingers (**Fig. 15.5 b**). When the patient's elbow is fully extended and supinated, with his wrist dorsiflexed and fingers and thumb in extension, the therapist moves his arm away from his body to abduct the shoulder. The movement of her thigh beneath his upper arm dictates the amount of shoulder extension and abduction (**Fig. 15.5 c**).

Sensitising additions: Turning the head away from the therapist; depression of the shoulder girdle and abduction of the shoulder.

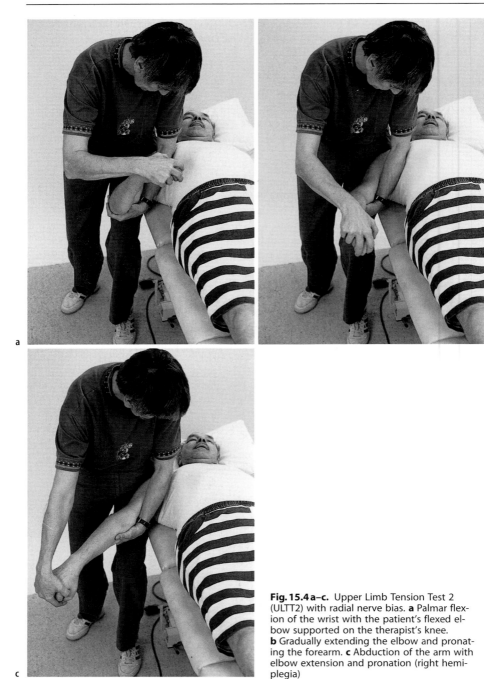

a

b

c

Fig. 15.4 a–c. Upper Limb Tension Test 2 (ULTT2) with radial nerve bias. **a** Palmar flexion of the wrist with the patient's flexed elbow supported on the therapist's knee. **b** Gradually extending the elbow and pronating the forearm. **c** Abduction of the arm with elbow extension and pronation (right hemiplegia)

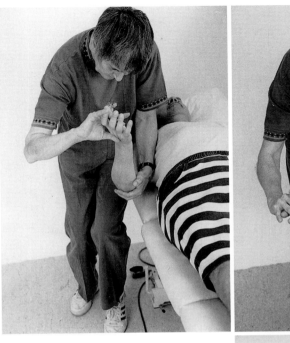

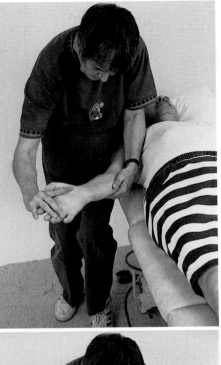

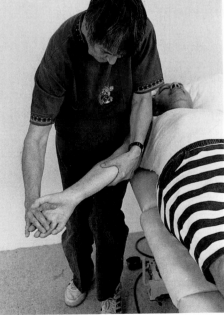

Fig. 15.5 a–c. Upper Limb Tension Test 2 (ULTT2) with median nerve bias. **a** Dorsiflexion of the wrist with the elbow still flexed. **b** Gradual extension of the elbow with supination of the forearm. **c** With the elbow fully extended and supinated, the therapist uses her thigh to support the patient's arm and to move it away from his side (right hemiplegia)

a

b

c

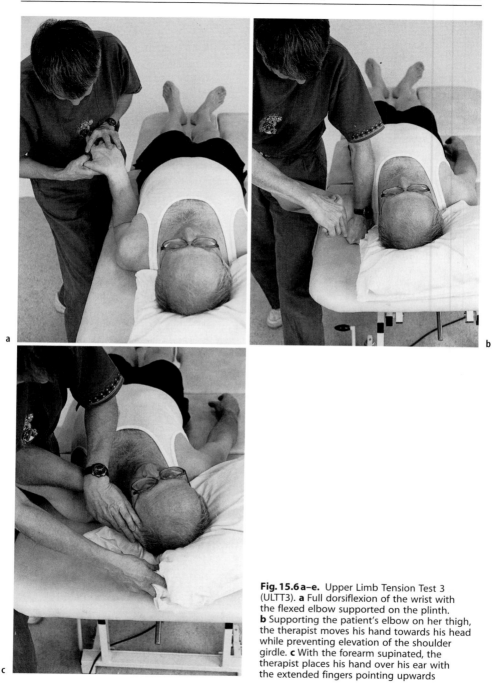

a

b

c

Fig. 15.6 a–e. Upper Limb Tension Test 3
(ULTT3). **a** Full dorsiflexion of the wrist with
the flexed elbow supported on the plinth.
b Supporting the patient's elbow on her thigh,
the therapist moves his hand towards his head
while preventing elevation of the shoulder
girdle. **c** With the forearm supinated, the
therapist places his hand over his ear with
the extended fingers pointing upwards

Upper Limb Tension Test 3 (ULTT3)

Starting position: The patient lies supine with his head on a pillow.

- The therapist stands beside him in a stride-standing position while his flexed elbow is still resting on the plinth, as she eases his forearm into supination and his wrist into dorsiflexion **(Fig. 15.6 a)**.
- Once the patient's fingers can be extended passively, the therapist moves his hand towards his head with the position of his elbow and wrist maintained. During the whole sequence, she uses her other hand to keep his shoulder girdle in a neutral position, by pressing her clenched fingers firmly down against the plinth **(Fig. 15.6 b)**.
- Supporting the patient's elbow in her groin, the therapist transfers her weight over the leg which is in front as she places his hand flat against the side of his head as if to cover his ear. His fingers remain extended with the tips pointing towards the top of his head **(Fig. 15.6 c)**. The effect is increased when the therapist moves the pillow, and thus the head, towards the opposite side.

Sensitising additions: Lateral flexion of the neck by moving the head towards the contralateral side.

Variation: Pronation of the forearm may reveal more significantly increased tension than with supination and should be included in the assessment. The therapist commen-

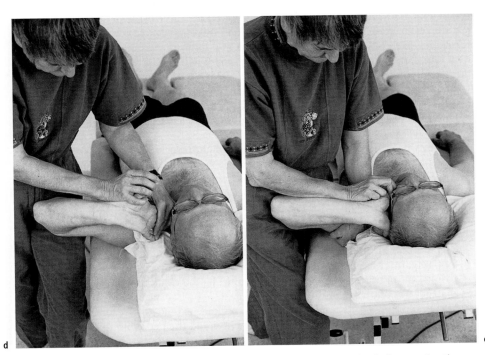

d   e

Fig. 15.6 d, e. d The therapist changes the position of the forearm to pronation before moving the patient's hand towards his head. **e** In pronation, his hand rests against the side of his head with the fingers pointing down towards his chest and his thumb in the direction of his nose (left hemiplegia)

ces the ULTT3 test movements in the same way as before, but, as the patient's hand nears his head with wrist and fingers extended, she pronates his forearm (**Fig. 15.6 d**). The hand is placed so that it lies flat against the side of his head with the fingers pointing towards the shoulder girdle and the thumb towards his nose (**Fig. 15.6 e**). If the fingers remain sufficiently relaxed, the therapist leaves them in place and can use her hand to adjust the position of the shoulder girdle or even add the component of depression.

NB: During all upper limb tension tests, the addition of lateral flexion of the neck to the contralateral side increases tension to a marked degree. Not only does depression of the shoulder girdle increase tension markedly, but full abduction of the shoulder is mechanically no longer possible.

Straight Leg Raise Test (SLR)

The straight leg raise test is not a new discovery but has been used for the differential diagnosis of sciatic nerve involvement for over a century, according to Dyck (1984). Many therapists and doctors will be familiar with the term "Leseague's test", named after its initiator, and dating back to 1864, but the term "straight leg raise test" has far wider use and merit (Butler 1991). In the field of orthopaedics, the SLR is usually associated with assessing and treating patients with back pain. For the patient with hemiplegia, the test is more important for assessing and treating adverse neural tension which is restricting mobility and activity in the trunk and limbs. For example, if the SLR is limited, knee extension at the end of the swing phase will not be possible and step length therefore reduced.

Starting position: The patient lies supine in a relaxed and comfortable position, with his head on a pillow.
- The therapist stands at his side and supports his leg from below, with one of her hands just proximal to his heel.
- She lifts his sound leg off the bed like a straight lever with no rotation of the hip, using her other hand on his thigh to prevent the knee from flexing (**Fig. 15.7 a**). The leg is raised as far as possible, the therapist noting if there is any resistance or significant loss of range and if the patient experiences any pain, which will usually be felt behind his knee.
- To differentiate between the hamstring muscles and neural tension, the therapist holds the leg at the exact level where the pain or resistance was first felt. With his heel supported on her shoulder, she uses her free hand to dorsiflex the patient's foot (**Fig. 15.7 b**). Because there has been no alteration in the length of the hamstrings, an increase in pain or resistance must be the result of the elongation of neural structures and not the muscles.
- The amount of hip flexion possible with the knee extended is recorded. A measurement of the distance between the patient's heel and the bed is useful for the records, or a diagram of the position of the leg can be drawn.
- The therapist moves the patient's hemiplegic leg in the same way and once again notes the degree of resistance and pain and the effect of dorsiflexing the foot (**Fig. 15.7 c**). If she continues to stand on the sound side while testing the affected

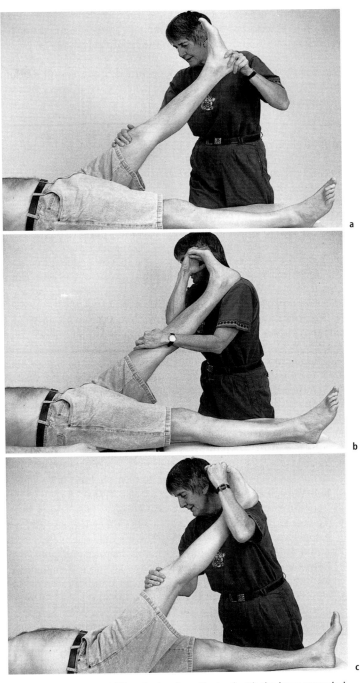

Fig. 15.7 a–c. The Straight Leg Raise Test (SLR). **a** Lifting the leg from the heel with the knee extended. **b** Dorsiflexion of the foot increases tension. **c** When testing the hemiplegic leg the therapist has to use her hand to prevent knee flexion (right hemiplegia)

leg or vice versa, she must be careful that she does not introduce additional abduction, adduction or rotation of his hip. Interestingly, the SLR is very often more limited on the sound side than on the hemiplegic side.

Sensitising additions: Dorsal flexion of the ankle is one way of increasing tension, but plantar flexion with inversion may have a greater effect in some cases. Hip adduction is another possible addition.

Because the SLR tests aspects of nervous system mechanics from the "toes to the brain", passive neck flexion will frequently cause signs of a further increase in tension, and headache or foot symptoms may be the result of tensing the sympathetic trunk.

The Slump Test

Although the slump test is one of the newer tension tests in manual therapy, its components of knee extension with spinal flexion have actually been suggested and used for many years, for example by Cyriax (1942) and Inman and Saunders (1942). It was Maitland (1979), however, who gave the test its name, when he published the results of testing a group of normal subjects. The test is one of the most comprehensive for both assessment and treatment purposes, because it tenses the whole neuraxis as well as peripheral components and thus includes many structures.

Starting position: The patient sits on the plinth with his thighs well supported and his knees together. He sits as far back as possible so that the edge of the supporting surface touches the back of his lower leg muscles.

- The therapist stands beside the patient on his hemiplegic side and asks him to let his trunk sag or slump down so that his spine flexes without changing the angle of his hips.
- She then lift his hemiplegic foot to extend his knee passively and notices any changes in the position of his hips and trunk (**Fig. 15.8 a**). Holding his foot in dorsiflexion, she uses her other arm to flex his trunk forwards until pain or resistance is felt The therapist presses her knee down on the thigh of the patient to maintain extension of his knee as the tension increases (**Fig. 15.8 b**).
- At first, the patient will probably extend his neck to reduce the tension, but as tension decreases, the therapist uses her arm behind his occiput to tip his head forward and thus flex his cervical spine as well (**Fig. 15.8 c**). Her hand behind his shoulder maintains the flexion of his trunk.
- The same procedure is followed for the other leg, but the patient may well be able to extend his sound knee and dorsiflex his ankle actively, which allows the therapist to remain on his affected side to support balance and prevent escaping movements.
- Releasing one of the distal components of the test enables the therapist to differentiate between muscular, articular and neural limitation. For example, if the knee extension is limited and pain is felt behind the knee, she can reduce the amount of dorsiflexion of the foot and ascertain whether the knee extension becomes full and free as a result. Likewise, she can let the patient extend his neck and assess whether the knee extension becomes possible or if the range of motion improves.
- Mobilising the slump test is very important in the treatment because it not only improves the movements of the lower limb but, through the continuum effect of the nervous system, helps to restore the mobility of the neuraxis, normalises tone and improves activity in the upper limb as well.

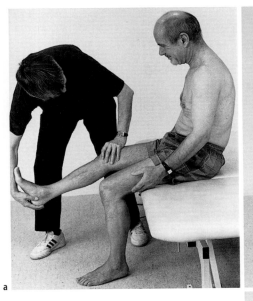
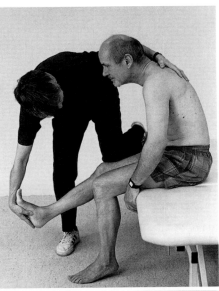
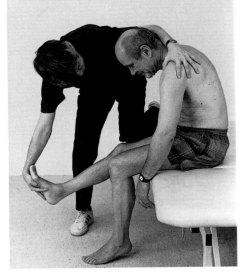

Fig. 15.8 a–c. The Slump Test (right hemiplegia). **a** When the patient's foot is dorsiflexed and his knee extended, his trunk moves back from the hips. **b** Flexion of the trunk while the therapist maintains knee extension with her knee on the patient's thigh. **c** She tips his head forward with her arm to flex his neck (right hemiplegia)

The Slump in Long Sitting (Slump LS)

The slump test can be performed in long-sitting, and is a useful method of assessment as well as a treatment technique in this position. Many patients have difficulty in sitting up from lying and maintaining an upright position when their legs are extended in front of them **(Fig. 15.9 a)**. If the therapist moves the patient's trunk further forwards with her

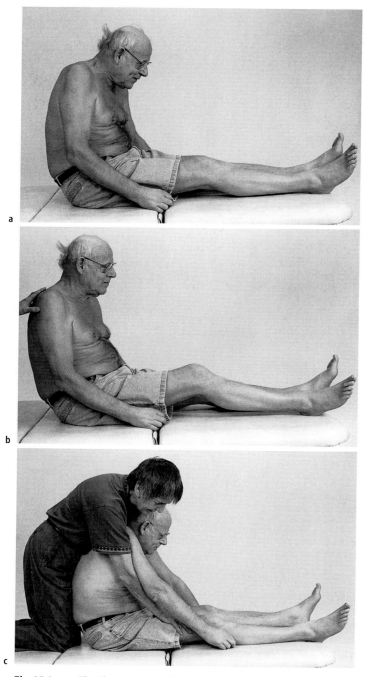

a

b

c

Fig. 15.9 a–e. The Slump in Long-Sitting (Slump LS). **a** Difficulty in sitting upright with the knees extended. **b** The patient cannot extend his knee actively when the therapist moves his trunk forwards.
c Kneeling behind the patient, the therapist flexes his whole trunk and uses her hands to extend his
knees

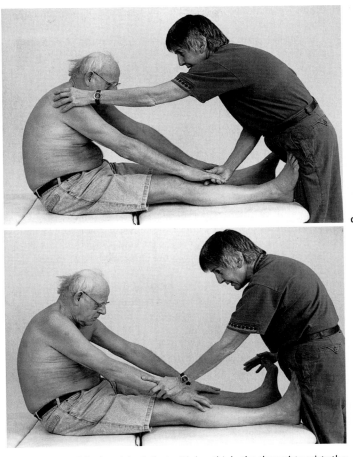

Fig. 15.9 d, e. d Maintaining dorsiflexion of the hemiplegic foot with her thigh, the therapist assists the forward movement of his scapula and arm. **e** Dorsiflexion of the sound foot increases tension; the patient's trunk is pushed further back and his neck extends (right hemiplegia)

hand, she encounters a marked resistance and he is unable to prevent flexion of his knee or knees or plantar flexion of his foot **(Fig. 15.9 b)**. To assess or mobilise the slump test in long-sitting, the therapist will usually have to kneel behind him at first, so that she can use her body to flex his whole trunk and her hands to extend his knees **(Fig. 15.9 c)**.

Starting position: The patient sits on the plinth or bed with his legs extended in front of him.

- The therapist stands at his feet and faces towards him. She asks him to slide his hands down his legs towards his feet, as far as he can. She will usually have to assist the movement of his hemiplegic hand by bringing the scapula forward.
- The therapist holds the patient's hemiplegic foot in full dorsiflexion with her thigh, while helping him to flex forwards as far as possible **(Fig. 15.9 d)**. The range of possi-

ble movement can be recorded by marking or measuring how far the tips of his fingers have reached.

• The patient is then asked to dorsiflex his sound foot actively, while the therapist continues to keep the other in position. Invariably, the patient is unable to bring his trunk and hands as far forward as he could before, and his neck extends to relieve the increased tension (**Fig. 15.9 e**).

Sensitising additions: Dorsiflexion of the sound foot increases tension to a marked degree, as does dorsiflexing the hemiplegic ankle, particularly with extension of the toes. In nearly all cases, further neck flexion will have a significant effect on tension, because the central and peripheral nervous systems are already in a stretched position.

Variations: In long-sitting rotation the slump test can be performed with rotation of the trunk, which will enhance the mobilisation of the neuraxis and the sympathetic chain in the thorax.

Abduction of the legs is a useful variation, particularly for patients troubled by hip adduction in all positions where the legs are extending, which can easily lead to loss of range and pain when the legs are passively abducted. The patient can be helped to part his legs so that his heels are over the sides of the plinth and the test is done in this position.

Working to regain the full mobility of the slump test in long-sitting is imperative, because the whole nervous system is mobilised in this position and many activities improve as a result. For example, the patient will be able to sit up from lying more easily, activity in the abdominal muscles will be facilitated and the range of motion in the legs necessary for walking regained.

The patient should be encouraged to mobilise his nervous system in long-sitting in bed on his own each morning before dressing. It is a movement that is easy for patients to understand and learn because it is such a classic exercise and familiar to most people. Athletes and football players are frequently seen performing the action before a competition, either live or on television.

The Prone Knee Bend (PKB)

Tension in the femoral nerve and lumbar nerve roots 2, 3 and 4 can be assessed and mobilised by the PKB test, but the transmission of tension causes movement of the neuraxis and meninges as well. The PKB is an important test and treatment modality because it mobilises knee flexion with hip extension, a movement component of normal walking. Most patients with hemiplegia have difficulty in flexing their knee sufficiently for the initiation of the swing phase of gait and for the normal 60° of flexion at midswing. Previously, the reason for the difficulty was immediately interpreted as being a tight or shortened rectus femoris muscle or hypertonicity of the quadriceps, but it may well be that increased tension in the neural structures, in particular the femoral nerve via its attachments to the muscle and surrounding fascia, causes a loss of their adaptive lengthening properties. Normally in prone, it is possible to flex the knee so that the heel touches the buttock, but for most patients the movement is grossly limited before specific mobilisation has been included in the treatment.

Starting position: The patient lies prone with his head turned towards the therapist each time to standardise the test for future comparison.

- The therapist holds the lower leg with her hand either just above the ankle or supporting the foot in a neutral position.
- She flexes the patient's knee and notes any resistance or pain which the flexion produces. The distance between the patient's heel and his buttock on that side can be measured and recorded for future comparison.
- If necessary, the therapist presses one hand firmly down over the patient's buttock to prevent any flexion of the hips or rotation of the pelvis from occurring due to the pull of increased tension or pain avoidance movements on his part **(Fig. 15.10)**. Care must also be taken that the hips do not abduct during the test, as they will often tend to do.
- The test is performed on the sound leg in the same way.

Sensitising additions: Hip extension can increase the effect on tension, and the therapist can place her knee on the plinth underneath the patient's thigh to extend his hip during the testing or mobilising movements. The addition of dorsal flexion with eversion or plantar flexion with inversion may also alter the response, particularly in patients with hemiplegia.

NB: There is an extreme variation in the normal range of extensibility of the rectus femoris muscle and, together with the powerful leverage provided when flexing the knee from the lower leg, soft tissues could easily be traumatised unwittingly without the necessary feedback from the patient. In prone, it is difficult for the therapist to see changes in his facial expression which would indicate that the movement is causing pain. If the patient is aphasic and cannot protest verbally, is unable to express himself nonverbally due to sensory-motor involvement of the facial muscles, and is unable to move to escape the painful movements, the PKB test should not be performed in prone until he has made sufficient progress.

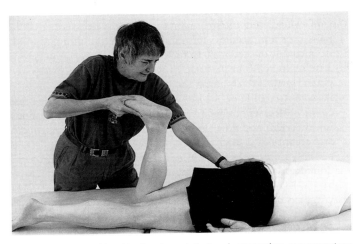

Fig. 15.10. Testing the prone knee bend (PKB), with the therapist's hand preventing compensatory movements of the pelvis (left hemiplegia)

Variations: If the patient's lumbar spine extends excessively when his knee is flexed in prone lying, the slump position can be added to flex the spine. The patient lies on his side with the leg on that side fully flexed at the hip and knee. An assistant holds his trunk and neck in a flexed position while the therapist lifts the leg which is uppermost and carefully adds the components of the PKB.

With more advanced patients it is useful to mobilise the PKB in standing as well, to facilitate knee flexion during walking. The patient stands with a table in front of him and his arms supported, while the therapist flexes his knee from behind him. To avoid compensatory extension of his lumbar spine, the patient is asked to tense his abdominal muscles actively, or he can place his elbows on the table so that his trunk remains flexed.

Using the Tension Tests as Treatment Techniques

The tension tests play an important role in the assessment of patients who have suffered a lesion of the central nervous system, because abnormal tension in neural structures is invariably found to be present. Butler (1991) describes adverse neural tension as being "abnormal physiological and mechanical responses produced from nervous system structures when their normal range of movement and stretch capabilities are tested". To optimise the recovery of voluntary activity and functional movement, specific treatment is required to reduce the tension and restore mobility to the nervous system. Using the tension tests as treatment techniques has proved to be most successful in this respect.

The tests are a powerful tool, because they have an effect on the whole nervous system. For example, the SLR moves and tensions the nervous system from the foot and along the neuraxis to the brain, which includes the lumbar sympathetic trunk and the sympathetic chain, according to Breig (1978). When mobilising the nervous system the following considerations are therefore important:

- Causing pain is not the aim, as Butler himself points out. He stresses that no force should be applied, but instead the therapist should always think of mobilising the nervous system and the structures around it rather than stretching it (Butler 1991). In addition, he advises that, "Any symptoms provoked during treatment should subside immediately the treatment technique is released", with reference to symptoms of pain, pins and needles and numbness. The symptoms should in fact, disappear within "a couple of seconds". In fact, eliciting pain is counterproductive, because it causes a reflex increase in the tone of those muscles which oppose the movement, and the patient may actively resist the painful motion if he is in the position to do so.
- Passive stretching of neighbouring muscles increases the pressure on nerves, and mechanical stresses applied to nerves evoke physiological responses such as alterations in intraneural blood flow, impulse traffic and axonal transport (Shacklock 1995). Stretch and compression alter circulation because the diameter of the vessel is decreased and possibly closed off altogether, with resultant ischaemia. Excessive and sustained elongation of nerves can seriously impede their essential blood flow, and elongation of a nerve by 15.7% has been shown to arrest its circulation completely (Ogata and Naito 1986).
- What has been called "component thinking" by Butler is advised, because it enables the therapist to mobilise the nervous system without stretching it and without causing undue pain. When a tension test is used as a mobilising procedure, the different components of the test movement are gradually added or subtracted according to the response of the individual patient, instead of the final position being attempted immedi-

ately. For instance, with the patient' s arm in abduction, the therapist first flexes and extends his elbow until the range of movement is full and pain free before adding the component of dorsal flexion of the wrist. She can also move one component until pain or resistance is encountered, retreat slightly until the symptom is eliminated, and then mobilise another component until that, too, is free before combining the different components. Any of the test components can be changed, or the order in which they are added varied. For example, the ULTT1 can be commenced from the hand and wrist, and tension then added by tightening the proximal components. Using the patient's other limbs can be a useful way of adding tension components, for example by placing the contralateral arm in the test position too, or supporting his leg on a stool with the knee extended to replicate the components of the SLR during the ULTT1.

- Although separate components and variations of the test can be useful during preparatory mobilisation, for optimal results the therapist must work towards making the final test position possible by gradually eliminating any limitations caused by pain or resistance. Careful observation of the patient's whole body is necessary, because abnormal tension can cause evasive deviations that may mislead the therapist. To attain an exact and fully mobile end position of a test, she will need to prevent parts of the patient's body from being pulled into postures which reduce or escape tension. Escaping or evasive movements occur either through the patient's consciously trying to avoid pain or, more often, because the powerful pull of the tension makes it impossible for him to prevent them actively.
- The therapist should always assess and reassess the effects of whichever treatment procedure or activity she has performed with the patient. If an improvement of some sort is not immediately noticeable, no matter how slight, it indicates that she has not found or had an effect on the cause of the problem she was trying to solve and will have to search further for a solution. The sequence in which the tests are mobilised, the speed and the force used will vary from patient to patient. There is no fixed recipe for nervous system mobilisation, and only by trial and observation can the therapist discover which way is the most beneficial for a particular patient and his individual needs.

Combining the Tension Tests and Their Components with Other Therapeutic Activities

To regain full mobility of the nervous system the tests must be mobilised exactly in the positions which have been described. In the correct test position, movements to escape tension can best be observed and more effectively prevented. In addition, however, the imaginative and resourceful therapist can find many different activities which will move the nervous system while at the same time helping the patient to regain functional skills and independence. "A technique is the brain child of ingenuity", according to Maitland (1986), and discovering ways in which mobilisation can be combined with the activities to regain motor control or improve perception certainly requires ingenuity but is well worthwhile. Not only is valuable therapy time saved, but the patient can understand the aim of such activities more clearly and perceive the improvement in his ability that they make possible. Mobilising the nervous system improves the desired activity, and the activity improves the mobility of the nervous system.

A few ways in which the nervous system can be mobilised during activities to regain or improve motor control are suggested and explained in the following examples.

ULTT1 and Selective Arm Activity

When voluntary activity in the hemiplegic arm starts to return, movements can be performed only in total mass synergies. Almost all patients are unable to move their arm selectively and demonstrate typical patterns of movement. For example, when a patient lifts his arm, from the very beginning of the movement, the shoulder girdle elevates and the scapula retracts. He is unable to reach forwards with his hand because the shoulder abducts with the elbow flexing simultaneously, and the wrist and fingers flex as well (**Fig. 15.11 a**). Invariably, the patient who can lift his arm only in this way will have abnormally increased tension revealed by ULTT1. There is a marked limitation of lateral flexion of the neck to the sound side, and if the therapist prevents elevation of the shoulder girdle and tries to move the patient's head passively sideways, the tension in the nerve plexuses and roots is obvious (**Fig. 15.11 b**). Intensive mobilisation of the nervous system in lying and sitting improves selective movement of the arm considerably, sometimes after only one treatment session (**Fig. 15.11 c**). The patient illustrated in **Fig. 15.11** received the following sequence of treatment during the 30 minutes between **Fig. 15.11 a** and **Fig. 15.11 c**.

- It is usually necessary to treat the patient in supine first, if the shoulder girdle is elevated at rest as well as when he tries to move his arm, as it was in this case (**Fig. 15.12 a**).
- The therapist mobilises the patient's thorax by pressing his sternum down in the direction of his umbilicus, because elevation of the shoulder girdle is usually associated with elevation of the rib cage and hypotonic abdominal muscles (**Fig. 15.12 b**).
- With the starting position corrected, the therapist mobilises the component of shoulder girdle depression, while preventing the patient's head from being pulled sideways (**Fig. 15.12 c**).
- As tension releases, she holds the shoulder girdle in position with one hand and mobilises lateral flexion of his neck towards the sound side, repeating the sideways movement until the movement feels free and relaxed (**Fig. 15.12 d**).
- The patient sits up and is helped to place both hands flat on the plinth on his hemiplegic side. His hands are shoulder-width apart and his elbows extended (**Fig. 15.13 a**).
- Keeping his arm in position with one hand, the therapist uses her other hand to show him exactly how he should move his sound arm back and forth on his own, namely, with lateral rotation of the shoulder, extension of the elbow and extension of his hand and fingers (**Fig. 15.13 b**).
- Once the patient understands his role, the therapist places one hand on each of his shoulders to correct their position during the movement. She needs to prevent their being pulled forward by the tension which increases when the sound arm moves back in outward rotation, while at the same time using her forearm to maintain extension of his hemiplegic elbow (**Fig. 15.13 c**). Because she is standing behind the patient, she should lean her head forwards so that she can see from his facial expression if any pain is caused.

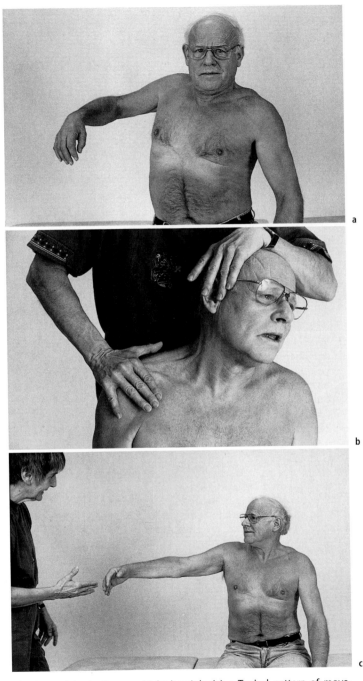

Fig. 15.11 a–c. Regaining selective activity in the arm (right hemiplegia). **a** Typical pattern of movement when the arm is lifted before selective movement is possible. **b** Lateral flexion of the neck reveals increased neural tension. **c** Selective movement possible following nervous system mobilisation

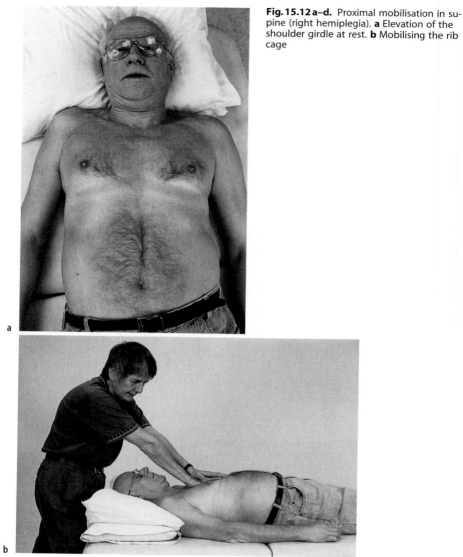

Fig. 15.12 a–d. Proximal mobilisation in supine (right hemiplegia). **a** Elevation of the shoulder girdle at rest. **b** Mobilising the rib cage

a

b

ULTT2 and Moving the Trunk in Standing

For a patient who is able to walk, but whose arm has hypertonus with associated reactions which pull his arm into a flexed position in upright postures, inhibition of tone can be combined with ULTT1 mobilisation in standing.

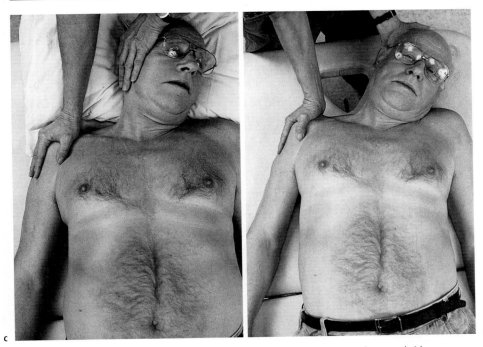

Fig. 15.12 c, d. **c** Depression of the shoulder. **d** Lateral flexion of the neck to the sound side

- The patient stands with his hemiplegic side to a wall and the therapist places his hand against the wall beside and slightly behind him, with his arm extended and outwardly rotated (**Fig. 15.14 a**).
- Keeping his hand in position on the wall with one hand and using her body to support extension of his elbow, the therapist moves the patient's sound arm to show him exactly how he should move it on his own for the best results (**Fig. 15.14 b**).
- The patient then moves his sound hand forwards to touch the wall by rotating his trunk without moving his feet (**Fig. 15.14 c**).
- The therapist continues to maintain the position of the patient's extended fingers and hand on the wall and his elbow in extension with her body. In addition, she uses her other hand to prevent his shoulder from being pulled forwards by tension during the movement (**Fig. 15.14 d**).

Not only does the combined activity inhibit hypertonus in the hemiplegic arm and overcome associated reactions; it also enables the patient to adduct his scapula and thus allow his arm to remain at his side in a normal position when he walks, instead of protraction with medial rotation of the shoulder causing his hand to be constantly in front of his crutch.

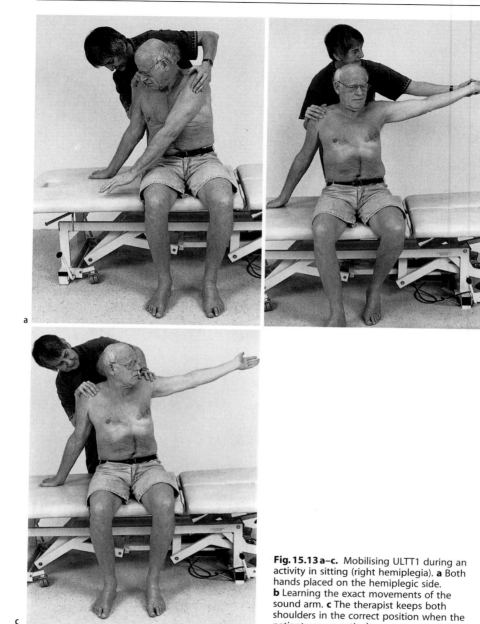

Fig. 15.13 a–c. Mobilising ULTT1 during an activity in sitting (right hemiplegia). **a** Both hands placed on the hemiplegic side. **b** Learning the exact movements of the sound arm. **c** The therapist keeps both shoulders in the correct position when the patient moves actively

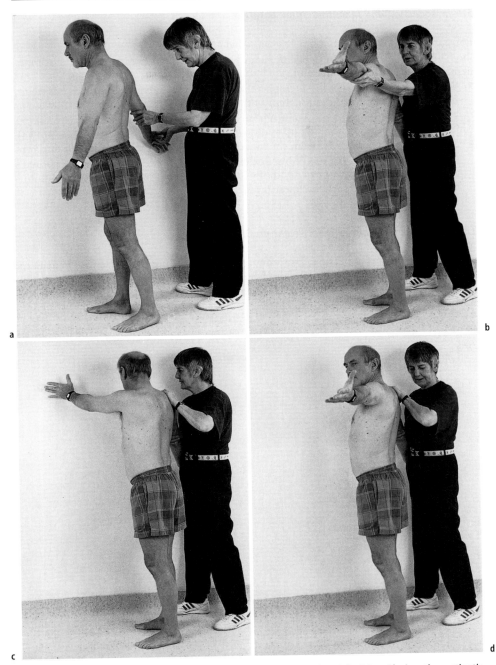

Fig. 15.14a–d. Mobilising ULTT1 by moving in standing (right hemiplegia). **a** Placing the patient's hand on the wall. **b** Guiding the movements of the sound arm. **c** Turning to touch the wall with the sound hand. **d** Preventing the hemiplegic shoulder from being pulled forwards

SLR in Adduction and Inhibitory Trunk Rotation

For patients who walk with the pelvis retracted and the extended leg outwardly rotated, the trunk is rotated forwards while the hemiplegic leg is mobilised by using the components of the SLR test in adduction.

- With the patient supine, the therapist stands on his sound side and holds his hemiplegic leg in flexion and adduction with his foot in dorsal flexion. She moves his knee towards her and back again repeatedly, and when she feels that it is more relaxed, she moves the lower leg up and down to mobilise knee extension (**Fig. 15.15 a**).
- Maintaining full knee extension, she moves the extended leg back and forth into progressively increasing degrees of hip flexion and adduction (**Fig. 15.15 b**). The patient's pelvis moves forwards together with the leg, and the resulting trunk rotation inhibits hypertonicity throughout the lower limb.

The Slump and Learning to Take Weight on One Leg

The combination of mobilising the slump test while standing on one leg is particularly useful for the patient who can walk, but who has difficulty in shifting weight sufficiently over one leg and in extending his knee at the end of the swing phase to take a step of normal length.

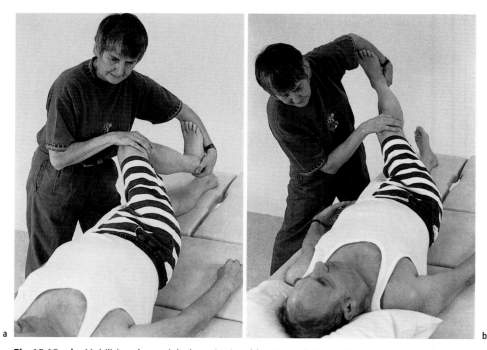

a   b

Fig. 15.15 a, b. Mobilising the straight leg raise in adduction (right hemiplegia). **a** Mobilising the component of knee extension with the hip adducted. **b** Increasing hip flexion with the knee extended and the foot dorsiflexed

- The therapist stands at the patient's hemiplegic side and helps him to place his hemiplegic foot on a step directly in front of him.
- The patient slides his hands down the front of the shin of his hemiplegic leg as far as he can, moving his hands down and then up again repeatedly (**Fig. 15.16 a**).
- When the movement becomes more relaxed and the patient feels secure, he lifts his hemiplegic leg again after a short interval, but this time he places his foot so that

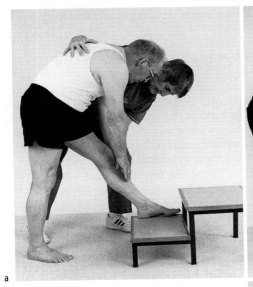 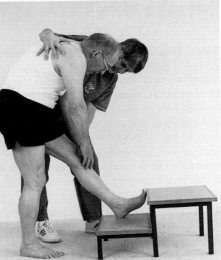

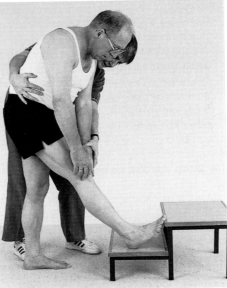

Fig. 15.16 a–c. Standing on one leg and mobilising the slump test (left hemiplegia).
a Standing on the sound leg with the hemiplegic foot on a step, moving the trunk forwards. **b** Dorsiflexion of the foot maintained by the step above during forward flexion of the trunk. **c** Standing on the hemiplegic leg with the sound foot on the step and sliding the hands down over the knee

the second step holds it mechanically in a dorsiflexed position. The therapist helps him to flex his trunk and move his hands further and further down his extended leg towards his foot (**Fig. 15.16 b**). The range of movement is more limited with his foot in dorsiflexion, but the movement needs to be mobilised. The range is that required for the heel to contact the ground with the knee extended at the end of the swing phase of gait.

- Standing on his hemiplegic leg, the patient performs the same mobilising movement by sliding his hands down the front of his sound leg (**Fig. 15.16 c**). The activity improves selective extension in the hemiplegic leg while reducing the tension that is often more restricting in this position than when he is standing on his sound leg.

Slump, Long-Sitting in Abduction and Inhibition of Extensor Hypertonus in the Leg

Mobilisation of the slump test with the patient's legs abducted reduces extensor hypertonicity in the hemiplegic leg considerably and can be most useful in overcoming the increased tone or shortening of the adductors of his hip. Raised tension in the neuraxis is also reduced, allowing more fluid trunk flexion, rotation and the recovery of activity in the oblique abdominal muscles. The mobilisation has a positive effect on the upper limb as well, and some patients have regained activity in their hand as a result. The mobilisation can be performed in two ways, either by moving the distal components of the slump test from the foot end or by moving the trunk proximally against the lengthened neural structures in the straight leg.

- The patient sits astride the plinth with his hands on the surface between his legs. If he has marked hypertonus or some shortening of his adductors, the therapist will need to mobilise abduction in supine before helping him to part his legs sufficiently in sitting. With his knees flexed, his legs are eased down over the sides of the plinth and gradually relax. The therapist places one of her hands beneath his heel and holds his foot in dorsal flexion by pressing against it with her forearm, as she moves his lower leg up and down to mobilise extension of his knee. Her other hand presses down on his thigh to prevent it from lifting off the bed, and the patient maintains the flexed position of his trunk and hips actively to avoid being pushed backwards as tension increases (**Fig. 15.17 a**).
- When knee extension is full and painless, the therapist supports the leg in the correct position by pressing her thigh against his foot and asks the patient to move his trunk back and forth. She uses one of her hands to keep his knee straight while with the other she assists the flexion of his trunk and neck (**Fig. 15.17 b**).

The Slump and Retraining Weightbearing on The Hemiplegic Leg

Instead of the therapist lifting the patient's extended leg passively in supine or sitting, or his flexing his trunk in long-sitting, he can stand with a table in front of him and move his elbows down to touch it and stand upright again. The movement components entailed are very similar with regard to the lengthening required of the nervous system and its tissues. More positive, however, is the fact that the patient is taking weight on his hemiplegic leg and using active hip extension to come upright again each time.

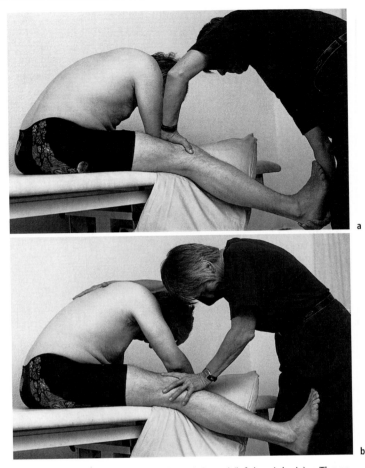

Fig. 15.17 a, b. Mobilising the slump in long-sitting with the legs abducted (left hemiplegia). **a** The patient maintains flexion of his trunk and hips while the therapist extends and flexes his knee. **b** Moving the trunk proximally with the knee held in extension and the foot dorsiflexed

- The patient stands with a plinth or table in front of him and the therapist stands close beside him on his hemiplegic side.
- He clasps his hands together and flexes his elbows to place his thumbs against his forehead before bending forward until his forearms are resting on the table. In this position, the therapist ensures that the whole spine is flexed evenly, by using her arm beneath his trunk to mobilise any stiff areas (**Fig. 15.18 a**). If the patient has difficulty in maintaining extension of his hemiplegic knee actively when the nervous system is elongated, a back slab bandaged on behind his leg helps him to keep his knee straight.
- The patient stands upright again, and by keeping his forehead in contact with his clasped hands he ensures that his neck automatically remains flexed. The common

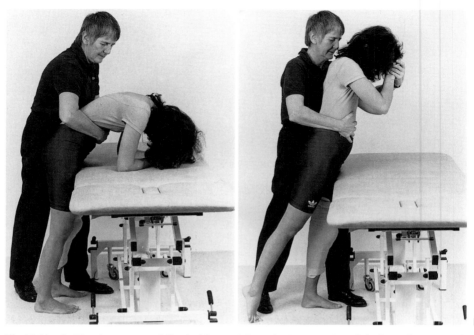

Fig. 15.18 a, b. The slump test mobilised while retraining selective extension of the hemiplegic leg (left hemiplegia). (From Davies 1994) **a** Trunk flexion with both knees extended. The therapist ensures that the whole spine is flexing, and a knee splint is used if the patient is unable to maintain knee extension actively. **b** With the weight on the hemiplegic leg, bending forwards to place the elbows on the plinth. The patient keeps her forehead in contact with her clasped hands to avoid extending her neck

tendency to use cervical extension when coming upright is thus avoided, and the therapist facilitates the upward movement with her hand beneath his hands.

- When the patient can flex forward and come upright again with relative ease, he places his sound foot behind him with his toes resting on the floor. With all his weight on his hemiplegic leg he repeats the mobilising movements, bending forward to touch the table with his elbows and then standing up again as he did before (**Fig. 15.18 b**). Throughout the activity, both of the patient's thighs should remain in contact with the edge of the table, and at first, the therapist will need to use her body to prevent their moving backward.

Once the patient has made progress and can maintain the extension of his knee actively and without too much effort, the extension splint to support his knee is no longer required.

To enhance the mobilising effect of the activity, the height of the plinth can be gradually lowered or the patient's foot held in more dorsiflexion. To increase the angle of dorsiflexion, the patient stands on a wedge-shaped board, with the plinth directly in front of him. He stands on his hemiplegic leg with a rolled bandage beneath his toes to hold them in extension, and places his sound foot behind him with only the toes touching

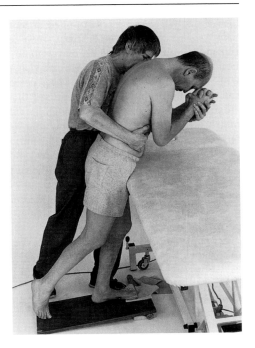

Fig. 15.19. Standing on an inclined surface enhances the effect of the mobilisation by increasing dorsal flexion of the ankle (left hemiplegia)

the surface. From this starting position he bends forward until his elbows reach the plinth before returning to standing again (**Fig. 15.19**). The therapist can help him to come upright more easily by placing her hand beneath his clasped hands and supporting some of his weight when he lifts his elbows off the plinth.

Mobilising the nervous system while standing on the hemiplegic leg will improve the patient's walking pattern to a remarkable degree by overcoming many different problems. Active dorsiflexion of the ankle often becomes possible without supination so that the patient can manage without a brace, and clonus in hypertonic plantar flexors is eliminated. It is a valuable activity for patients at all stages of their rehabilitation, ranging from those who are just starting to walk with the help of the therapist to those who can walk independently and have only slight problems.

Mobilising Peripheral Nerves Directly

Transverse movements of peripheral nerves can mobilise the nervous system directly and are a useful adjunct to mobilisation via the tension tests. When pain due to abnormal tension is in the foreground, using the tension tests as treatment techniques can magnify the pain if involved nerves are not free to move distally. In such cases the elongation of the system proximally can exert a shearing stress distally on the tethered nerves that fail to move when pulled or tensed, and they must therefore be freed locally before the tests are implemented. Adverse tension in peripheral nerves hampers impulse transport, and distal muscles may remain inactive because of their impeded innervation. The disturbed innervation can also precipitate abnormal tone, which interferes with selective limb movements. Many peripheral nerves are surprisingly accessible and can therefore be moved and mobilised directly by the therapist, once she has studied an anatomy book and rediscovered where exactly they are located. The nerve itself can be treated by moving it transversely in a way similar to friction, or the surrounding interface can be moved in relation to the nerve. G. Rolf (personal communication 1997, cited in Davies 1997) describes the direct mobilisation of the nerves as being "accessory movements" of the nervous system, because the movements cannot be performed actively and do not occur during active physiological movements of the body. Maitland (1986) used the term originally with reference to joints: "Accessory movements are those movements of his joints that a person cannot perform himself actively, but which can be performed on him by another person."

Examples of how direct peripheral nerve mobilisation can help to overcome two typical problems are illustrated and explained in **Figs. 15.20** and **15.21**.

Example 1

The patient suffered from marked hypertonus in the flexors of his fingers with loss of extension, a common problem for many patients, which impedes both active and passive movements and is distressing from a cosmetic point of view (**Fig. 15.20 a**). With the patient seated and his hemiplegic arm supported on a table, the therapist supinates his forearm and holds his thumb in abduction/extension. With the fingers of her other hand she feels for and locates the median nerve and, with some downward pressure applied, moves it firmly from side to side (**Fig. 15.20 b**). Immediately afterwards, without any other therapeutic procedures having been performed, the patient's fingers are seen to be relaxed and remain in a position of extension and abduction (**Fig. 15.20 c**)

Example 2

The patient is unable to dorsiflex his foot or extend his toes actively. The therapist uses her fingers to palpate the lateral popliteal nerve below the head of the fibula. She then moves it firmly from side to side in relation to the surrounding tissues along its course towards the foot (**Fig. 15.21 a**).The transverse movements are continued, moving the nerve where it lies superficially on the lateral aspect of the foot (**Fig. 15.21 b**). Following the direct mobilisation of the nerve, the patient is able to extend his toes actively as well as to dorsiflex his foot a little (**Fig. 15.21 c**).

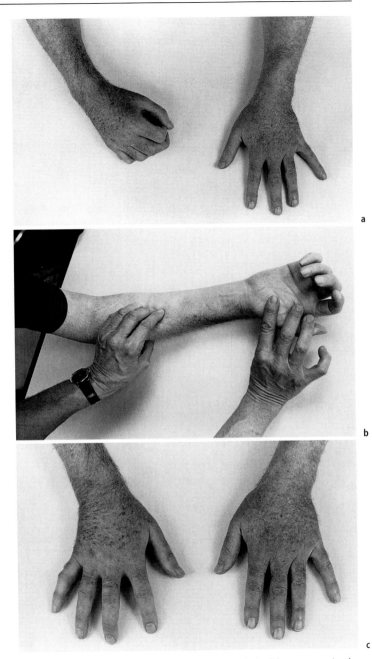

Fig. 15.20 a–c. Mobilising the median nerve directly (right hemiplegia). **a** Marked hypertonus in the flexors of the wrist and fingers. **b** Moving the median nerve transversely with the forearm held in supination. **c** With hypertonicity inhibited, the fingers remain in extension and abduction

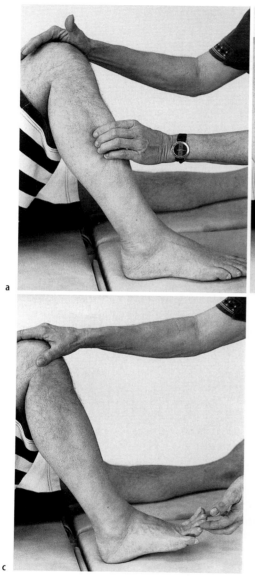
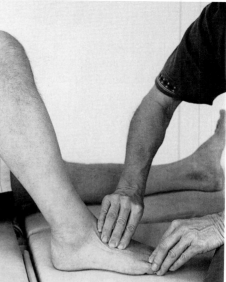

Fig. 15.21 a–c. Direct mobilisation of the lateral popliteal nerve to improve active movements of the foot (right hemiplegia). **a** Palpating and moving the nerve transversely. **b** Mobilising the nerve on the lateral aspect of the foot. **c** Active extension of the toes and dorsiflexion of the ankle become possible

Conclusion

It is most important for nervous system mobilisation to be included in the treatment of all patients with hemiplegia, in the most effective way possible, because "a muscle can only be as good as the nerve that supplies it" (Rolf 1999 b). Any form of treatment which the physiotherapist prefers to use will move and thus mobilise nerves either inadvertently or by design, to a greater or lesser degree. Even the gentlest of breathing exercises moves the neural structures of the thoracic spine and the brachial plexus, according to McLellan and Swash (1976), while the connective tissue massage described by Gifford and Gifford (1988), the transverse frictions advocated by Cyriax (1959), and muscle mobilising techniques will inevitably move nerves as well. Other concepts, such as proprioceptive neuromuscular facilitation (Knott and Voss 1968; Adler et al. 1993) and functional kinetics (Klein-Vogelbach 1991), move the limbs and trunk in combination and through a large range of motion which mobilises the nervous system indirectly. Many of the successful activities developed by Berta Bobath and illustrated in the final edition of her book on the treatment of hemiplegia (1990) incorporate the components of many of the tension tests. For example, those of the ULTT1, PKB and SLR are repeated in several of the figures. Through her long and fruitful clinical experience she had realised, even without the help of scientific explanations now available, that such movements normalised tone and facilitated the return of voluntary activity. As she once confessed to this author (1989), "I don't know why trunk rotation inhibits spasticity; I only know that it does!", but clearly, in her wisdom, she had instinctively used a movement which mobilises the neuraxis and the sympathetic chain and observed the positive effects of rotating the trunk when treating adults with hemiplegia and children with cerebral palsy.

Although the nervous system is moved during all forms of physiotherapy, for the restoration and maintenance of its full mobility and ability to transport nerve impulses, direct mobilisation is essential, and successful treatment involves a continuous interplay between direct and indirect mobilisation. Direct mobilisation entails mobilising the tension tests or moving nerves transversely, and for both of these specific procedures based on the systems anatomy and biomechanics must be used. Indirect mobilisation is the result of active movements and correction of abnormal postures.

However, there is no recipe for success, no cut-and-dried sequence of direct mobilisation techniques to be performed routinely with each and every patient. On the contrary, which will be the most effective is very individual, because different movements and combinations of movements help some patients more than others. Only careful assessment and reassessment, observation of the patient's response to the treatment, and improvement in his condition following each session can guide the therapist. The principle to be followed is much the same as that which Berta Bobath taught on so many occasions with regard to her concept of treatment: "The only reply to the question as to whether what you are doing is right for the patient is the reaction of the patient to what you are doing."

In this respect, the reaction of patients to mobilisation of the nervous system has shown it to be unquestionably "right"! Surprising results have been achieved through its inclusion in the treatment program, in that some patients have been helped to regain functional activity even many years after the onset of hemiplegia and the walking ability of others has improved remarkably. In addition, teaching the patient how he can maintain the restored mobility of his nervous system on his own after leaving the hospital or rehabilitation centre will prevent his condition from deteriorating when he no longer has therapy. With so many advantages for the patient, and because each and every therapist is already mobilising neural structures in some way, it would seem logical to include more thorough and effective means of mobilisation of the nervous system in the treatment. Only when the patient's nervous system is fully mobile and pain free at the limit of its possible range will he be able to move freely, without resistance or pain in the mid-range required for the activities of daily living.

16 Maintaining and Improving Mobility at Home

Even today, no one can say with certainty for how long patients with hemiplegia will continue to recover or regain useful motor function. Many hypotheses as to the probable outcome of rehabilitation have been put forward, but all provide only a statistical probability which has nothing to do with individual possibility, and there have been many surprising exceptions to the prognostic results. It is certainly not true that after 3 months, or 6 months or even a year no further improvement in a patient's condition is possible. Improvement continues far longer, with recovery of function occurring more than 5 years after the onset of hemiplegia (Bach-y-Rita 1981b; Kaste 1995). Because of the present-day financial limitations in health insurance, many patients will have to stop receiving treatment before they have achieved their full potential or even regained independence in activities of daily life. For some patients cessation of treatment means that they will not have the chance to achieve what might otherwise have been possible, such as being able to walk, to go out and about with others and to enjoy life more fully. It would be a great pity to stop too soon after spending so much time, effort and money on expensive diagnostic measures such as magnetic resonance imaging (MRI) or positron emission tomography (PET) and on the costly, comprehensive treatment during the intensive care and rehabilitation stages. With regard to how long treatment should continue, the same principles as for other medical, surgical and traumatic conditions should be followed and the same reasons considered valid. Treatment should certainly not be curtailed on the grounds that it is taking too long or is considered to be too expensive. If a patient with hemiplegia is still making progress because of the treatment, it should definitely be continued, just as a patient with tuberculosis who requires 2 years of hospital care with expensive medication before he is cured has the necessary treatment financed without question. Similarly, a patient with a fractured femur that has failed to unite would not be denied prolonged treatment on the grounds that it was taking longer than expected or that surgery to make walking possible would be too expensive.

Obviously, an extended period of intensive treatment would be ideal for all patients to allow optimal recovery. A recent study has shown that even elderly patients in nursing homes respond well and benefit from high-intensity treatment and that "advanced age, activities of daily living status and cognitive impairment were not associated with poor physiotherapy outcomes" (Chiodo et al. 1992). Elderly patients and those severely affected can be effectively rehabilitated; with systematic stroke management they have the potential for recovering, becoming independent and living at home but they may not do so without such rehabilitation, according to Kaste (1995).

However, it must be taken into account that it would be impossible to treat all the patients forever because there are just too many worldwide and too few therapists available for the task, and because the financial resources of most health-care systems would be placed under too great a strain. Some criteria are therefore necessary to guide the doctor or therapist responsible for deciding whether further treatment is necessary or should be recommenced later. In conjunction with several experts experienced in the field of stroke rehabilitation, the following list has been compiled.

Treatment should always be continued if any of the following apply:

1. The patient is still making progress because of the treatment.
2. The patient is unable to maintain the level of function and mobility on his own without treatment.
3. The patient cannot walk at all, even with the help of aids or with assistance from another person.
4. The patient has pain and/or loss of range of movement.
5. The patient falls frequently, is afraid to fall and is in real danger of falling and injuring himself.
6. The patient cannot eat and drink with enjoyment and in the company of others.
7. The patient has such dysarthria that others cannot understand him and no alternative form of communication has been provided.
8. The patient has no hobby or recreational activity which he enjoys and never leaves the house at all.

Treatment should be recommenced if and when:

1. Further return of active movement occurs which could be enhanced and used functionally and thus lead to greater independence.
2. The patient's level of performance deteriorates, perhaps as the result of an accident that hurt his arm or leg, or an operation or an illness. He therefore requires an intensive period of treatment to regain his previous status.

To ensure that the transition from intensive rehabilitation to managing at home without formal therapy is proceeding well, regular check-ups are necessary to assess how the patient is managing and whether he is maintaining his physical condition. The patient should also be able to contact the doctor or therapist if problems arise or if he feels that he needs a refresher course of treatment. It is important to offer a review service to patients in order to maintain functional levels and prevent deterioration (Lennon and Hastings 1996). All too often, treatment stops completely after 6–8 weeks without the patients being offered continuing support or therapy (Tyson 1995). As a result, patients frequently feel abandoned and think that the reason for their being discharged is that there is no hope of further recovery in the future (Greveson and James 1991), which is not the case at all. Ideally, the patient should continue to have outpatient treatment, and experience has shown that a 3-week period of intensive daily therapy benefits the patient far more than does having a treatment once a week for 3 months, which would involve the same number of actual sessions. In Switzerland, where most patients with hemiplegia are able to have twice-yearly periods of rehabilitation covered by their medical insurance, the results have been surprisingly good. The patients make considerable progress during the 2-to 3-week period and are given activities to practise at home before their next visit. Kaste (1995) also recommends that, "After the active rehabilitation programme has come to an end, the patient with stroke needs a long-term rehabilitation programme which should include a twice-yearly series of 15–20 physiotherapy sessions". The Sätra Brunn stroke program in Sweden, organised by Uppsala University, has been most successful and rewarding for all concerned (Lind and Loid 1995). Since

1987, approximately 200–250 patients from different parts of the country attend one of three 4-week periods each summer at the Sätra spa, which is a kind of holiday rehabilitation centre. The patients accepted for the programme all live at home during the rest of the year and have had their hemiplegia for a long time. During the summer "holiday", each patient participates in an intensive therapy programme based on the Bobath concept, which consists of individual treatment sessions and various group treatments. Self-care activities are stressed, with physiotherapists and occupational therapists working in close harmony. The patients live very closely together and enjoy social, cultural and sporting activities, and picnics and walks in the forest. Realistic goals are set, and the patient is expected to work towards them at home before he returns for treatment the following summer. All the patients have been able to learn new abilities and make further progress during the short time, and an evaluation of the program showed that the positive results had been maintained 6 months later (Carlsson 1988).

However, such ongoing treatment possibilities are not always available or financially feasible, and there may be no therapist in the patient's vicinity to treat him on an outpatient basis. At some stage, every patient will have to continue to work on his own at home, either between the periods of rehabilitation or when treatment is discontinued altogether for whatever reason. He has no option, because otherwise his condition will deteriorate and the level of performance achieved during his rehabilitation will decline. A large group of patients who had suffered a stroke were assessed at the time of their discharge from treatment, 1 year after they had returned home, and again after 5 years. The patients' functional level had been maintained for the first year but during the following 4 years a significant decrease in functional level occurred, especially in the ability to perform active movements, to maintain balance and to walk (Lindmark 1995) Clearly, no patient can maintain or improve his level of mobility and function after discharge from treatment if he has not been carefully and adequately taught how and what he can do to maintain and improve his present condition.

Maintaining Mobility Without the Help of a Therapist

Most important for the patient after being discharged from the hospital or rehabilitation centre, or when outpatient therapy ceases, is his 24-hour way of life, rather than having a long list of exercises which he has to perform each day. The activities of his daily life, when carried out correctly and without eliciting hypertonicity, will help him to maintain his mobility and will also encourage further improvement. During his rehabilitation he should have learned how to turn over in bed on his own and position himself correctly on his side, how to dress himself without associated reactions, how to stand up symmetrically with his weight on both legs, etc. By moving in more therapeutic ways and by avoiding prolonged abnormal postures in sitting and lying, much can be done to maintain mobility. There are, however, certain movements which do not occur in his daily life, and the patient must therefore carry out specific exercises or activities regularly to prevent loss of range of motion in muscles and joints or an increase in spasticity.

Common Sites of Increased Hypertonicity and/or Loss of Range of Motion

The following problems are those most frequently seen when patients who have not had adequate instruction or who have failed to perform a home exercise programme return for a check-up or a further period of intensive treatment, or are referred from another hospital where they did not have informed treatment.

- The shoulder no longer has full range of motion and may have become painful.
- The elbow flexors have shortened and are hypertonic.
- There is loss of full dorsal flexion of the wrist with full extension of the fingers.
- Full supination of the arm is not possible, even passively.
- The full range of abduction of the arm in outward rotation with elbow extension has not been maintained.
- The knee is spastic in extension and the patient has trouble releasing the spasticity for functions such as crossing his legs to put on his shoe, walking or climbing the stairs.
- The Achilles tendon has shortened and the patient cannot bear weight with his heel on the floor. Clonus may have developed.
- The toes are flexed strongly and adducted, and sometimes corns have developed or there are painful areas on the pads of the toes from the pressure against the floor.
- In addition, the nervous system has lost the property of adaptive lengthening, which is a contributory factor to the above problems, and the patient has increasing difficulty in moving freely and maintaining his level of performance in daily life. A vicious circle ensues, in that the less he moves the more immobile he becomes and the less the nervous system is moved.

Ensuring the Patient's Participation

As do most people, patients require a great deal of will power and self-discipline to practise alone in the long term without the guidance of a trainer, a teacher or a therapist. It is well known that most back patients fail to carry out their home exercise program once the pain has gone. But for the patient with hemiplegia, his active participation is essential if he is to stay mobile and make further progress. Bach-y-Rita and Balliet (1987) stress the need to "train the patient to be his/her own best therapist as soon as possible". Making the exercises physically possible for the patient through adequate instruction and practice and his being convinced of the necessity to do them are the secrets to success. All who work with him must give him hope and encouragement and convince him of the active role he himself has to play.

If the therapists, the doctors, the neuropsychologist, the speech pathologist and the nurses have a negative attitude about the possibility of further improvement and this is conveyed to the patient, then it is unlikely that he will feel motivated to keep on working for improvement on his own, or be convinced of how important it is to maintain the mobility of his body. It should be explained to him that doing his exercises regularly is an investment in his health, as it is for other people who go to the fitness club or take part in some active sport. He should set aside an appropriate time each day to exercise, a time that fits in with his normal routine. First thing in the morning would perhaps suit a pensioner, but a patient who works might find a later time more appropriate. Whichever time is chosen, performing the exercises must become a routine like brushing the teeth and not just left to chance and whim, because they will otherwise be performed less and less frequently and later be left out altogether.

Some useful hints for selecting and teaching the exercises follow.

- The number of activities included in the recommended home programme should be reduced to a minimum, as very few people would be prepared to practise a long list of exercises every day.
- The activities must be possible for the patient to perform without having preparatory treatment from the therapist.
- The therapist should avoid the necessity of the patient's wife or other family members having to help him perform the exercises whenever possible, because the relationship can easily change to one of therapist and patient instead of man and wife, father and son, etc.
- The exercises should not require special apparatus but be possible with the support of normal furniture, so that the room does not resemble a gymnasium.

The activities described below have proved to be suitable and are considered to be necessary for the majority of patients; they should be carefully taught from the beginning so that the patient knows them well and can perform them accurately and independently before he goes home or stops having outpatient treatment. The activities are gradually prepared from the first treatment onwards and then included regularly in the treatment sessions, whether the patient is being treated in the ICU or comes later for rehabilitation or a second period of treatment. As a final test, the patient should be able to go right through the list of required activities without the therapist having to prompt him in any way or correct part of his performance. To avoid his wasting time by practising an incorrect or useless activity, he should have points of reference that enable him to check that he is performing each exercise correctly on his own. For example, in **Fig. 16.4a**, the patient mobilises supination of his forearm until he sees and feels that his hemiplegic thumb is against the surface of the table.

The therapist should provide some way to assist the patient in remembering each activity with its key points and the sequence in which to carry out the exercises. A list of the activities and how they are carried out can be written by the therapist, but such a description is confusing, particularly if the patient has a language problem. Pre-printed booklets, illustrated with diagrams or drawings of various exercises and some of them ticked off for the patient to do, are very impersonal and uninspiring, as well as being unclear. The most useful aid has proved to be a video of the patient performing his exercises if he has a recorder at home, or a photograph of himself practising each activity with the most important features written on or next to it. A Polaroid camera is very useful for this purpose because the photo can be checked immediately and the white border provides space for a pertinent comment. For example, a picture showing the activity illustrated in **Fig. 16.2** might require a comment such as: "Keep your elbows straight and the balls of your hands together. Continue until your thumbs touch the mattress beyond your head." Arrows can be drawn on the photographs with a marking pen to indicate deviations which must be avoided.

Specific Exercises for Muscles and Joints

There is no absolute prescription applicable to all patients, but the following activities have proved to be possible and beneficial for most. The exercises which have been selected are those considered essential for preventing the most common complications. Performing them daily will prevent the development of painful and unsightly contractures that cause the patient additional suffering and could prevent further recovery of activity in the future (**Fig. 16.1**)

To Prevent Shoulder Stiffness

The patient lies on his bed or on the floor and clasps his hands with the fingers interlaced so that the hemiplegic thumb is uppermost and the balls of his hands fit against each other exactly. He pushes his clasped hands away from him until his elbows are straight and moves his arms towards his sound side to bring the scapula well into protraction.

He then lifts his arms up over his head until his hands touch the supporting surface, with his elbows remaining extended (**Fig. 16.2**). He lowers and raises them a few times until the hemiplegic arm lies relaxed above his head.

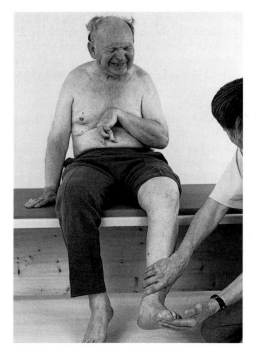

Fig. 16.1. A home programme is essential because it prevents the development of problems like these. Such contractures and deformities of the limbs are painful and unsightly and impede the return of functional activity (left hemiplegia)

To Inhibit Extensor Hypertonus in the Lower Limb

Lying on his back, the patient clasps his hands together and encircles his flexed knees with both arms. He draws his knees up to his chest and lifts his head at the same time. He then allows the hips to extend somewhat, until his elbows are straight and his shoulders have been drawn well forward in protraction. He then repeats the movement by flexing his legs again (**Fig. 16.3**). The activity can also be practised with only the hemiplegic leg flexed and the other leg remaining flat on the bed.

To Maintain Supination of the Forearm

The patient sits at a table with his hands clasped and his arms stretched out in front of him. He leans toward his hemiplegic side, pushing his affected arm into supination until the thumb is pressed onto the table (**Fig. 16.4 a**). Moving from side to side, he releases the spasticity until he can place the sound hand flat on the other hand, holding the fingers in extension (**Fig. 16.4 b**).

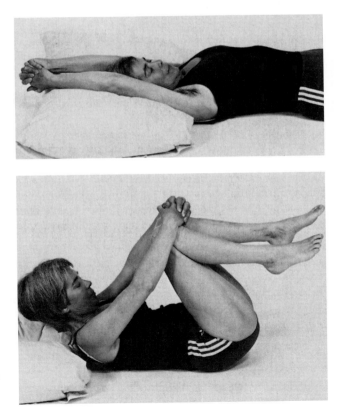

Fig. 16.2. Maintaining full, pain-free range of motion of the shoulder (right hemiplegia)

Fig. 16.3. Inhibiting extensor spasticity in the leg (right hemiplegia)

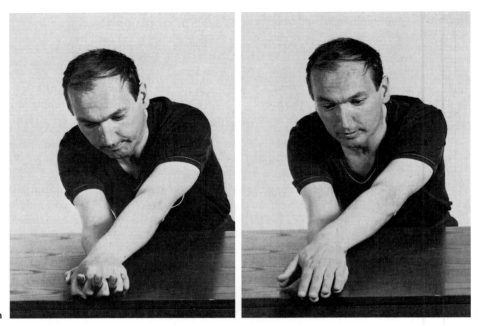

a   b

Fig. 16.4 a, b. Mobilising supination of the forearm (right hemiplegia) **a** leaning towards the hemiplegic side with the hands clasped. **b** Extending the fingers with the sound hand

To Maintain Full Dorsal Flexion of the Wrist

The patient clasps his hands together, and with both elbows supported parallel on a table in front of him he brings his hands towards his face. Using his sound hand, he dorsiflexes the hemiplegic wrist fully and then repeatedly moves the wrist into the corrected position. The activity can be repeated often during the day, and the position adopted
when the patient is sitting and talking or watching television (**Fig. 16.5**).

To Prevent Shortening of the Flexors of the Wrist and Fingers

The flexors of the fingers and wrist are often markedly spastic and can easily become
shortened. The patient must be taught a method of maintaining their full length. It
may be difficult for him to achieve at first, but one of the following three ways is essential.

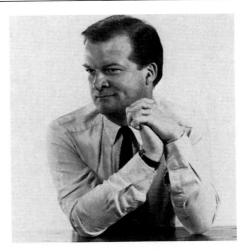

Fig. 16.5. Full dorsiflexion of the wrist with the elbows supported on a table (right hemiplegia)

Method 1

Sitting on a chair, the patient turns his clasped hands over as far as is possible for him. He breathes out and places the heels of his hands on his sound thigh with the elbows still flexed. When he feels that his fingers have relaxed somewhat, he pronates his forearms further until the palms are facing downward and slides his hands slowly down between his legs towards the floor. With his fingers extended, he places the palms of both hands on the floor between his feet(**Fig. 16.6 a**). An advantage of this method is that if the patient still has too little voluntary activity in the extensor muscles, his legs pressing against his arms will help him to keep his elbows straight.

At first, pronating the forearms and turning the clasped hands over so that the palms face downward may be difficult for the patient, and the movement will need to be carefully practised with the help of the therapist. It is, however, particularly important for him to learn to do so on his own, because it is almost the only way in which he can elongate the flexors of his wrist and fingers fully without assistance when his hemiplegic elbow is extended. It is also an excellent way to inhibit spasticity in the hand and, when performed during treatment sessions, will frequently unveil activity in the fingers immediately afterwards.

Learning to pronate the forearms with the hands clasped is usually easier in a sitting position. To help the patient, the therapist stands in front of him and places her thumbs on the dorsal aspect of his wrists. She asks him to breathe out, relax and just let his hands sink down forwards. If he struggles to push his hands down with overactivity of the sound arm the movement is blocked, because the hemiplegic shoulder retracts and the forearm fails to pronate. Instead, the therapist facilitates the pronation of both forearms by turning the patient's hands over with her thumbs and draws them gradually forwards and downwards onto her thigh. Only when his hands are relaxed and comfortable should he attempt to place them first on his own knee and then onto a supporting surface such as a stool in front of him or the floor. Only when he can move his hands easily in sitting should he attempt placing them on the table while standing.

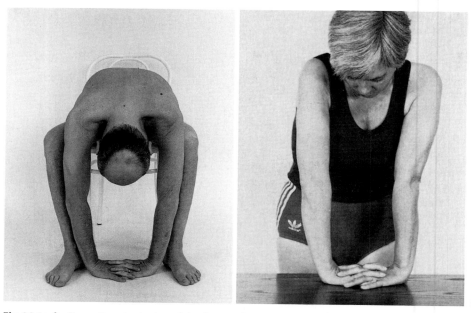

Fig. 16.6 a, b. Preventing shortening of the flexors of wrist and fingers **a** In sitting, placing the hands on the floor with wrist and fingers extended. The patient's legs help to keep the elbows extended (left hemiplegia). **b** In standing, the hands are placed flat on a table (right hemiplegia)

Method 2

In standing, the patient claps his hands together, turns them over and places the palms on a table or some other firm surface with his fingers extended. Keeping his elbows straight, he moves his weight forwards until the wrists are in as full dorsal flexion as possible (**Fig. 16.6 b**). He can also shift his weight gently from one side to the other, which inhibits the flexor hypertonus considerably.

Method 3

Some patients find it easier to place their hemiplegic hand flat on a supporting surface beside them, but the method takes longer and the passive movement needs quite some practice before it can be performed successfully. The patient sits on a table, or on a chair with another chair right next to it. Using his sound hand he passively extends the fingers and wrist of his hemiplegic hand. The supination of the forearm will help to relax the finger flexors but if there is marked hypertonus in his hand, he will need to use his sound leg to give counterpressure against the dorsal aspect of the wrist while extending his fingers passively (**Fig. 16.7 a**).

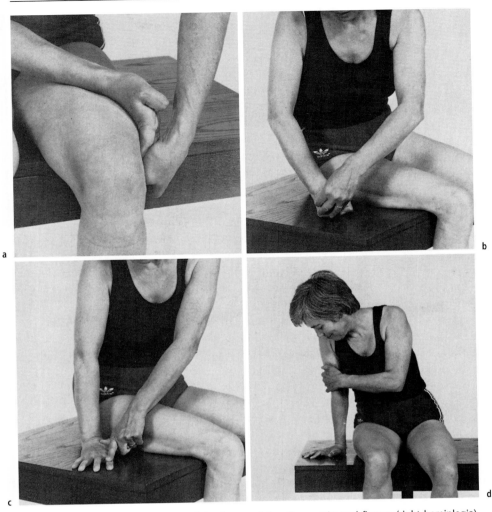

Fig. 16.7 a–d. Preventing shortening of the flexors of the elbow, wrist and fingers (right hemiplegia). **a** Passively extending the fingers with the sound hand, using the sound leg to provide counterpressure; **b** placing the hemiplegic hand at the side with the fingers kept in extension; **c** bringing the flexed thumb into extension and abduction; **d** extending the elbow with the sound hand when weight is taken through the arm

Once the fingers and wrist are extended, he places his hand on the firm surface at his side, leaving his elbow still in some degree of flexion (**Fig. 16.7 b**). With the hand resting on the table, he carefully moves his thumb into abduction (**Fig. 16.7 c**). Using his sound hand to hold the affected elbow in full extension, he moves his body weight over the affected arm, taking care that the fingers do not flex as he does so (**Fig. 16.7 d**).

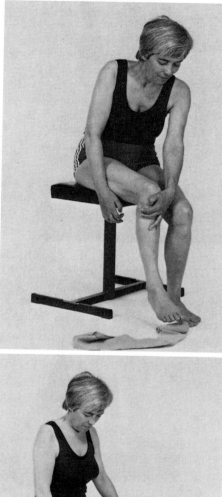

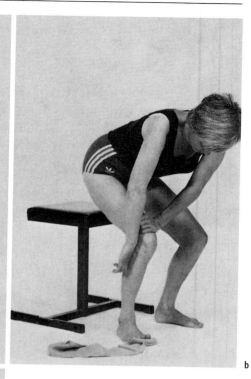

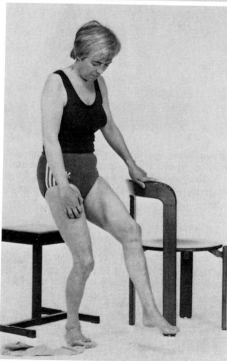

Fig. 16.8 a–c. Preventing shortening of the Achilles tendon and toe flexors (right hemiplegia). **a** The patient places her foot carefully on a rolled bandage, so that the bandage lies directly under all her toes. **b** She presses down on her knee until the heel is on the floor and then lifts her buttocks off the stool. **c** Standing with all her weight on the hemiplegic leg, the patient flexes and extends her knee and holds on lightly to the back of a chair for safety

To Prevent Shortening of the Achilles Tendon and Toe Flexors

The patient puts a rolled bandage in position on the floor in front of him and places his foot so that his toes are supported on it in extension (**Fig. 16.8 a**). He stands up and, if necessary, pushes on the affected knee with his sound hand to ensure that the heel maintains contact with the floor (**Fig. 16.8 b**). Standing erect, he brings his weight over his hemiplegic leg and lifts the other leg into the air. Supporting himself lightly on the back of a chair, a chest of drawers or the washbasin to maintain balance, the patient stands on the bandage and bends and straightens his knee, keeping his hips forward as he does so (**Fig. 16.8 c**).

The patient is advised to do this important exercise in the bathroom every day, because there he is already barefooted and the bandage can be kept in the cupboard above the basin. He can, for example, stand on the bandage routinely while he is shaving (**Fig. 16.9 a**). The basin provides a stable support, and the patient's head automatically moves freely during the activity, while the mirror enables him to check that his trunk and shoulders are symmetrical and his posture correct. A female patient can do the same while she is brushing her hair or putting on her make-up. This simple activity will ensure that the foot remains fully mobile even after many years (**Fig. 16.9 b**). It also prevents the shortening of the calf muscles or painful clawing of the toes, which can otherwise so easily occur and make walking precarious and uncomfortable (**Fig. 16.9 c**).

To Maintain the Full Range of Horizontal Abduction with the Elbow Extended

If patients carry out these exercises regularly and correctly, the full range of movement in the hypertonic or paralysed muscles as well as in the joints will be maintained.

Independently

The patient places the fingers of his hemiplegic hand around the handle of a cupboard door and slowly moves his feet away so that his elbow is passively extended and the shoulder laterally rotated. With the hand thus stabilised, he stretches his sound arm out sideways as well, and rests the dorsal aspect of the hand against the cupboard door behind him. Keeping his feet stationary and parallel to one another, he moves his chest and buttocks away from the cupboard as far forwards as he can with the hands remaining in position (**Fig. 16.10 a**). Different fixtures can serve to keep the affected hand in place, such as a door handle or the handle of the refrigerator, and if none can be found, a suitable disc can be screwed onto a wall for the purpose.

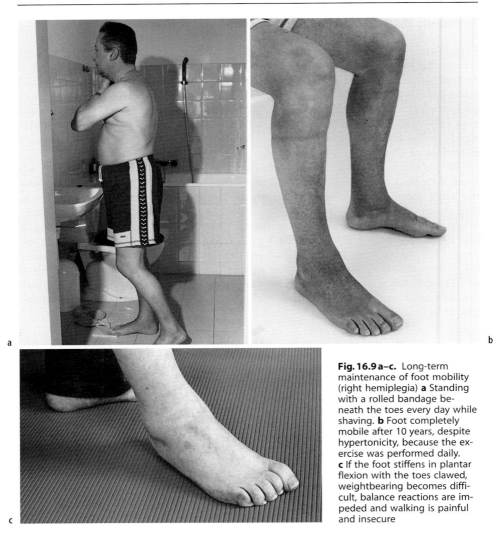

Fig. 16.9 a–c. Long-term maintenance of foot mobility (right hemiplegia) **a** Standing with a rolled bandage beneath the toes every day while shaving. **b** Foot completely mobile after 10 years, despite hypertonicity, because the exercise was performed daily. **c** If the foot stiffens in plantar flexion with the toes clawed, weightbearing becomes difficult, balance reactions are impeded and walking is painful and insecure

With Help

If the patient is not yet able to perform the activity in standing on his own, he requires the help of another person to maintain the range of movement until he has made sufficient progress. It can be one of the family or a neighbour who has been taught the movement.

The patient first inhibits hypertonicity by clasping his hands together and lifting them above his head (right hemiplegia) The helper then takes his hemiplegic arm and, holding the elbow in extension, moves it slowly sideways until it lies flat on the bed,

Fig. 16.10 a, b. Maintaining range of horizontal abduction with elbow extension (right hemiplegia). **a** With his hemiplegic hand held in place by a door handle, the patient's arm abducts when he moves his body away from the cupboard door. **b** A patient who is not yet able to move in standing needs the assistance of her husband to maintain the range of abduction of her arm with her elbow, wrist and fingers extended

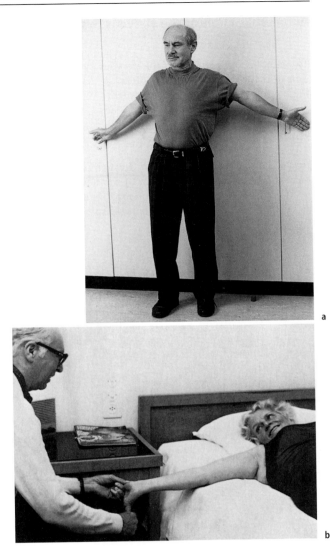

a

b

with the palm of the hand facing upward. The arm lies at an angle of 90° to the body. The thumb is drawn out of the hand in extension and abduction, and with his other hand the helper extends all the fingers (**Fig. 16.10 b**). The activity continues until the wrist, fingers and thumb are fully extended. A pillow placed under the patient's chest during the activity will increase the effect, and will also maintain extension of the patient's thoracic spine.

Automobilisation of the Nervous System

To maintain full mobility of the nervous system, specific activities are required in addition to those for muscles and joints, so that the escaping movements caused by abnormally increased tension are prevented.

Rotating the Neuraxis

In combination with the activity to maintain full range of motion at the shoulder, the patient can include mobilisation of the neuraxis as well. When his arms are above his head with his hands correctly clasped together, he moves them as far over to one side as he can with rotation of his thoracic spine (**Fig. 16.11**).

Mobilising the ULTT1

In addition to ensuring the elasticity of the adductors and medial rotators of the shoulder, the patient must also mobilise the neural structures of the whole upper limb to maintain their property of adaptive lengthening. To do so on his own, he moves both his arms into abduction and lateral rotation while his hemiplegic hand is held in a stationary position, and includes as many of the components of the ULTT1 as possible in the mobilisation:

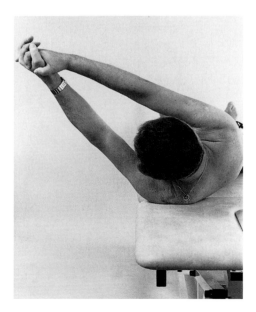

Fig. 16.11. Rotation of the thorax mobilises the neuraxis (right hemiplegia)

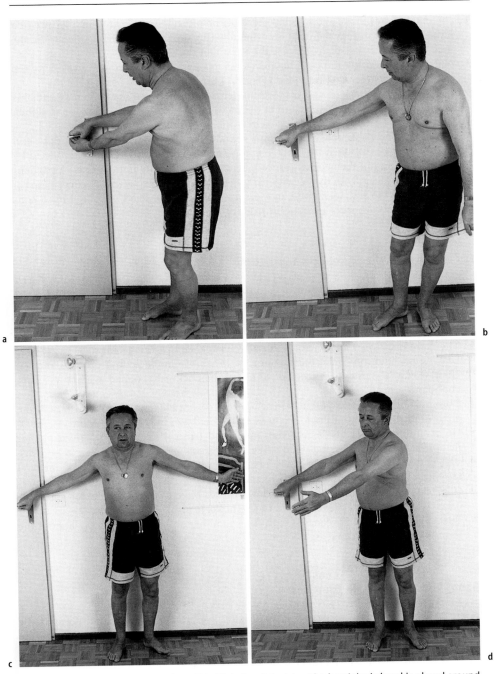

Fig. 16.12 a–d. Automobilisation for ULTT1 (right hemiplegia). **a** The hemiplegic hand is placed around the door handle. **b** Moving the body away to extend the hemiplegic arm passively; **c** moving the thorax away from the wall with both arms abducted and laterally rotated; **d** bringing the sound arm forwards with trunk rotation

- The patient uses his sound hand to place his hemiplegic fingers around a fixture of a suitable height, such as a doorknob or handle (Fig. 16.12 a). With hypertonicity in the arm, the elbow is left flexed, as are the wrist and the fingers.
- With his hand firmly in place, he moves his feet and his trunk slowly away from the handle until his elbow is extended (Fig. 16.12 b).
- With his back to the wall and his feet in line with one another, the patient extends his sound arm and places the dorsum of the hand against the wall on that side, and then brings his chest and his seat forward over his feet (Fig. 16.12 c).
- Keeping his pelvis in line, he moves his sound hand repeatedly towards the door and then back again to touch the wall (Fig. 16.12 d). Not only is the ULTT1 mobilised by this movement but the neuraxis as well, through the rotation of the thorax. A particular benefit derived from the activity is that when walking the patient's arm remains at his side with the shoulder girdle in the correct position, instead of being pulled constantly into flexion with his hand in front of his crotch.

Mobilisation of the Slump in Long-Sitting

Automobilisation of the slump in long-sitting will help the patient to maintain a good walking pattern and the mobility of almost his whole nervous system via the neuraxis as well. The greatest difficulty for most patients is keeping the foot dorsiflexed when they lean forwards to touch their toes with their knees straight.
- The patient sits on a chair with his seat well back against the backrest.
- Leaving his sound foot flat on the floor, he lifts his hemiplegic foot up onto another chair which is standing in front of him with its backrest propped against a wall or cupboard.
- With his knee still flexed, the patient places the sole of his foot against the back of the chair and uses his sound hand to press the ankle down into dorsiflexion.
- He carefully extends his knee, using his sound hand if necessary to avoid plantar flexion of his foot occurring with active knee extension.
- The patient slides his hands down his leg towards his foot, flexing his trunk and moving repeatedly back and forth to mobilise rather than to stretch the structures (Fig. 16.13). His sound hand presses down on his knee if it tends to flex off the chair or assists the forward movement of the hemiplegic arm.
- The same movement is repeated with the sound leg on the chair and the hemiplegic foot resting on the floor.

Some Additional Active Exercises

Some patients may wish to be taught additional exercises to practise actively on their own. An individual selection should then be provided by the therapist, one appropriate to the patient's needs and ability. Many of the activities with a gymnastic ball as described by Klein-Vogelbach (1991) in her well-illustrated book on the subject and demonstrated in an excellent video (Klein-Vogelbach 1992) have proved to be very useful for many patients. The ball adds interest and makes the exact activation of specific muscle groups possible. Not only do patients enjoy exercising with the ball, but the ball also

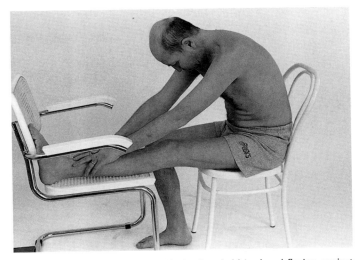

Fig. 16.13. Automobilisation of the slump in long-sitting with the foot held in dorsal flexion against the backrest of a chair (left hemiplegia)

provides them with information as to whether the exercise is being performed correctly or not, because it either moves in a certain direction or does not move as specified by the activity. Many of the activities have been adapted and used successfully with patients of different ages and at different stages of rehabilitation (Davies 1990). The following are some useful examples.

Lifting the Ball Up with the Heels and Straightening the Knees

The patient lies supine and places his heels one on either side of the ball. With his arms remaining relaxed at his sides, he lifts the ball off the ground, keeping his hips abducted and outwardly rotated and the ball in the midline of his body (**Fig. 16.14a**). He lifts the ball further up into the air by extending his knees, which not only enhances selective knee extension but also mobilises the straight leg raise (**Fig. 16.14b**).

Extension of the Legs with Rotation of the Trunk

In supine, the patient puts both his legs onto the ball and lifts his buttocks and trunks off the supporting surface. Keeping the ball absolutely stationary, he then tries to maintain the position while lifting his sound arm off the floor (**Fig. 16.15a**).

With both shoulders remaining flat on the floor and his arms at his sides, the patient rotates his pelvis and lower trunk until his hemiplegic leg is lying on top of his sound leg (**Fig. 16.15b**). He then turns his pelvis towards the opposite side until the sound leg rests on the other one, with his knees extended and without the pelvis sinking down at all (**Fig. 16.15c**).

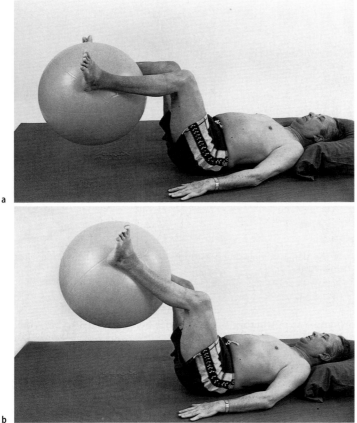

Fig. 16.14 a, b. Furthering selective activity in the leg by lifting a gymnastic ball with both feet (right hemiplegia). **a** The patient presses his heels against the ball and flexes his hips and knees to lift it into the air. **b** Extending both knees selectively to lift the ball higher

Training Selective Abdominal Muscle Activity

Lying supine, the patient rests his hemiplegic leg on the ball and lifts his sound leg into the air, with the hip flexed to approximately 90° and the knee somewhat extended. He adducts and abducts the sound leg, and as a result the ball supporting his hemiplegic leg moves reactively from one side to the other in the contralateral direction to the sound leg (**Fig. 16.16 a**). The patient tries to leave the hemiplegic leg lying relaxed in extension, inhibiting the tendency for the knee to flex when the abdominal muscles are activated.

With the sound calf resting on the ball, the patient lifts up his hemiplegic leg and moves it from one side to the other, trying not to use his sound leg actively as the ball

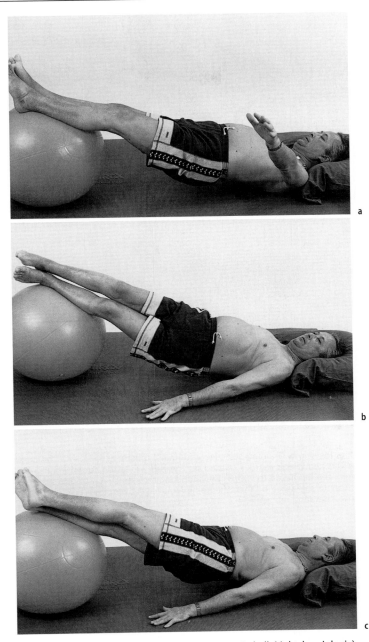

Fig. 16.15 a–c. Improving hip extension and trunk control with a gymnastic ball (right hemiplegia). **a** With both legs supported on the ball, the patient lifts his seat into the air and tries to maintain the position when he raises his sound arm. **b** Rotating the pelvis forwards until the hemiplegic leg is resting on the other one. **c** The patient keeps his seat off the floor and rotates his lower trunk and pelvis towards the hemiplegic side

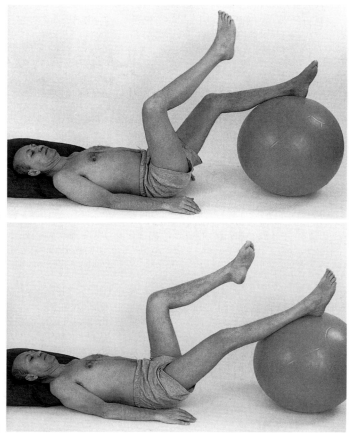

Fig. 16.16 a, b. Training selective abdominal muscle activity with the gymnastic ball (left hemiplegia).
a The hemiplegic leg lies relaxed on the ball, while the sound leg moves from one side to the other
with the hip flexed to 90°. As the sound leg moves actively to one side, the hemiplegic leg moves reactively to the other. **b** When the hemiplegic leg moves sideways through the air the patient tries not to
use his sound leg actively

moves in the opposite direction each time (**Fig. 16.16 b**). Because the thoracic spine is
supported in extension while the legs move, selective abdominal muscle activity is stimulated and retrained.

Leisure Activities and Hobbies

Before the patient is discharged from treatment, therapists and other care givers must
realise that there is more to life than performing a list of exercises. Tyson (1995) stresses

the importance of social activity being included as part of the rehabilitation programme, the aim being "to return people to an active life style, not merely an existence". Great care must be taken that when treatment ceases, the patient does not just sit at home all day with nothing to do to fill the long hours. There is a real danger that, apart from watching television, his only pleasure will be eating and drinking, which could lead to his gaining weight if combined with lack of active exercise and enforced immobility. Obesity not only makes walking and self-care activities more difficult but also is a known risk factor for raised blood pressure. Aesthetically, if the patient is overweight, his appearance does not please him, his clothes no longer fit and the loss of self-esteem can be an additional reason why he does not like to leave the house. A study on the long-term outcome of stroke patients revealed that although 90% of the patients were able walk indoors and climb stairs independently, many in fact were effectively housebound and never went out of doors (Thorngren et al. 1990) Hobbies and leisure activities help to keep the patient mobile and encourage him to go out of the house and to meet other people. However, it has been found that few patients return to their previous activities and even fewer take up new activities on their own (Jongbloed and Morgan 1991). Moreover, patients are unable to modify or replace their leisure activities without help. Just as they cannot teach themselves how to walk and dress themselves after the stroke, many will need guidance, information and encouragement to take up new interests and activities (Drummond 1990).

It therefore becomes an integral part of successful rehabilitation for the therapist to advise the patient on which activities would be possible, to help him to choose one after trying out a few practically, and to teach him how to succeed with his final choice. Without such help and guidance the patient may lack the confidence to go out, and will gradually become withdrawn, socially isolated and less and less active.

People have very different interests, and not all patients will wish to take up some form of sport even though the movements might be therapeutic and beneficial. A sense of well-being seems to be related to participation in leisure activities and, according to Tyson (1995): "It does not matter what the patients do, or how well they do it – just to be actively involved in something is important."

Interests Other than Sport

Owning a Dog

A dog can be a wonderful companion for the patient, and having one as a pet will encourage him to go out of the house for walks. A young engineer in Austria had a stroke and was still in a wheelchair 2 years later when he returned home from the rehabilitation period. He had grave problems with eating and speaking and had to be fed by his wife and daughters. At the end of his rehabilitation he asked what he could do to improve his condition further and was advised by his doctors to "move as much as possible because the whole brain takes part in the process of walking". He had the idea that having a dog might encourage him to move more, and he later wrote a touching letter that explains just how valuable having a dog can be for someone with hemiplegia.

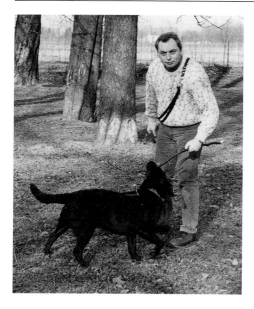

Fig. 16.17. Going for a walk with Cassy

*Since August we have had a Labrador retriever, dogs of this breed being particularly suitable for disabled people because they are most intelligent and good-natured. I am so very happy to have 'Cassy', because I am no longer alone when the family leaves the house (work or school). In addition, I must go out with her regularly, and when I do, I meet and have conversations with other people, mostly other dog owners. This strengthens my self-confidence, is a pleasure for me and 'rescues' me from the inevitable isolation caused by my illness (**Fig. 16.17**). My wife and both my daughters are also delighted with Cassy; she really 'enriches' the lives of the whole family (H. Sobotha, personal communication, 1996, translated from the German).*

Even a small dog can make a big difference, as one tiny dachshund did when she helped an aphasic patient to enjoy life again, understanding his voice without words, encouraging him to take her for walks and playing endlessly with the ball he threw for her to catch.

Singing

Some patients have found singing in a choir stimulating and enjoyable, and their voice and breath control has improved as well.

Gardening

Seeing plants grow and tending them can be most satisfying, and many patients have become ardent gardeners even if they were not interested before their stroke. For those without a garden, balcony plants and window boxes suffice. One patient took to cultivating orchids in his apartment and became quite an expert in the field.

Painting

Surprising results have been demonstrated by patients in this creative field after attending group art classes, which are thoroughly enjoyed by all who participate. A 70-year-old lady who had never drawn or painted before she suffered her stroke, displayed considerable talent and had much success with her work.

Sporting Activities

Many different types of sport and active movement have been tried successfully and enjoyed by disabled people, ranging from yoga and aerobics (Rasmussen 1995) to archery and horse riding (Malmström et al. 1995). Many patients of different ages and at various stages of rehabilitation have been able to master and enjoy the following, readily available activities.

Swimming

Learning to swim is possible and pleasurable for almost all patients even if they were not able to swim before their hemiplegia. Instruction is necessary, however, and the Halliwick method is recommended. The patient benefits from moving while supported by the water, and it is an activity that he can enjoy together with his family and friends. Weber-Witt (1994) describes and illustrates how patients can be taught to swim safely and therapeutically despite marked weakness or paralysis. Ways to solve problems such as how to enter and leave the swimming pool are also explained.

Cycling

The patient can be taught to ride a bicycle with both his hands on the handlebars or, if he is not yet able to manage on a two-wheeler, there are many attractive tricycles for adults on the market at present. According to the needs of the patient, these are fitted with a saddle or a seat with a backrest. Particularly for patients who can walk only very slowly, the tricycle allows them to move freely and confidently and to keep up with those accompanying them. Some patients ride a tandem cycle with a friend or partner and can manage considerable distances on interesting outings even with a marked disability.

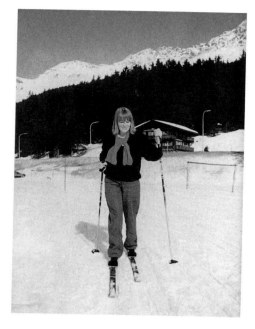

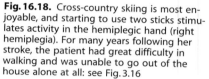

Fig. 16.18. Cross-country skiing is most enjoyable, and starting to use two sticks stimulates activity in the hemiplegic hand (right hemiplegia). For many years following her stroke, the patient had great difficulty in walking and was unable to go out of the house alone at all: see Fig. 3.16

Cross-country Skiing

Even a patient who has difficulty in walking alone can learn cross-country skiing and benefit from the activity considerably, improving his walking ability while enjoying the experience (Gerber 1995). If the patient has no return of motor control in his hemiplegic arm he skis without ski sticks, but should activity be present, it can be enhanced by practising with two sticks **(Fig. 16.18)**.

Golf

The movements of the golf swing are very beneficial for the patient because they include weight transference, trunk rotation and hand-eye coordination. In addition, playing 18 holes entails walking more than 5 kilometres, a distance that few would walk without the stimulus of the game. The patient's stamina is improved, as is his walking ability. Golf is also a game that can be played rather well with one hand **(Fig. 16.19)**. Dr Mueller, a neurologist who suffered a left hemiplegia after a skiing accident, is the patient illustrated in **Fig. 16.19**. He has already achieved a handicap of 32 and plans to compete in the international games in Australia in the year 2000. So enthralled was he with the physical progress he made through playing golf and the enjoyment he experienced, that he has now set in motion a project for building and financing a golf course for disabled players in Northern Germany, which has come close to realisation; its motto "Trotz

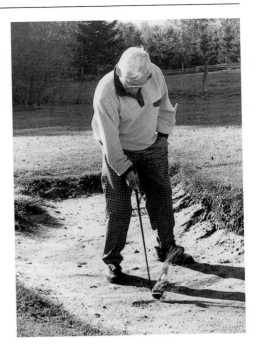

Fig. 16.19. A handicap of 32 despite his handicap! Getting out of a bunker successfully and onto the green with only one active hand (left hemiplegia)

Handicap zum Handicap" means approximately "towards a handicap despite a handicap" (*Kurier am Sonntag*, 9 February, 1997). Dr. Mueller recommends that other patients also take up a sport that they had not participated in prior to their hemiplegia, so as to avoid a disappointing comparison with previous prowess. He, himself, having been an avid football player and downhill skier, chose golf and started to learn the game together with his wife. Not only did he reduce his handicap; his gait also improved amazingly as a result of playing golf and the physical activity that it entails. He also enjoys cross-country skiing in winter, has lost weight and is fit, sun-tanned and healthy.

Conclusion

Performing the activities recommended for maintaining the elasticity of muscles, the range of motion in joints, and the mobility of the nervous system will prevent the development of painful and unsightly contractures and keep the doors open for further recovery in the future. Not only will the patient be able to maintain the level of performance which he achieved during his rehabilitation, but voluntary activity will be improved and functional use enhanced. It is most important for the patient to keep on keeping on – setting realistic goals for himself, no matter how small they may seem, and then working hard to attain them. He should be adventurous and – when the moment feels right – find new, more active ways to perform certain everyday activities, ways that previously were not possible but, due to gradually improving motor control, have become possible, like crossing his legs without the help of the sound hand or using the stairs instead of the lift. For example, Andreas furthered control of his hemiplegic leg by practising putting on and taking off his shoes in standing, with a stool in front of him to support his foot (**Fig. 16.20**).

With regard to regaining the activity in his affected arm, it is even more important for the patient to find tasks in his daily life for which he uses his hemiplegic hand in some way, although he could quite easily perform the tasks with his sound hand on its own. He has to set rules for himself and then adhere to them, regarding a steadily increasing number of activities that he will always perform with his hemiplegic hand playing a part, and thus try to extend the repertoire of the activities. For example, he can always open the door or eat a piece of apple or a biscuit with his affected hand or pick up his shoe from the floor with it before passing it to the other hand to put on.

Finding activities for the hemiplegic arm is essential for improvement because it really is a case of "use it or lose it", as the saying goes. Paolo, for instance, improved the sensation and movement in his hemiplegic arm by deciding that he would always use it when putting on his hat, which was difficult for him and at first required the help of his sound hand (**Fig. 16.21 a**). But, after continuing to practise the activity for some time, quite unexpectedly one day he took his hat in his hemiplegic hand and proudly lifted it onto his head without any assistance (**Fig. 16.21 b, c**).

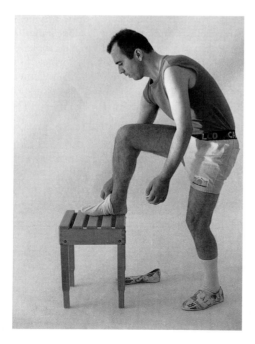

Fig. 16.20. Putting on a sock in standing improves balance and active control of the hemiplegic leg (left hemiplegia)

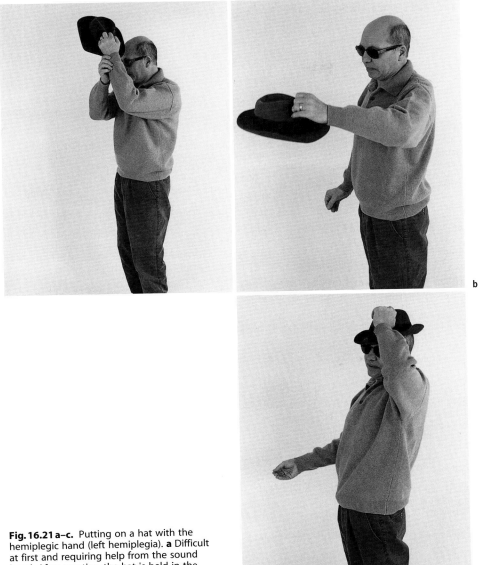

Fig. 16.21 a–c. Putting on a hat with the hemiplegic hand (left hemiplegia). **a** Difficult at first and requiring help from the sound hand. After practice, the hat is held in the hemiplegic hand (**b**) and lifted into place (**c**) without any assistance

Making progress brings a sense of achievement and enables certain tasks to be performed more easily. Every gain in functional activity, no matter how small it may seem, will be a big bonus for the patient himself, will encourage him to continue exercising on his own and will enhance his quality of life in some special way.

17 References

Abend W, Bizzi E, Morasso P (1982) Human arm trajectory formation. Brain 105: 331–348
Ackerman S (1992) Discovering the brain. National Academic Press, Washington
Adams GF, Hurwitz LJ (1963) Mental barriers to recovery from stroke. Lancet 14: 533–537
Adams C, Logue V (1971) Studies in cervical spondolytic myelopathy. Brain 94: 557–568
Adler MK, Brown CC, Acton P (1980) Stroke rehabilitation – is age a determinant? J Am Geriatr Soc XXVIII: 499–503
Adler SS, Beckers D, Buck M (1993) PNF in practice. An illustrated guide. Springer, Berlin Heidelberg New York
Affolter F (1981) Perceptual processes as prerequisites for complex human behaviour. Int Rehabil Med 3: 39
Affolter F, Bischofberger W (1996) Gespürte Interaktion im Alltag. In: Lipp B, Schlaegel W (eds) Wege von Anfang an: Frührehabilitation schwerst hirngeschädigter Patienten. Neckar-Verlag, Villingen-Schwenningen
Affolter F, Stricker E (eds) (1980) Perceptual processes as prerequisites for complex human behaviour. A theoretical model and its application to therapy. Huber, Bern
Andrews K, Brocklehurst JC, Richards B, Laycock PJ (1982) The recovery of the severely disabled stroke patient. Rheumatol Rehabil 21: 225–230
Ashburn A, Partridge C, De Souza LH (1993) Physiotherapy in the rehabilitation of stroke: a review. Clin Rehabilitation 7: 337–345
Atkinson HW (1986) Aspects of neuro-anatomy and physiology. In: Downie, PA (ed) Cash's textbook of neurology for physiotherapists, 4th edn. Faber and Faber, London, p 73

Bach-y-Rita P (ed) (1980) Brain plasticity as a basis for therapeutic procedures. Recovery of function: theoretical considerations for brain injury rehabilitation. Huber, Bern
Bach-y-Rita P (1981a) Central nervous system lesions: sprouting and unmasking in rehabilitation. Arch Phys Med Rehabil 62: 413–417
Bach-y-Rita P (1981b) Brain plasticity as a basis of the development of rehabilitation procedures for hemiplegia. Scand J Rehabil Med 13: 73–83
Bach-y-Rita P, Balliet R (1987) Recovery from stroke. In: Duncan PAW, Bradke MB (eds) Stroke rehabilitation. The recovery of motor control. Year Book Medical, Chicago
Bannister D (1974) Personal construct theory and psychotherapy. In: Bannister D (ed) Issues and approaches to psychotherapy. Wiley, New York
Basmajian JV (1979) Muscles alive. Their functions revealed by electromyography, 4th edn. Williams and Wilkins, Baltimore
Basmajian JV (1981) Biofeedback in rehabilitation: a review of principles and practices. Arch Phys Med Rehabil 62: 469–475
Bateman JE (1963) The diagnosis and treatment of ruptures of the rotator cuff. Surg Clin North Am 43: 1523–1530
Bernstein NA (1967) The co-ordination and regulation of movements. Pergamon, Oxford
Bernstein NA (1996) On dexterity and its development. In: Latash ML, Turvey MT (eds) Dexterity and its development. Lawrence Erlbaum Associates, Mahwah, NJ
Biewald F (1989) Krankengymnastik. In: Mäurer H-C (ed) Schlaganfall. Rehabilitation statt resignation. Thieme, Stuttgart
Biguer B, Donaldson IML, Hein A, Jeannerod M (1988) Neck muscle vibration modifies the representation of visual motion and direction in man. Brain 111: 1405–1424
Bobath B (1971) Abnormal postural reflex activity caused by brain lesions. Heinemann Medical Books, London
Bobath B (1977) Treatment of adult hemiplegia. Physiotherapy 63: 310–313
Bobath B (1978) Adult hemiplegia: evaluation and treatment. Heinemann Medical Books, London
Bobath B (1990) Adult hemiplegia: evaluation and treatment, 3rd edn. Heinemann Medical Books, Oxford

Bobath K (1971) The normal postural reflex mechanism and its deviation in children with cerebral palsy. Campfield, St Albans (reprinted from Physiotherapy, November 1971, pp 1–11)

Bobath K (1974) The motor deficit in patients with cerebral palsy. Medical education and information unit of the spastics society. Heinemann Medical Books, London

Bobath K (1976–1982) Unpublished lectures given during courses on the treatment of adult hemiplegia. Postgraduate Study Centre Hermitage, Bad Ragaz

Bobath K (1980) Neurophysiology, part 1. Videofilm recorded at the Postgraduate Study Centre Hermitage, Bad Ragaz

Boivie J, Leijon G (1991) Clinical findings in patients with central post stroke pain. In: Casey KL (ed) Pain and central nervous system disease: the central pain syndromes. Raven, New York

Bojsen-Moller F, Lamoreux L (1979) Significance of dorsiflexion of the toes in walking. Acta Orthop Scand 50: 471–479

Bowsher D (1992) Neurogenic pain syndromes and their management. In: Wells JCD, Woolf CJ (eds) Pain mechanisms and management. Churchill Livingstone, Edinburgh (British Medical Bulletin series, vol 47, no 3)

Boyle JJW (1999) Is the pain and dysfunction of shoulder impingement lesion really second rib syndrome in disguise? Manual Ther 4: 44–48

Brandt T, Dietrich M (1987) Pathological exe-head coordination in roll. Tonic occular tilt reaction in mesencephalic and medullary lesion. Brain 110: 649–666

Braun RM, West F, Mooney V, Nickel VL, Roper B, Caldwell C (1971) Surgical treatment of the painful shoulder contracture in the stroke patient. J Bone Joint Surg 53-A: 1307–1312

Braus DF (1990) Schmerzsyndrome nach Schlaganfall. Praev Rehabil 2: 73–77

Braus DF, Krauss JK, Strobel J (1994). The shoulder-hand syndrome after stroke: a prospective trial. Ann Neurol 36: 728–733

Breig A (1978) Adverse mechanical tension in the nervous system. Almquist and Wiksell, Stockholm

Breig A, Marions O (1963) Biomechanics of the lumbosacral nerve roots. Acta Radiologica 4: 602–604

Breig A, Troup J (1979) Biomechanical considerations in the straight-leg raise test. Cadaveric and clinical studies of the effects of medial hip rotation. Spine 4: 242–250

Brodal A (1973) Self-observations and neuroanatomical considerations after a stroke. Brain 96: 675–694

Brooks VB (1986) The neural basis of motor control. Oxford University Press, New York

Brunnstrom S (1970) Movement therapy in hemiplegia. A neurophysiological approach. Harper and Row, Hagerstown

Burl M, Williams JG, Nayak USL (1992) The effect of cervical collars on walking balance. Physiotherapy 78: 19–22

Butler DS (1989) Adverse mechanical tension in the nervous system: a model for assessment and treatment. Aust J Physiother 35: 227–238

Butler DS (1991) Mobilisation of the nervous system. Churchill Livingstone, Melbourne

Butler PB, Major RE (1992) The learning of motor control: biomechanical considerations. Physiotherapy 78: 6–11

Cailliet R (1980) The shoulder in hemiplegia. Davis, Philadelphia

Cain HD, Liebgold HB (1967) Compressive centripetal wrapping technic for reduction of edema. Arch Phys Med Rehabil 48: 420–423

Caldwell CB, Wilson DJ, Braun RM (1969) Evaluation and treatment of the upper extremity in the hemiplegic stroke patient. Clin Orthop 63: 69–93

Carlsson M (1988) Effekter av behandling enlight Bobath konceptet. Untvärdering av strokebehandling på Sätra Hälsobrunn sommaren 1987. FoU-rapport Vårdhögskolan, Uppsala

Carr JH, Shepherd RB (1982) A motor relearning programme for stroke. Heinemann, London

Carr JH, Shepherd RB (1996) "Normal" is not the issue: it is "effective" goal attainment that counts. Commentary/Latash & Hanson: Movements in atypical populations. Behav Brain Sci 19: 72–73

Carslöö S (1966) The initiation of walking. Acta Anat 65: 1–9

Carterette EC, Friedman MP (eds) (1973) Handbook of perception, vol 3. Academic, New York

Charlton JE (1991) Management of sympathetic pain. Br Med Bull 47, 3: 601–618

Chiodo LK, Gerety MB, Mulrow CD, Rhodes MC, Tuley MR (1992) The impact of physical therapy on nursing home patient outcomes. Phys Ther 72: 168–175

Christensen K, Jensen EM, Noer I (1982) The reflex dystrophy syndrome response to treatment with systemic corticosteroids. Acta Chir Scand 148: 653–655

Codman EA (1934) The shoulder. Todd, Boston

Coombes K (1977 1983) Unpublished lectures and demonstrations given during courses on the rehabilitation of the face and oral tract. Postgraduate Study Centre Hermitage, Bad Ragaz

Coughlan AK, Humphrey M (1982) Presenile stroke: long-term outcome for patients and their families. Rheumatol Rehabil 21: 115–122

Cyriax J (1942) Perineuritis. Br Med J 1: 578–580

Cyriax J (1959) Text-book of orthopaedic medicine, vol II: Treatment by manipulation and massage, 6th edn. Cassell, London

Cyriax J (1978) Textbook of orthopaedic medicine, vol 1, 7th edn. Balliere Tindall, London

Damasio AR (1994) Descartes' error. Emotion, reason and the human brain. G. P. Putnam's Sons, New York

Davenport M, Hall P (1981) Speech therapy. In: Evans CD (ed) Rehabilitation after severe head injury. Churchill Livingstone, Edinburgh

Davies PM (1980) Physiotherapeutische Maßnahmen im Umgang mit der Problematik der hemiplegischen Schulter. Der Physiotherapeut [Suppl] „Die Schulter", National Congress, pp 106–108

Davies PM (1990) Right in the middle. Selective trunk activity in the treatment of adult hemiplegia. Springer, Berlin Heidelberg New York

Davies PM (1994) Starting again. Early rehabilitation after traumatic brain injury or other severe brain lesion. Springer, Berlin Heidelberg New York

Davies PM (1997) Taking a new look at spasticity. Proceedings of the South African Physiotherapy Society International Congress in Cape Town, pp 209–214

Davis SW, Petrillo CR, Eichberg RD, Chu DS (1977) Shoulder-hand syndrome in a hemiplegic population: a 5-year retrospective study. Arch Phys Med Rehabil 58: 353–356

Dennet DC (1991) Consciousness explained. Allen Lane/Penguin, London

Dewar R (1983) Personal communication

Diethelm U, Davies PM (1985) Die Schulter beim Hemiplegiker. Schweiz Rundsch Med Prax 74: 177–179

Dimitrijevic MR, Faganal J, Sherwood AM, McKay WB (1981) Activation of paralysed leg flexors and extensors during gait in patients after stroke. Scand J Rehabil Med 13: 109–115

Drillis RJ (1958) Objective recording and biomechanics of pathological gait. Ann N Y Acad Sci 74: 86–109

Drummond A (1990) Leisure activities after stroke. Int Dis Studies 12: 157–160

Duncan PAW, Bradke MB (1987) Stroke rehabilitation. The recovery of motor control. Year Book Medical, Chicago

Dyck P (1984) Lumbar nerve root: the enigmatic eponyms. Spine 9: 3–6

Elvey R (1986b) Treatment of arm pain associated with abnormal brachial plexus tension. Aust J Physiother 32: 225–230

Elvey RL (1979) Brachial plexus tension tests and the pathoanatomical origin of arm pain. In: Aspects of manipulative therapy. Lincoln Institute of Health Sciences, Melbourne, pp 105–110

Elvey RL (1984) Abnormal brachial plexus tension and shoulder joint limitation. In: Gilraine F, Sweeting L (eds) Proceedings of the International Federation of Orthopaedic Manipulative Therapists. Fifth International Seminar, Vancouver, pp 132–139

Elvey RL (1986a) The investigation of arm pain. In: Grieve GP (ed) Modern manual therapy of the vertebral column. Churchill Livingstone, Edinburgh, pp 530–535

Elvey RL (1988) The clinical relevance of signs of brachial plexus tension. Papers & Poster Abstracts of the Congress of the International Federation of Orthopaedic Manipulative Therapists (IFOMT). Cambridge, September, pp 14–20

Evans CD (1981) Rehabilitation after severe head injury. Churchill Livingstone, Edinburgh

Evans P (1980) The healing process at cellular level: a review. Physiotherapy 66: 256–259

Fields HL (1987) Pain. McGraw-Hill, New York

Fiorentino MR (1981) A basis for sensorimotor development – normal and abnormal. Thomas, Springfield

Friedland F (1975) Physical therapy. In: Licht S (ed) Stroke and its rehabilitation. Williams and Williams, Baltimore, pp 246–248

Gabell A, Nayak USL (1984) The effect of age on variability in gait. J Gerontol 39: 662–666

Garland DE (1995) Reconstructive surgery for residual lower extremity deformities. In: Montgomery J (ed) Physical therapy for traumatic brain injury. Churchill Livingstone, New York

Geary J (1997) A trip down memory's lanes. Time 149 (18): 39–45

Geisseler T (1993) Halbseitenlähmung. Hilfe zur Selbsthilfe. Springer, Berlin Heidelberg New York

Gibson JJ (1966) The senses considered as perceptual systems. Houghton Mifflin, Boston

Gifford J, Gifford L (1988) Connective tissue massage. In: Wells P, Frampton V, Bowsher D (eds) Pain: management and control in physiotherapy. Heinemann Physiotherapy, London

Gresty MA, Bronson AM, Brandt T, Dietrich M (1992) Neurology of otolith function. Peripheral and central disorders. Brain 115: 647–673

Greveson G, James O (1991) Improving long-term outcome after stroke: the views of patients and carers. Health Trends 23: 161–162

Grieve GP (1970) Sciatica and the straight-leg-raising test in manipulative therapy. Physiotherapy 56: 337–346

Griffin J, Reddin G (1981) Shoulder pain in patients with hemiplegia. A literature review. Phys Ther 61: 1041–1045

Grillner S (1981) Control of locomotion in bipeds, tetrapods and fish. In: Geiger SR (ed) Handbook of physiology, vol 2. American Physiological Society, Bethesda, Md.

Gerber M (1995) Cross-country skiing and the Bobath concept. In: Harrison MA (ed) Physiotherapy in stroke management. Churchill Livingstone, Edinburgh

Grillner S, Zangger P (1979) On the central control of locomotion in the low spinal cat. Exp Brain Res 34: 241–261

Gunn CC, Milbrandt W (1977) Tenderness of motor points: an aid to the diagnosis of shoulder pain referred from the cervical spine. J Am Osteopath Assoc 77: 196–212

Guymer AJ (1988) The neuromuscular facilitation of movement. In: Wells PE, Frampton V, Bowsher D (eds) Pain. Management and control in physiotherapy. Heinemann Physiotherapy, London

Halligan PW, Marshall JC, Wade DT (1990) Do visual field defects exacerbate visuo-spatial neglect? J Neurol Neurosurg Psychiatry 53: 487–491

Hesse S, Lücke D, Malezic M, Bertelt C, Friedrich H, Gregoric M, Mauritz KH (1994) Botulinum toxin treatment for lower limb extensor spasticity in chronic hemiparetic patients. J Neurol Neurosurg Psychiatry 57: 1321–1324

Hornby AS (1975) Oxford advanced dictionary of current English, 4th edn. Oxford University Press, London

Houtz SJ, Fischer FJ (1961) Function of leg muscles acting on foot as modified by body movements. J Appl Physiol 16: 597–605

Hurd MM, Farrell KH, Waylonis GW (1974) Shoulder sling for hemiplegia: friend or foe? Arch Phys Med Rehabil 55: 519–522

Inman VT, Saunders JB (1942) The clinico-anatomical aspects of the lumbosacral region. Radiology 38: 669–678

Irwin-Carruthers S, Runnalls MJ (1980) Painful shoulder in hemiplegia prevention and treatment. S Afr J Physiother March: 18–23

Isaacs B (1977) Stroke research and the physiotherapist. Physiotherapy 83: 366–368

Jacobs HE (1988) Yes, behaviour analysis can help, but do you know how to harness it? Brain Inj 2: 339–346

Jeannerod M (1990) The neural and behavioural organisation of goal-directed movements. Clarendon, Oxford

Jeffrey DL (1981) Cognitive clarity: key to motivation in rehabilitation. J Rehabil 47: 33–35

Jimenez Y, Morgan P (1979) Predicting improvement in stroke patients referred for inpatient rehabilitation. Can Med Assoc J 121: 1481–1484

Johnston TB, Willis J (eds) (1954) Gray's anatomy. Longmans, Green and Co., London

Johnstone M (1978) Restoration of motor function in the stroke patient. Livingstone, New York, pp 15–177

Jongbloed L, Morgan D (1991) An investigation of involvement in leisure activities after a stroke. Am J Occup Ther 45: 420–427

Joynt RL (1992) The source of shoulder pain in hemiplegia. Arch Phys Med Rehabil 73: 409–413

Jull GA (1996) Clinical tests for active spinal stabilisation. Keynote lecture at the Biennial Conference of the New Zealand Society of Physiotherapists, March 29–April 1, Dunedin

Kamal A (1987) A colour atlas of stroke. Cerebrovascular disease and its management. Wolfe Medical Publications, London

Karnath H-O (1994) Subjective body orientation in neglect and the interactive contribution of neck muscle proprioception and vestibular stimulation. Brain 117: 1001–1012

Kaste M (1995) Early and late rehabilitation of stroke: current approaches including assessment of the quality of outcome. In: Harrison MA (ed) Physiotherapy in stroke management. Churchill Livingstone, Edinburgh

Katz RT, Rymer WZ (1989) Spastic hypertonia: mechanisms and measurement. Arch Phys Med Rehabil 70: 144–158

Kesselring J (1994) Rotation-induced change of muscle tone (letter to the editor). Eur Neurol 905: 300

Kesselring J, Calame C, Zweifel H-J (1992) Ganganalyse – eine Voraussetzung fur eine allgemeine Bewegungsanalyse. Schweiz Rundsch Med Prax 81: 1495–1499

Kim JS, Choi Kwon S (1996) Discriminative sensory dysfunction after unilateral stroke. Stroke: 27: 6777–6782

Kinsella G, Ford B (1985) Hemi-inattention and the recovery patterns of stroke patients. Int Rehabil Med 7: 102–106

Klein-Vogelbach S (1976) Funktionelle Bewegungslehre. Rehabilitation und Prävention, vol 1, 1st edn. Springer, Berlin Heidelberg New York

Klein-Vogelbach S (1984) Funktionelle Bewegungslehre. Rehabilitation und Prävention, vol 1, 2nd edn. Springer, Berlin Heidelberg New York Tokyo

Klein-Vogelbach S (1990) Functional kinetics. Observing, analyzing and teaching human movement. Springer, Berlin Heidelberg New York

Klein-Vogelbach S (1991 a) Therapeutic exercises in functional kinetics. Analysis and instruction of individually adaptable exercises. Springer, Berlin Heidelberg New York

Klein-Vogelbach S (1991) Ball exercises in functional kinetics. Springer, Berlin Heidelberg New York

Klein-Vogelbach S (1992) Functional kinetics: ball exercises. Video VHS 45 min. Springer, Berlin Heidelberg New York

Klein-Vogelbach S (1995) Gangschulung zur funktionellen Bewegungslehre. Springer, Berlin Heidelberg New York

Knott M, Voss DE (1968) Proprioceptive neuromuscular facilitation. Patterns and techniques, 2nd edn. Hoeber Medical Division, Harper & Row, New York

Knuttson E (1981) Gait control in hemiparesis. Scand J Rehabil Med 13: 101–108

Kottke FJ (1978) Coordination training. IRMA III Congress Lecture, Basel (unpublished)

Kottke FJ (1980) From reflex to skill: the training of coordination. Arch Phys Med Rehabil 61: 551–561

Lance JW (1980) Symposium synopsis. In: Feldman RG, Young RR, Koella WT (eds) Spasticity: disordered motor control. Year Book Medical, Chicago

Landau WM (1988) Clinical mythology 11. Parables of palsy pills and PT pedagogy: a spastic dialectic. Neurology 38: 1496–1499

Latash ML, Anson JG (1996) What are „normal movements" in atypical populations? Behav Brain Sci 19: 55–106

La Vigue J (1974) Hemiplegia sensorimotor assessment form. Phys Ther 54: 128–134

Lehmann JF, Delateur BJ, Fowler RS, Warren CG, Arnold R, Schertzer G, Hurka R, Whitmore JJ, Masock AJ, Chambers KH (1975) Stroke: does rehabilitation affect outcome? Arch Phys Med Rehabil 56: 375–382

Lehmann JF, Condon SM, de Lateur BJ, Smith JC (1985) Ankle-foot orthoses: effects on gait abnormalities in tibial nerve paralysis. Arch Phys Med Rehabil 66: 212–218

Lennon S, Hastings M (1996) Key physiotherapy indicators for quality of stroke care. Physiotherapy 82: 655–661

Leviton-Rheingold N, Hotte EB, Mandel DR (1980) Learning to dress: a fundamental skill to independence for the disabled. Spec Articl Rehabil Lit 41: 72–75

Lind S, Loid M (1995) Rehabilitation of chronic stroke patients – experiences from Sätra Brunn. In: Harrison MA (ed) Physiotherapy in stroke management. Churchill Livingstone, Edinburgh

Lindmark B (1995) A 5-year study of stroke patient recovery. In: Harrison MA (ed) Physiotherapy in stroke management. Churchill Livingstone, Edinburgh

Lipp B (1996) Frührehabilitation aus medizinischer Sicht: Hauptstörungen, Komplikationen und therapeutische Möglichkeiten. In: Lipp B, Schlaegel W (eds) Wege von Anfang an: Frührehabilitation schwerst hirngeschädigter Patienten. Neckar-Verlag, Villingen-Schwenningen

Louis R (1981) Vertebroradicular and vertebromedullar dynamics. Anat Clin 3: 1–11

Luria AR (1978) The working brain. An introduction to neuropsychology. Penguin, London

MacKenzie CL (1994) The grasping hand, Advances in Psychology, vol 104. North-Holland, Amsterdam

Mahoney FI, Barthel DW (1965) Functional evaluation: the Barthel index. Md State Med J 14: 61–65

Maitland GD (1973) Peripheral manipulation, 2nd edn. Butterworths, London

Maitland GD (1979) Negative disc exploration: positive signs. Aust J Physiother 25: 129–134

Maitland GD (1985) The slump test: examination and treatment. Aust J Physiother 31: 215–219

Maitland GD (1986) Vertebral manipulation, 5th edn. Butterworths, London

Maitland GD (1991) Peripheral manipulation, 3rd edn. Butterworth-Heinemann, London, p 70

Maki BE (1997) Gait changes in older adults: predictors of falls or indicators of fear? J Am Geriatr Soc 45: 313–320

Maki BE, McIlroy WE (1997) The role of limb movements in maintaining upright stance: the change in support strategy. Phys Ther 77: 488–507

Malmström K, Johansson S, Sallnäs M (1995) Volleyball, music and balance, archery and riding with stroke patients. In: Harrison MA (ed) Physiotherapy in stroke management. Churchill Livingstone, Edinburgh

Marquardsen J (1969) Natural history of acute cerebrovascular disease: retrospective study of 769 patients. Acta Neurol Scand 45 [Suppl 38]: 56–59

Massey AE (1986) Movement of pain-sensitive structures in the neural canal. In: Grieve GP (ed) Modern manual therapy of the vertebral column. Churchill Livingstone, Edinburgh

Mathiowetz V, Bolding DJ, Trombly CA (1983) Immediate effects of positioning devices on the normal and spastic hand measured by electromyography. Am J Occup Ther 37: 247–254

McCarthy GT, Atkinson HW (1986) The development of the nervous system, chap 3. In: Downie PA (ed) Cash's textbook of neurology for physiotherapists, 4th edn. Faber and Faber, London

McKibbin H (1995) Neurodynamics related to the treatment of patients following a cerebrovascular accident. In: Harrison MA (ed) Physiotherapy in stroke management. Churchill Livingstone, Edinburgh

McLellan DL, Swash M (1976) Longitudinal sliding of the median nerve during movements of the upper limb. J Neurol Neurosurg Psychiatry 39: 556–570

McMaster W, Liddle S, Waugh T (1978) Laboratory evaluation of various cold therapy modalities. Am J Sports Med 6: 291–294

Melzack R (1991) Central pain syndromes and theories of pain. In: Casey KL (ed) Pain and central nervous system disease: the central pain syndromes. Raven, New York

Michels E (1959) Evaluation of motor function in hemiplegia. Phys Ther Rev 39: 389–395

Millesi AJ (1986) The nerve gap. Hand Clin 2: 651–663

Montgomery J (1987) Assessment and treatment of locomotor deficits in stroke. In: Duncan PW, Badke MB (eds) Stroke rehabilitation. The recovery of motor control. Year Book Medical, Chicago

Moore J (1980) Neuroanatomical considerations relating to recovery of function following brain in jury. In: Bach-y-Rita P (ed) Recovery of function: theoretical considerations for brain injury rehabilitation. Huber, Bern

Morasso P (1981) Spatial control of arm movements. Exp Brain Res 42: 223–227

Morasso P (1983) Three-dimensional arm trajectories. Biol Cyber 48: 187–194

Morasso P, Sanguinetti V (1995) Self-organizing body schema for motor planning. J Motor Behav 27: 62–66

Morris D (1987) Manwatching. A field guide to human behaviour. Grafton, London

Moskowitz E, Bishop HF, Pe H, Shibutani K (1958) Posthemiplegic reflex sympathetic dystrophy. JAMA 167: 836–838

Moskowitz E, Lightbody FE, Freitag S (1972) Long-term follow-up of poststroke patient. Arch Phys Med Rehabil 53: 167–172

Mossmann PL (1976) A problem-orientated approach to stroke rehabilitation. Thomas, Springfield

Mountcastle VB (1978) Brain mechanisms for directed attention. J R Soc Med 71: 14–28

Mulder T, Pauwels J, Nienhuis B (1995) Motor recovery following stroke: towards a disability-orientated assessment of motor dysfunctions. In: Harrison MA (ed) Physiotherapy in stroke management. Churchill Livingstone, Edinburgh

Mulley G (1982) Associated reactions in the hemiplegic arm. Scand J Rehabil Med 14: 117–120

Murray PM, Drought AB, Kory RC (1964) Walking patterns of normal men. J Bone Joint Surg Am 46: 335–360

Najenson T, Pikielni SS (1965) Malalignment of the gleno-humeral joint following hemiplegia. A review of 500 cases. Ann Phys Med 8: 96–99

Najenson T, Yacubovich E, Pikielni SS (1971) Rotator cuff injury in shoulder joints of hemiplegic patients. Scand J Rehabil Med 3: 131–137

Newell KM (1996) Change in movement and skill: learning, retention and skill. In: Latash ML, Turvey MT (eds) Dexterity and its development. Lawrence Erlbaum Associates, Mahwah, NJ

Nyburg L, Gustafson Y (1995) Patient falls in stroke rehabilitation: a challenge to rehabilitation strategies. Stroke 26: 838–842

Ofir R, Sell H (1980) Orthoses and ambulation in hemiplegia: a ten-year retrospective study. Arch Phys Med Rehabil 61: 216–220

Ogata K, Naito M (1986) Blood flow of peripheral nerve. Effects of dissection stretching and compression. J Hand Surg 11B: 10–14

Paillard J (1986) Cognitive versus sensorimotor encoding of spatial information. In: Eilen P, Thinus-Blanc C (eds) Cognitive processes and spatial orientation in animal and man. Martinus Nijhoff, Dordrecht, pp 1–35

Palastanga NP (1988) Heat and cold. In: Wells PE, Frampton V, Bowsher D (eds) Pain. Management and control in physiotherapy. Heinemann Physiotherapy, London

Pedersen PM, Wandel A, Jorgensen HS, Nakajama H, Raaschou HO, Olsen TS (1996) Ipsilateral pushing in stroke: incidence, relation to neuropsychological symptoms, and impact on rehabilitation. The Copenhagen stroke study. Arch Phys Med Rehabil 77

Perry J (1969) The mechanics of walking in hemiplegia. Clin Orthop 63: 23–31

Perry J (1992) Gait analysis: normal and pathological function. Slack Inc., Thorofare, NJ

Polya G (1973) How to solve it. A new aspect of mathematical method. Princeton University Press, Princeton

Raibert MH, Sutherland IE (1983) Maschinen zu Fuss. Spektrum der Wissenschaft 3: 30–40

Rasmussen G (1995) Aerobics with hemiplegic patients: results of physical aerobic fitness training in stroke rehabilitation. In: Harrison MA (ed) Physiotherapy in stroke management. Churchill Livingstone, Edinburgh

Reason JT (1978) Motion sickness adaptation. A neural mismatch model. J R Soc Med 71: 819–829
Riddoch G, Buzzard EF (1921) Reflex movements and postural reactions in quadriplegia and hemiplegia, with special reference to those of the upper limb. Brain 44: 397
Riddoch J, Humphreys GW, Bateman A (1995) Stroke. Issues in recovery and rehabilitation. Physiotherapy 81: 689–694
Ring H, Tsur A, Vashdi Y (1993) Long-term follow-up and electromyographical (EMG) follow-up of hemiplegic's shoulder. Eur J Phys Med Rehabil 3: 137–140
Roland PE (1993) Brain activation. Wiley-Liss, New York
Rolf G (1997a) Bedeutung der Mobilität des Nervensystems für ein gesundes Bewegungsverhalten. Krankengymnastik. [Sonderdruck] 49: 608–613
Rolf G (1997b) Unpublished lecture given during a course on the treatment of abnormal neurodynamics in neurologically impaired patients. Albertinen Haus, Hamburg
Rolf G (1999a) Die neuralen Spannungsteste für die obere Extremität. Unpublished lecture given during the course: Aspekte der Neurodynamik bei der Befundaufnahme und Behandlung von Patienten mit einer Läsion des zentralen Nervensystems. Therapie Zentrum Burgau, Germany, April 6–17
Rolf G (1999b) Patho-neurodynamics following lesions of the central nervous system. Unpublished lectures during the information course for IBITAH instructors and instructor candidates. Therapy Centre Burgau, Germany, September 20–25
Roper BA (1975) Surgical procedures in hemiplegia. Unpublished lecture to the Hemiplegic Interest Group, London
Roper BA (1982) Rehabilitation after a stroke. J Bone Joint Surg 64-B: 156–163
Ruskin AP (1982) Understanding stroke and its rehabilitation. Current concepts of cerebrovascular disease. Stroke XVII: 27–32
Russel WR, Dewar AJ (1975) Explaining the brain. Oxford University Press, London
Ryerson S, Levit K (1997) Functional movement reeducation. A contemporary model for stroke rehabilitation. Churchill Livingstone, New York

Sachs O (1985) The man who mistook his wife for a hat. Picador Edition, Pan Books, London
Saeki S, Ogata H, Hachisuka K, Okubo T, Takahashi K, Hoshuyama T (1994) Association between location of the lesion and discharge status of ADL in first stroke patients. Arch Phys Med Rehabil 75: 858–860
Sagan C (1977) The dragons of Eden. Speculations on the evolution of human intelligence. Ballantine, New York
Satterfield WT (1982) Hemiplegia – an 11-year summary. J Tenn Med Assoc 75: 525–529
Saunders M, Imman VT, Eberhart HD (1953) The major determinants in normal and pathological gait. J Bone Joint Surg 35: 543–557
Searle J (1984) Minds, brains and science. Penguin, London
Semans S (1965) Treatment of neurological disorders, concept and systems. J Am Phys Ther Assoc 45: 11–16
Seyffarth H, Denny-Brown D (1948) The grasp reflex and the instinctive grasp reaction. Brain 71: 109–183
Shacklock M (1995) Neurodynamics. Physiotherapy 81: 9–16
Sherrington C (1947) The integrative action of the nervous system, 2nd edn. Yale University Press, New Haven
Shumway-Cook A, Woollacott M (1995) Motor control. Theory and practical applications. Williams and Wilkins, Baltimore
Skilbeck CE, Wade DT, Hewer RL (1983) Recovery after stroke. J Neurol Neurosurg Psychiatry 46: 58
Smith JL (1980) Programming of stereotyped limb movements by spinal generators. In: Stellmach GE, Requin J (eds) Tutorials in motor behaviour. Adv Psychol 1: 95–115
Smith RG, Cruikshank JG, Dunbar S, Akhtar AJ (1982) Malalignment of the shoulder after stroke. Br Med J 284: 1224–1226
Sodring KM (1980) Upper extremity orthosis for stroke patients. Int J Rehabil Res 3: 33–38
Sonderegger H (1997) Wiedererkennen sukzessiver auditiver, visueller und vibratorischer Muster bei Erwachsenen mit Hirnverletzung und Aphasie und Erwachsenen mit Hirverletzung ohne Aphasie. APW-Informationsblatt 4: 20–52

Taub E (1980) Somato-sensory deafferentiation research with monkeys: implications for rehabilitation medicine. In: Ince LP (ed) Behavioural psychology in rehabilitation medicine: clinical applications. Williams and Wilkins, Baltimore
Thilmann AF, Fellows SJ, Ross HP (1991) Biomechanical changes at the ankle joint after stroke. J Neurol Neurosurg Psychiatry 54: 134–139
Thorngren M, Westling B, Norrving B (1990) Outcome after stroke in patients discharged to independent living. Stroke 21: 236–240
Todd JM, Davies PM (1986) Hemiplegia – assessment and approach, chap 10; Hemiplegia – physiotherapy, chap 11. In: Downie PA (ed) Cash's textbook of neurology for physiotherapists, 4th edn. Faber and Faber, London

Tubiana R (1981) The hand, vol 1. W.B.Saunders, Philadelphia

Tuchmann-Duplessis H, Auroux M, Haegel P (1975) Nervous system and endocrine glands. Springer, Berlin Heidelberg New York (Illustrated human embryology, vol 3)

Turvey MT, Carello C (1996) Dynamics of Bernstein's level of synergies. In: Latash ML, Turvey MT (eds) Dexterity and its development. Lawrence Erlbaum Associates, Mahwah, NJ

Tyson SF (1995) Stroke rehabilitation: what is the point? Physiotherapy 81: 430–432

Van Cranenburgh B (1995) Schmerz zwingt zum Nachdenken: eine neurophysiologische Betrachtung von Schmerzen. SVMP/ASPM/ASFM Bulletin 3-4: 6–15

Van Ouwenaller C, Laplace PM, Chantraine A (1986) Painful shoulder in hemiplegia. Arch Phys Med Rehabil 67: 23–26

von Randow G (1991) Die Erfindung der Hand. Geo 11: 110–136

Voss DE (1969) What's the answer? Phys Ther 49: 1030

Waddell G, Newton M, Henderson I, Somerville D, Main CJ (1993) A fear avoidance beliefs questionnaire (FABQ) and the role of fear avoidance beliefs in chronic low back pain and disability. Pain 52: 157–168

Wall JC, Ashburn A (1979) Assessment of gait disability in hemiplegics. Hemiplegic gait. Scand J Rehabil Med 11: 95–103

Wall PD (1987) Foreword. In: Fields HL (ed) Pain. McGraw-Hill, New York

Wall PD (1991) Neuropathic pain and injured nerve: central mechanisms. Br Med Bull 47: 631–643

Wall PD (1995) Placebo und Placeboeffekt. SVMP/ASPM/ASFM Bulletin 2: 5–21

Walmsley RP (1977) Electromyographic study of the phasic activity of peroneus longus and brevis. Arch Phys Med Rehabil 58: 65–69

Walshe FMR (1923) On certain tonic or postural reflexes in hemiplegia with special reference to the so-called "associated movements". Brain 46: 1

Waters RL, Hislop HJ, Perry J, et al (1978) Energetics: application to the study and management of locomotor disabilities. Orthop Clin North Am 9: 351–377

Weber-Witt H (1994) Erlebnis Wasser. Therapeutische Übungen und Schwimmen. Springer, Berlin Heidelberg New York

Wells P (1988) Manipulative procedures. In: Wells PE, Frampton V, Bowsher D (eds) Pain. Management and control in physiotherapy. Heinemann Physiotherapy, London

Werner D (1996) Disabled village children: a guide for community health workers, rehabilitation workers and families. The Hesperian Foundation, Palo Alto, Calif.

Wilson P (1989) Sympathetically maintained pain: diagnosis, measurement, and efficacy of treatment. In: Stanton-Hicks M (ed) Pain and the sympathetic nervous system. Kluwers, Boston, pp 91–123

Winter DA (1988) The biomechanics and motor control of human gait. University of Waterloo Press, Waterloo, Ontario, Canada

Wolff T, Schiffter R, Finck G-A (1991) Das sogenannte „Pusher-Syndrom". In: Mauritz K-H, Neinberg V (eds) Neurologische Rehabilitation. 1. Huber, Bern

Woodworth CN (1899) The accuracy of voluntary movements. Psychol Rev Monogr [Suppl 3] (cited in Jeannerod 1990)

Wyke B (1983) Clinical neurology of the spine, part 2. 7th international congress for manual medicine, Zurich, 9 September

Wyke BD (1985) Articular neurology and manipulative therapy. In: Glasgow EF, Twomey LT, Scull ER, Kleynhans AM, Idczak RM (eds) Aspects of manipulative therapy. Churchill Livingstone, Edinburgh

Yaxley GA, Jull GA (1991) A modified upper limb test: an investigation of normal responses in normal subjects. Aust Physiother 37: 1435–1500

Zinn WM, Mason RM, Currey HLF (1973) Einführung in die Klinische Rheumatologie. Huber, Bern

Zittlau J (1996) Das äussere Gehirn. Medizin und Umwelt, Nürnberger Zeitung, no 101, p 22

Zorowitz RD, Idank D, Ikai T, Hughes MB, Johnston MV (1995) Shoulder subluxation after stroke: a comparison of four supports. Arch Phys Med Rehabil 76: 763–771

18 Subject Index